# INDEX TO

# SPEECH, LANGUAGE, AND HEARING

# JOURNAL TITLES, 1954-78

**PAUL H. PTACEK**

*Case Western Reserve University*

**PATRICIA B. KRICOS**

*University of Akron*

**MELVIN HYMAN**

*Bowling Green State University*

**JOHN W. BLACK**

*The Ohio State University*

**COLLEGE-HILL PRESS**

HOUSTON/BOMBAY 1979

College-Hill Press
P.O. Box 35728
Houston, Texas 77035

Library of Congress Cataloging in Publication Data
Ptacek, Paul H.

  Index to Speech, Language, and Hearing Journal Titles, 1954-78

  Bibliography: p.
  1. Communicative disorders—Bibiography.  2. Communicative disorders—Code words.  3. Speech—Bibliography.  4. Language and languages—Bibliography.  5. Hearing—Bibliography.

I. Ptacek, Paul H., 1918–
Z6675.S55152 [RC423]  016.6168'55  79-20058

ISBN 0-933014-54-6

Printed in the United States of America

# CONTENTS

# PREFACE

It is almost universally stated and practiced by researchers and scholars that the prelude of a research project is a review of pertinent literature. But often this necessary prelude is difficult to achieve. For example, Kent (1959) reported that an executive of a large steel company insisted that it is cheaper to repeat an experiment, if the cost does not exceed $100,000, than to search to determine if it has been done. In the same article, a vice-president of Colgate-Palmolive suggested that if easier access to library materials could cut only one percent of a researcher's time, American industry might save $20,000,000 a year. The inaccessibility of library holdings is not a new problem. Dewey (1927) developed his plan for improving the efficiency of the use of libraries and their materials early in 1873 because the need became apparent to him as a result of over 50 personal visits to libraries. He stated,

> Only a fraction of the servis posibl cud be got from them without clasification, catalogs, indexes and other aids, to tel librarians and readers what they containd on any givn subject; yet, by methods then uzed, this cud be dun satisfactorily only at a cost so great as to be prohibitiv to all but a few wealthy libraries (p. 67). [Both Melvil Dewey (Dewey decimal system) and his brother, Godfrey (word and sound tally) used "reformed spelling".]

One attempt to keep up with ever increasing literature in the medical field is the *Index Medicus*. Durack (1977) found that for the first 60 years the average weight of the *Index Medicus* was 4 pounds per annum. Now the weight of the yearly *Index* is about 66 pounds. This is an indication, in only one field, of the enormity of the problem of searching the literature. Although library computer systems have been a boon to searchers of literature, many complain about the large number of irrelevant references they receive and the delay in receiving the helpful material. Moreover, the cost for the searches usually available in university libraries becomes prohibitive if several searches are made and many of the references turn out to be irrelevant. It was because of problems like these that the need for an index to literature in the field of speech and hearing became apparent.

The very nature of the field of speech and hearing cuts across many disciplines; thus, relevant literature can be found in many journals in diverse fields. That is one reason the authors selected as many as 31 journals to cover the field of speech, language, and hearing. They excluded some otherwise important journals because they were peripheral to the defined field or indexed elsewhere. More specifically, most medical journals and psychological journals were excluded not only because of the large number of journals, but also because of the long standing bibliographic aids such as the *Index Medicus* and *Psychological Abstracts*. However, not all is lost because of these exclusions. The references listed in the journals covered by this index will lead the searcher to pertinent articles in many of the journals indexed elsewhere. This index serves as an *entry* index to articles in other subject-related journals.

The codes in this index were developed from a project in which the theses and dissertations in speech and hearing of six Ohio universities from 1954 through 1974 were compared with articles appearing in 18 national and international journals in the field of speech, language, and hearing for the same period. Since the authors wished to have comparable data for the period covered, some of the more recent journals were not included because of their late arrival in the field, not for their lack of substance. Since 1974, 13 journals have been added to the original 18 to cover the more recent journals in the field, for example, *The Cleft Palate Journal*, and to add to the international dimension, for example, *Phonetica*.

This index to the literature in normal and disordered language, speech, and hearing from 1954 to 1978 is broad in scope covering 31 national and international journals. Yet, it has focus in that only those titles judged to be clearly relevant to the field of speech, language, and hearing are included. This provides economy not only in size, but also results in a practical index for workers in speech pathology, audiology, and related professions. The major categories and subcategories of this index provide a first order screening not expected in other indexes; consequently, there is an economy of time and effort in finding the relevant literature sought on a target topic. The use of this index will prove of value to the researcher who wants to review pertinent literature, and to the "in-the-field" practitioner who is eager to keep abreast of specific disorder-areas in speech and hearing.

Earlier attempts to develop codes applicable to searching literature have not been wholly successful or sufficiently effective. The KWIC (Key Word in Context) in psychology was tested by Brandhurst (1970). He found "... in general a research worker will fail to retrieve a minimum of about 40% of the papers of interest to him that are covered by such a service" (p. 427). The development of Rehabilitation Codes was an N.I.H. project directed by Maya Riviere. It never came to fruition because professional workers could not agree on a proposed code for any of the fields covered, including speech pathology and audiology.

The codes of this index, 10 categories and 100 subcategories, were agreed upon through empirical observation of the tables of contents of journals selected. Dewey (1927) in his introduction to the twelfth edition of his well known *Decimal Classification and Relativ Index* system developed to facilitate the use of libraries and materials therein made this comment, "Practical utility and economy ar its keynotes and no theoretic refinement has been allowd to modify the skeme, if it wud detract usefulness or ad to cost" (p. 67). A similar approach was used in developing this index which has its major emphasis in speech, language, hearing and variations thereof. The authors met frequently and after many discussions agreed upon 10 major categories and 100 sub-categories which were coded for computer use. Frequent meetings were held so that the authors could keep themselves "calibrated" in assigning the codes to the titles of the specific articles comparing multi-judge codings of the same titles. The process was similar to training judges in scaling studies. However, one author served as final arbitrator to increase reliability in assigning the codes to the titles.

Some observations have been made about the changes in journals over time. First, there has been a substantial increase in the number of journals since 1954. Second, some journals are now published more often and more regularly. Third, the number of articles in the journals has increased. Fourth, there has been an increase in the percentage of multiple authors in later years. Fifth, there have been changes and increases in the subheadings within the individual journals. Sixth, a higher percentage of titles in recent journals could only be appropriately classified under multiple codes, limited to three. These observations may reflect:

   (a) An increase in instrumentation and technology.
   (b) An increase in the number of persons involved and interested in the field of speech, language, and hearing and their spin-offs.
   (c) An increase in specialization in the field leading to an increase in the number of journals.
   (d) An increase in awareness of the inter-connections among the various fields, leading to the need for multiple coding of more recent titles.
   (e) An increase in the number of people wanting quick publication, creating an apparent need for a new journal.

The authors of this index recognize that the categories developed may not be the ultimate categories and are aware of the difficulties inherent in achieving agreement for any scheme of categorizing topics of speech, language, and hearing. However, they have found that the present categories are workable and facilitate searches in gaining access to the literature of their general areas of interest and frequently to the specific areas. While the KWIC, according to Brandhurst's evaluation, led to 40% of the papers relevant to the search, 87% accuracy was found in trial uses of the codes developed in this index.

Students who have had access to a preliminary form of the index have made extensive use of it in their searches of the literature. In short, they have found it a highly practical and useful index that saves the user considerable time in the quest for pertinent literature. For example, a student whose term paper or independent study is due soon, may have a limited amount of time and can not wait for the output of computer searches provided by many libraries. And those students not having access to computer searches will find this index especially useful. Moreover, students seeking topics for independent study, theses, dissertations, or term papers may find the index particularly helpful as they peruse the general categories of interest to them and then narrow their search to more specific areas through the subcategories. This will provide a quick overview of what has or has not been done in their areas of potential study during the past 25 years. Clinicians, researchers, specialists in the use of instrumentation and amplification, and other professional workers and scholars will find the index useful in similar pursuits or when they have a pressing need for information on topics related to their work of the moment or the near future.

**Paul H. Ptacek**

## REFERENCES

Brandhurst, W. T. 1970. The proposed KWIC Index for psychology: an experimental test of its effectiveness. *Journal of the American Society for Information Science*, 21: 427-28.

Dewey, Godfrey. 1950. *The relative frequency of English speech sounds.* Rev. ed. Cambridge: Harvard University Press.

Dewey, Melvil. 1927. *Decimal classification and relative index for libraries and personal use in arranging for immediate reference books, pamphlets, clippings, pictures, manuscript notes and other material.* 12th ed. Lake Placid Club, Essex County, N.Y.: Forest Press.

Durack, D. T. 1978. The weight of medical knowledge. *The New England Journal of Medicine*, April, 773-75.

Kent, A. 1959. A machine that does research. *Harper's Magazine*, April, 67-71.

# BASIC DATA REGARDING THE INDEX
# AND ITS USE

Before detailed instruction on the use of the index, certain basic information is necessary to facilitate the instruction. This information includes: (a) a schema of the index providing an overview, (b) a list of the journals covered and their codes, (c) a list of the abbreviations used in the index, and (d) a list of the major categories and subcategories with examples of titles fitting each category.

*Part 1*

## A SCHEMA OF THE INDEX

The schema of the index provides an overview of the basic components involved and their inter-relationships in the development of the index.

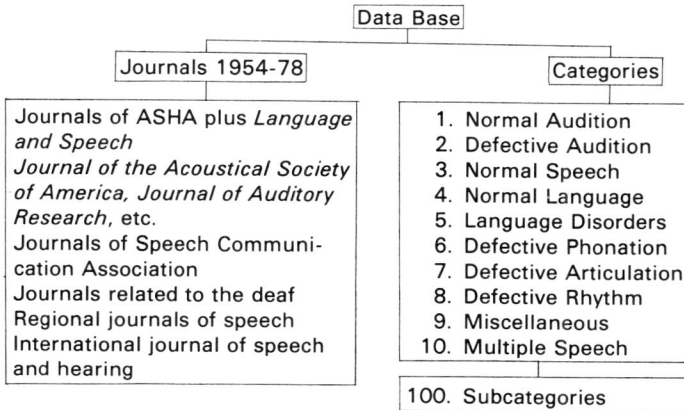

| Data Base | |
|---|---|
| Journals 1954-78 | Categories |
| Journals of ASHA plus *Language and Speech*<br>*Journal of the Acoustical Society of America, Journal of Auditory Research*, etc.<br>Journals of Speech Communication Association<br>Journals related to the deaf<br>Regional journals of speech<br>International journal of speech and hearing | 1. Normal Audition<br>2. Defective Audition<br>3. Normal Speech<br>4. Normal Language<br>5. Language Disorders<br>6. Defective Phonation<br>7. Defective Articulation<br>8. Defective Rhythm<br>9. Miscellaneous<br>10. Multiple Speech |
| | 100. Subcategories |

## Part 2
# THE JOURNALS COVERED AND THEIR CODES

In order to use the computer in the development of this index, it was necessary to assign code numbers to the journals covered. Each journal was assigned a two-digit number which permitted room on the computer cards for the lengthy titles of articles in the journals.

### Journals Covered and Their Codes

01  =  DELETED: THESES NOT INCLUDED
02  =  DELETED: DISSERTATIONS NOT INCLUDED
03  =  JSHD (JOURNAL OF SPEECH AND HEARING DISORDERS)
04  =  JSHR (JOURNAL OF SPEECH AND HEARING RESEARCH)
05  =  ASHA (A JOURNAL OF THE AMERICAN SPEECH AND HEARING
    =  ASSOCIATION)
06  =  JASA (JOURNAL OF THE ACOUSTICAL SOCIETY OF AMERICA)
07  =  ASHA REPORTS, MONOGRAPHS, AND SUPPLEMENTS
08  =  LANGUAGE, SPEECH, AND HEARING IN THE SCHOOLS
09  =  QUARTERLY JOURNAL OF SPEECH
10  =  SPEECH MONOGRAPHS (After 1975 = COMMUNICATION
    =  MONOGRAPHS)
11  =  JAR (JOURNAL OF AUDITORY RESEARCH)
12  =  ACTA SYMBOLICA
13  =  FOLIA PHONIATRICA
14  =  LANGUAGE AND SPEECH
15  =  VOLTA REVIEW
16  =  AMERICAN ANNALS OF THE DEAF
17  =  DELETED: JOURNAL NOT INCLUDED
18  =  WESTERN SPEECH COMMUNICATION JOURNAL
19  =  SOUTHERN SPEECH COMMUNICATION JOURNAL
20  =  CENTRAL STATES SPEECH JOURNAL
21  =  JOURNAL OF PHONETICS
22  =  BRAIN
23  =  JOURNAL OF CHILD LANGUAGE
24  =  CLEFT PALATE JOURNAL
25  =  CORTEX
26  =  JOURNAL OF PSYCHOLINGUISTIC RESEARCH
27  =  JOURNAL OF COMMUNICATION DISORDERS
28  =  JOURNAL OF FLUENCY
29  =  JOURNAL OF HUMAN COMMUNICATION

30  =  JOURNAL OF THE AMERICAN AUDITORY SOCIETY
31  =  JOURNAL OF THE ACADEMY OF REHABILITATIVE AUDIOLOGY
32  =  BRAIN AND LANGUAGE
33  =  PHONETICA
34  =  THE SPEECH TEACHER (after 1975 = COMMUNICATION EDUCATION)

## *Part 3*

# ABBREVIATIONS USED IN THE INDEX

Since many terms were frequently used and required considerable number of spaces on the computer cards, abbreviations were used to conserve space on the cards, when needed.

## *Abbreviations*

+ = and
acous = acoustic(al)
aud = auditory
audio= audiology
at = auditory training
ar = aural reflex

bs = brain stem

cp = cerebral palsy
char = characteristics
chil = children/child
clp = cleft palate
clin = clinical
coch pot = cochlear potential(s)
comm = communication

daf = delayed auditory feedback
dev = development
dis = disorder(s)

educ = education
eso = esophageal
eval = evaluation
ep = evoked potential(s)
er = evoked response(s)

freq = frequency(s)
ff = fundamental frequency(ies)

hng = hearing
ha = hearing aids
hi = hearing impaired/handicapped
hl = hearing loss(es)

lang = language
ld = learning disability(ies)

meas = measure(ment)
mem = memory
mr = mentally retarded

percep = perception
perf = performance
prod = production
pt = pure tone(s)

rehab = rehabilitation
rf = reinforcement(s)
rel = relation(s)
r = response(s)

sch = school
spl = sound pressure level
sp = speech
sp path = speech pathology

thr = threshold(s)
trng = training

## *Part 4*

# A LIST OF THE MAJOR CATEGORIES, SUBCATEGORIES, AND THEIR CODE NUMBERS WITH EXAMPLES OF TITLES FITTING EACH CATEGORY

Approximately 11,000 titles of articles in national and international journals were examined to determine the topics covered in the field of speech, language, and hearing in the years 1954-78. In attempting to handle this number of titles, the key words in the titles were determined. For example, a title such as "The Relationship Between Word Association and Grammatical Classes in Aphasia" was reduced to "Relationship Word Association Grammatical Classes Aphasia". However, key words were not adequate, because much of the meaningfulness of a key word was lost if viewed out of context. Therefore, key words were grouped into meaningful phrases, clauses, etc. A dollar sign ($) was used to link the key words in phrases and/or thought units. Initial or final words which were not of key importance were omitted and spaces were left for other omitted words such as prepositions and conjunctions. In this manner, the key-word analysis for the title above became: "Relationship Word$Association Grammatical$Classes Aphasia". This technique provided constraints on the meanings by adding a significant degree of context. The authors were limited to 66 spaces on each computer card, so occasionally key words may be omitted or cut short.

Another procedure found necessary was to do something quite similar to the training of judges in rating studies. The four authors first selected key words and phrases independently, and then met for many sessions to arrive at a general agreement. This process of calibrating the authors was time consuming, yet essential. The four authors had varied and extensive experience in the field of speech and hearing as well as familiarity with the literature. These characteristics were crucial in the development of the index, however short of perfection the outcome.

The major categories with 100 subcategories were used to classify the various titles. The subcategories divide the major categories for a finer discrimination of the topics. In some instances, titles could not be classified into a single major or subcategory and were classified under two or three categories. We chose arbitrarily to limit each title to three cards.

The categories and subcategories are presented below and each is illustrated by one title:

## *01 Normal Audition*

01 = DISCRIMINATION (e.g., frequency, intensity, duration, discrimination by normal ears): DETECTION DURATION$DISCRIMINATION NOISE$ INCREMENTS.

02 = AUDITORY LOCALIZATION: AUDITORY$LOCALIZATION SINGLE PAIRED$SOURCES.

03 = AURAL REFLEX AND IMPEDANCE: NOTES ARTIFACT MEASURING AURAL$REFLEX.

04 = AUDITORY FATIGUE (includes TTS, habituation, and adaptation studies): PRESTIMULATORY$AUDITORY$FATIGUE CONTINUOUS$ AND$INTERRUPTED$NOISE.

05 = ANATOMY AND PHYSIOLOGY: TONOTOPIC$ORGANIZATION CAT$ AUDITORY$CORTEX COMPLEX$STIMULI.

06 = HEARING CONSERVATION: ROCK-AND-ROLL$MUSIC DAMAGE-RISK$CRITERIA.

07 = NORMATIVE TESTING STUDIES: RELATION HEARING$THRESHOLD$ DURATION TONE$PULSES.

08 = ACOUSTICS: LOG$SPECTRA GAUSSIAN$SIGNALS.

09 = SPEECH PERCEPTION: PERCEPTION SIMULTANEOUS$DICHOTIC MONOTIC$MONOSYLLABLES.

10 = THEORIES OF HEARING: NEUROLOGICAL$THEORY BEAT$TONES.

11 = OTHER (besides including miscellaneous titles under normal audition, all animal studies relating to the study of normal hearing were also coded under this category in order to keep track of which studies employed the use of animals): KEYTAPPING DELAYED$AUDITORY$ FEEDBACK (DAF): UNDERWATER$AUDITORY$LOCALIZATION SEA$ LION.

12 = MASKING: EFFECT MASKING PITCH PERIODIC$PULSES.

13 = ELECTROENCEPHALIC HEARING TESTING: STUDIES AUDITORY$ ADAPTATION AMPLITUDE$DECLINE EVOKED$AUDITORY$ POTENTIAL.

14 = PSYCHOACOUSTICS: PARAMETERS PERCEPTION AMPLITUDE-MODULATED$SIGNALS.

15 = ENVIRONMENT (studies dealing with the sense of audition in varying environments): UNDERWATER$HEARING$THRESHOLD MAN FUNCTION WATER$DEPTH.

16 = ELECTROPHYSIOLOGICAL HEARING TESTING: CARDIAC$REFLEX TONES THRESHOLD$INTENSITY.

17 = LISTENING: RESPONSE AGE$GROUPS DICHOTIC$LISTENING.

18 = AUDITORY SKILLS OF EXCEPTIONAL PERSONS: AUDITORY$ ABILITIES BLIND.

## 02 Defective Audition

01 = HEARING TESTING: COMPARISON GROUP$PURE$TONE$HEARING$ TESTS INDIVIDUAL$HEARING$TESTS.

02  =  HEARING AIDS AND AMPLIFICATION: GROUP WEARABLE$HEAR-
       ING$AID RESIDENTIAL$SCHOOL$DEAF.
03  =  DEAF EDUCATION: TEACHING READING HEARING-IMPAIRED$
       CHILDREN.
04  =  SPEECHREADING: INVESTIGATION LEVEL ASPIRATION HARD-
       OF-HEARING$LIPREADERS.
05  =  AUDITORY TRAINING: PROGRAMMED$INSTRUCTION HEARING-
       IMPAIRED$CHILDREN AUDITORY$DISCRIMINATION VOWELS.
06  =  AURAL REHABILITATION: HEARING$THERAPY CHILDREN.
07  =  DEAF SPEECH AND LANGUAGE: ASSESSMENT VERBAL$LANGUAGE
       $DEVELOPMENT DEAF$CHILDREN.
08  =  HEARING LOSS: SUDDEN UNILATERAL$HEARING$LOSS MUMPS.
09  =  NOISE-INDUCED HEARING LOSS: HEARING$LOSS AIRCRAFT$
       REPAIR$SHOP$PERSONNEL.
10  =  SPEECH DISCRIMINATION TESTING: RELATIVE$INTELLIGIBILITY
       ITEMS CID$AUDITORY$TEST$W-1.
11  =  OTHER: VEIN$PLUG$STAPEDIOPLASTY BONE$CONDUCTION$
       ACUITY.

## 03 Normal Speech and Vocalization

01  =  ANATOMY AND PHYSIOLOGY: ROLE LARYNGEAL$VERTRICLE
       VOICE$PRODUCTION.
02  =  DESCRIPTIVE PHONETICS: ALLOPHONIC$PROBLEM AUSTRALIAN
       $ENGLISH.
03  =  VOCAL ATTRIBUTES (includes studies of fundamental frequency,
       formants, rate, duration of speech sounds, etc.): FORMANT
       BANDWIDTHS VOWELS$PREFERENCE.
04  =  ORAL READING: EFFECT INSTRUCTIONS RATE ORAL$READING.
05  =  METHODS OF STUDYING: BILABIAL$STOP$NASAL$CONSONANTS
       MOTION$PICTURE$STUDY ACOUSTIC$IMPLICATIONS.
06  =  X-RAY STUDIES: RADIOLOGICAL$ASPECTS EMOTIVE$SP.
07  =  SPECTROGRAPHIC STUDIES: SPECTROGRAPHIC$INVESTIGATION
       AUSTRALIAN$VOWELS.
08  =  CINEFLOUROGRAPHIC STUDIES: CINEFLOUROGRAPHIC STUDY
       ALLOPHONES ENGLISH /I/.
09  =  DEVELOPMENT OF SPEECH: ROLE DISTINCTIVE$FEATURES
       CHILDREN$ACQUISITION$PHONOLOGY.
10  =  NORMAL PHONATION: MYOELASTIC-AERODYNAMIC$THEORY
       VOICE$PRODUCTION.
11  =  GERONTOLOGY: CHANGES COMMUNICATION AGING.
12  =  DISTORTED SPEECH (includes distortions such as filtering, compres-
       sion, gating, etc.): EFFECTS INTERRUPTION INTERAURAL$
       ALTERNATION SPEECH$INTELLIGIBILITY.

13  =  DISTINCTIVE FEATURE ANALYSIS: INVESTIGATION DISTINCTIVE
       $FEATURE$CONFUSIONS PRODUCTION DISCRIMINATION$CON-
       SONANTS.
14  =  OTHER: EFFECTS VERBAL$PUNISHERS DISFLUENCIES NORMAL$
       SPEAKERS.
15  =  SYNTHETIC SPEECH: OBJECTIVE$TECHNIQUES SPEECH$
       SYNTHESIS.
16  =  ORAL OR TACTILE PERCEPTION: STUDY SCHOOL$CHILDREN ORAL$
       FORM DISCRIMINATION.
17  =  DIALECT (includes foreign, black, regional, etc.): INVESTIGATION
       PHONOLOGICAL$VARIATIONS BLACK$SCHOOL$CHILDREN.
18  =  SPEECH IMPROVEMENT: PRONUNCIATION AMERICAN$ENGLISH
       PHONETICS$THEORY APPLICATION SPEECH$IMPROVEMENT.
19  =  ORAL-BEHAVIORAL RESPONSE: ORAL$COPYING HEARD$PHRASES.
20  =  DELAYED AUDITORY FEEDBACK: EFFECT DELAYED$AUDITORY$
       FEEDBACK AGE SEX LENGTHS$INFANT$VOCALIZATIONS.
21  =  MACHINE-EAR SPEAKER RECOGNITION: SOLUTION FUNDAMENTAL
       $PROBLEMS MECHANICAL$SPEECH$RECOGNITION.
22  =  SPEECH INTELLIGIBILITY: EFFECT VISUAL$FACTORS SPEECH$
       INTELLIGIBILITY.
23  =  TESTING: SPEECH LANGUAGE$SCREENING PRESCHOOL$
       CHILDREN.


## 04 Language Disorders

01  =  APHASIA: SPELLING$ABILITY DYSPHASIC$SUBJECTS.
02  =  DELAYED LANGUAGE: COMPARISON OBTAINING LANGUAGE$
       SAMPLES CHILDREN$DELAYED$LANGUAGE.
03  =  DIAGNOSIS AND TESTS: DIFFERENTIAL$DIAGNOSIS APHASIC$
       SUBJECTS SCHIZOPHRENIC$LANGUAGE CHILDREN.
04  =  CULTURALLY DEPRIVED: LANGUAGE SPEECH$DEFICITS
       CULTURALLY$DISADVANTAGED$CHILDREN IMPLICATIONS.
05  =  MENTALLY RETARDED: COMPARISON ORAL$LANGUAGE$
       BEHAVIOR EDUCABLES$MENTALLY$RETARDED$CHILDREN.
06  =  THERAPY: CREATIVE$DRAMATICS IMPROVING LANGUAGE
       DEPRIVED$CHILDREN.
07  =  LEARNING DISABILITIES: INVESTIGATION PERCEPTION
       DYSLEXIC$CHILDREN.
08  =  OTHER: SOCIAL$PARTICIPATION NONLANGUAGE$CHILDREN.
09  =  LEARNING DISABILITIES: ALEXIA, IDEOGRAM READING.
10  =  EMOTIONALLY BASED LANGUAGE DISORDERS: VOCABULARY$
       DIVERSITY SCHIZOPHRENICS.

## 05 Normal Language

01 = DESCRIPTIVE LINGUISTICS: COMPARISON WORD$CLASSES CHILDREN.
02 = DEVELOPMENT OF LANGUAGE: RELATION SPEECH$LANGUAGE$ DEVELOPMENT INTELLIGENCE SOCIOECONOMIC$STATUS.
03 = VOCABULARY: VOCABULARY COLLEGE$STUDENTS CLASSROOM$ SPEECHES.
04 = AUDITORY PROCESSING SKILLS: IMMEDIATE$VERBAL$MEMORY LINGUISTIC$SOPHISTICATION CHILDREN.
05 = OTHER: LINGUISTIC$FUNCTIONING BILINGUAL$CHILDREN MONOLINGUAL$CHILDREN.
06 = TESTING: EFFECT RATE CONTROLLED$SPEECH AUDITORY$ RECEPTIVE$SCORES LANGUAGE$ABILITY.

## 06 Defective Phonation

01 = ALARYNGEAL (including esophageal)SPEECH: SOUND$ANALYSIS VOWELS ESOPHAGEAL$SPEAKERS.
02 = FUNCTIONAL DISORDERS OF INTENSITY, PITCH, AND QUALITY: INVESTIGATION VOICE$THERAPY$TECHNIQUES ADULTS PSYCHO-GENIC$VOICE$DISORDERS.
03 = LARYNGEAL AND OROFACIAL ANOMALIES: PATHOGENESIS TREATMENT VOCAL NODULES.
04 = OTHER: VOICE$PROBLEMS ACTOR$SINGER.
05 = VOICE THERAPY: SPEECH$REHABILITATION LARYNGOPLASTY.
06 = THEORY: SEE 0310.
07 = TESTING AND METHODS OF STUDYING: MERITS BACKWARD$ PLAYING$SPEECH SCALING VOICE$QUALITY$DISORDERS.

## 07 Defective Articulation

01 = FOREIGN ACCENTS: BILINGUAL PLUS BICULTURAL$EDUCATION SP$PATHOLOGIST
02 = ORGANIC: DYSARTHRIA AMYOTROPHIC$MYOTONIA.
03 = TESTING: INFLUENCE ORAL VERSUS PICTORIAL$PRESENTATION ARTICULATION$TESTING.
04 = ARTICULATION THERAPY: EFFECTIVENESS COMBINED$VISUAL-AUDITORY$STIMULATION IMPROVING$ARTICULATION.
05 = DEVELOPMENTAL DISORDERS: PARENTAL$ATTITUDES DEVELOP-MENTAL$SPEECH$PROBLEMS.
06 = OTHER: ARTICULATION$DISORDERS PERSONALITY.

## 08 Defective Rhythm

01  =  STUTTERING ETIOLOGIES: SIGNAL$DETECTION$HYPOTHESIS PERCEPTUAL$DEFECTS$THEORY STUTTERING.
02  =  STUTTERING THERAPY: USE MEBROBAMATE STUTTERING$ THERAPY.
03  =  STUTTERING DESCRIPTIONS: CHARACTERISTICS LINGUISTIC $OUTPUT STUTTERERS.
04  =  OTHER: AUDITORY$DISABILITY CLUTTERING$CHILDREN.

## 09 Miscellaneous

01  =  SPEECH CLINICIANS AND AUDIOLOGISTS: SERVICES$FUNCTIONS SPEECH$HEARING$SPECIALISTS$SCHOOLS.
02  =  SPEECH AND HEARING CENTERS, PROGRAMS, ETC.: MOBILE$ UNIT SPEECH$THERAPY$PROGRAM.
03  =  STATISTICS: LATIN$SQUARE$DESIGN SPEECH$HEARING$ RESEARCH.
04  =  OTHER: LIMITATIONS USE INTELLIGENCE$SCALES MENTAL$AGES CHILDREN.
05  =  PROFESSIONAL CONCERNS: SPEECH$HEARING$CERTIFICATION NEW$YORK$STATE.
06  =  PRIMARILY PSYCHOLOGICAL: EFFECT ULTRAVIOLET$LIGHT$ APPARATUS ATTENTIVE$BEHAVIOR$CHILDREN.
07  =  SPEECH AND HEARING PROBLEMS IN GENERAL: CLASSROOM $TEACHER$ATTITUDES ACTIVITIES$SPEECH$CORRECTION.
08  =  MEDICAL CONCERNS: SKELETAL$DENTAL$IRRGULARITIES RELATION NEUROMUSCULAR$DYSFUNCTIONS.
09  =  PSYCHOPHYSICS: RATING$SCALES$METHOD LOUDNESS$ MEASURE.
10  =  STUDIES ON THE NATURE OF SIGNALS: STUDY MAYDAY$SOS RADIOTELEPHONY$DISTRESS$SIGNALS.
11  =  COMMUNICATION MODELS: THEORY SPEECH$MECHANISM$ SERVOSYSTEM.
12  =  INSTRUMENTATION: EVALUATION ARTIFICIAL$MASTOID INSTRU-MENT$CALIBRATION AUDIOMETER BONES$CONDUCTION.

## 10 Multiple Speech Disorders

01  =  CEREBRAL PALSY: NONVERBAL$COMMUNICATION CHILDREN$ CEREBRAL$PALSY.

02  =  CLEFT PALATE: NASALITY ISOLATED$VOWELS CONNECTED$
       SPEECH CLEFT PALATE.
03  =  OTHER: MYASTHENIA$GRAVIS STUDY FUNDAMENTAL$
       FREQUENCY.

## Part 5
## HOW TO USE THE INDEX

The persons who use the index first identify the codes for the category and subcategory in which they are interested and then turn to that section which contains all the titles (reduced to key words) relevant to that topic. When a title of interest has been identified, the source of the title is determined by a four-digit number. The first two digits identify the year in which the article appeared, and the last two digits the journal.

Examples will clarify the use of the index. Should a speech pathologist be interested in literature related to emotionally based language disorders in children, she identifies the code for this category and subcategory (e.g., 0406: 04=Language disorders; 06=Emotionally based) and turns to the relevant section of the index containing these titles (See pages 248-250). She then identifies which titles appear specifically to be of interest to her and determines their source by use of the code numbers next to each title. For example, a code number of 7403 identifies the title as appearing in 1974 in the *Journal of Speech and Hearing Disorders*.

If interested in teaching reading to deaf children, the index user would identify the category and subcategory most relevant to this area (in this case, 0203, for Defective Audition (02), "deaf education" (03). The user turns to the section of the index labeled 0203 and notes titles in this section that appear to be related to teaching reading to deaf children. For example, one of the titles under 0203 is: 5415 TEACHING$READING HI$CHIL (Teaching Reading to the Hearing-Handicapped Child). This alerts the user to the existence of an article of interest to him in the 1954 issue of journal #15 (*Volta Review*). The authors acknowledge that literature searching will be easier for articles appearing in journals from 1975 to 1978 because of the inclusion of the first author's name in the index for these years. The last name of the first author listed will precede the title. With knowledge of the author's name, the index user can then go to the last issue of a particular year for a journal and look up the exact reference (issue number and pages in the annual index of the journal.

## Part 6

# EXAMPLES OF CATEGORIES, CODES, AND TITLES IN THE INDEX

The examples in the following table provide a guide to deciphering the coded entries of the Index. The first line of each example gives the information provided and the second line gives the code numbers and abbreviated authors' names and article's title for each item of information. The type of information given is indicated by the following columns from left to right: (a) major category, (b) sub-category, (c) year of publication, (d) journal in which the article appeared, (e) authors of the article, and (f) the title of the article.

| | MAJOR CATEGORY | SUBCATEGORY | YEAR | JOURNAL | AUTHOR | TITLE |
|---|---|---|---|---|---|---|
| *Example 1* | Defective Audition | Deaf Education | 1954 | Volta Review | [No Author Given Prior to 1974] | Teaching Reading to the Hearing Handicapped Child |
| *Code* | 02 | 03 | 54 | 15 | | TEACHING$READING HI$CHIL |
| *Example 2* | Miscellaneous | Professional Concerns | 1975 | Asha | Richard F. Curlee and Richard W. Israel | Training of Foreign Students in Speech-Pathology-Audiology in U.S. Colleges and Universities |
| *Code* | 09 | 06 | 75 | 05 | CURLEE | TRAINING FOREIGN$STUDENTS SP$ PATHOLOGY$AUD US$COLLEGES |
| *Example 3* | Normal Audition | Normative Testing Studies | 1976 | The Journal of the Acoustical Society of America | T. Houtgast | Subharmonic pitches of a puretone at low S/N ratio |
| *Code* | 01 | 07 | 76 | 06 | HOUTGAST | SUBHARMONIC$PITCHES PT LOW S/N RATIO |
| *Example 4* | Miscellaneous | Instrumentation | 1977 | Journal of Speech and Hearing Research | Carolyn H. Musket and Ross J. Roesser | Using Circumaural Enclosures with Children |
| *Code* | 09 | 12 | 77 | 04 | MUSKET | CIRCUMAURAL$ENCLOSURES CHILD |
| *Example 5* | Normal Speech and Vocalization | Normal Phonation | 1978 | Folia Phoniatrica | A.R. Mallard, R.L. Ringl, Y. Horii | Sensory Contributions to Control of Funda-mental Frequency of Phonation |
| *Code* | 03 | 10 | 78 | 13 | MALLARD | CONTROL FUNDAMENTAL$FREQ |

| | | | | | | |
|---|---|---|---|---|---|---|
| *Example 6* | Miscellaneous | Speech and Hearing Problems in General | 1976 | | Frank Parker | Distinctive Features in Speech Pathology: Phonology or Phonemics? |
| *Code* | 09 | 07 | 76 | 03 | PARKER | DISTINCTIVE$FEATURES SP$PATH |
| *Example 7* | Defective Articulation | Organic | 1976 | Journal of Speech and Hearing Disorders | Netsell, Ronald and Kent, Raymond D. | Paroxysmal Ataxic Dysarthria |
| *Code* | 07 | 02 | 76 | 03 | NETSELL | PAROXYSMAL$ATAXIA$DYSARTHRIA |
| *Example 8* | Normal Speech | Spectographic Studies | 1970 | Journal of the Acoustical Society of America | | Vowel Spectra, Vowel Spaces, and Vowel Identification |
| *Code* | 03 | 07 | 70 | 06 | | Vowel Spectra, Vowel Spaces, and Vowel Identification |
| *Example 9* | Language Disorders | Aphasia | 1955 | Journal of Speech and Hearing Disorders | | Auditory Dedifferentiation in the Dysphasic |
| *Code* | 04 | 01 | 55 | 03 | | AUD$DEDIFFERENTIATION A: HASIA |
| *Example 10* | Defective Articulation | Organic | 1970 | Journal of Speech and Hearing Research | | Phonemic Variability in Apraxia of Speech |
| *Code* | 07 | 02 | 70 | 04 | | PHONEMIC$VARIABILITY APRAXIA$SP |
| *Example 11* | Defective Rhythm | Stuttering Descriptions | 1971 | Asha | | The Fear of Stuttering |
| *Code* | 08 | 03 | 71 | 05 | | FEAR STUTTERING |
| *Example 12* | Normal Audition | Discrimination | 1961 | Journal of Auditory Research | | Auditory Discrimination and Sleep Deprivation |
| *Code* | 01 | 01 | 61 | 11 | | AUD$DISCRIM SLEEP$DEPRIVATION |

5406    INTENSITY$DISCRIM$THR PSYCHOPHYSICAL$PROCEDURES
5406    NOTE AUDIBILITY INTENSE$ULTRASONICS$SOUND
5406    PITCH$DISCRIM MELS KOCKS$CONTENTION
5506    AUD$TESTING VOWEL$ARTIC
5506    CHANNELS$RECEPTION PITCH$DISCRIM
5506    DL$INTENSITY VOWEL
5506    NOTE THR$PULSED$SIGNALS FUNCTION DUTY$CYCLE CARRIER
      $FREQ
5506    PITCH$PERCEP PERIODIC$AUD$STIMULI
5606    JND DICHOTIC$PHASE
5703    DL FORMANT$AMPLITUDE
5706    FREQ$DL NARROW$BAND$NOISE
5706    INTENSITY$DISCRIM$THR
5706    SIMULTANEOUS$TWO-TONE$PITCH$DISCRIM
5806    ADVANTAGES DISCRIMINABILITY$CRITERION LOUDNESS$SCALE
5806    AX$ABX$LIMENS
5806    DL TONE$DIMINUTION
5806    EFFECT AUD$CUE DISCRIM AUD$STIMULI
5806    EXPLANATION LIMENS$LOUDNESS
5806    PITCH$RATINGS VOICED$WHISPERED$VOWELS
5906    DISCRIM NUMBER SIMULTANEOUSLY$SOUNDING$TONES
5906    EFFECT BACKGROUND$NOISE AUD$INTEN$DL
5906    INTENSIVE$DIFFERENTIAL$THR OCTAVE-BAND$NOISE
6006    PITCH$DISCRIM TWO-FREQ$COMPLEXES
6106    APPLICATION THEORY$SIGNAL$DETECTABILITY AMP$DISCRIM
6106    COMBINATION INTENSITY FREQ$DIFFERENCES AUD$DISCRIM
6106    PROCEDURE CALCULATING LOUDNESS
6106    SIMULTANEOUS$DICHOTIC$FREQ$DISCRIM
6111    AUD$DISCRIM SLEEP$DEPRIVATION
6111    INTENSITY$DISCRIM NARROW$BANDWIDTHS$NOISE PULSE$LENGTHS
6206    AUD$INTENSITY$DISCRIM FUNCTION STIMULUS$PRESENTATION
      $METHOD
6206    EFFECTS AUD$FATIGUE INTEN$DISCRIM
6206    HUMAN$DISCRIM AUD$DURATION
6206    PERCEP TWO-COMPONENT NOISE$BURSTS
6206    PT$LOUDNESS REL
6206    TIME$INTEGRATION DISCRIM FREQ$R$PATTERNS
6211    REL FREQ$DISCRIM SP$PERCEP
6215    PITCH$DISCRIM
6304    MONAURAL$VS$BINAURAL$DISCRIM
6304    MONAURAL$VS$BINAURAL$DISCRIM
6306    AUD$INTEN$DISCRIM FUNCTION STIMULUS$PRESENTATION$METHOD
6306    CUMULATION DL INTENSITY$CHANGE LOW$SENSATION$LEVELS
6306    DETECTION DISCRIM LOUDNESS SHORT$TONES
6306    EFFECT PRACTICE FEEDBACK FREQ$DISCRIM
6306    FACTORS EFFECTIVE AUD INTENSIVE DL

```
6306   FREQ$DISCRIM PULSED$TONES
6306   INTEN$DISCRIM PEDESTAL$EFFECT NEGATIVE$MASKING WHITE-NOISE
       $STIMULI
6306   LOW-FREQ DL EFFECT HIGH-FREQ NOISE
6306   ONSET$DISCRIM WHITE$NOISE
6306   PERCEP TEMPORAL$ORDER LOUDNESS$JUDGMENTS DICHOTIC
       CLICKS
6306   SENSORY$THR R$BIAS
6306   SHORT-TERM AUD$FREQ$DISCRIM
6307   LOUDNESS$DISCRIM
6406   DL LOUDNESS RATES INTEN$CHANGE
6406   MINIMUM$DETECTABLE$CHANGE INTERAURAL$TIME INTENSITY
       $DIFFERENCE
6406   NOTE BUZZ-HISS$DETECTION
6406   PROCEDURAL$VARIABLES INFLUENCING ESTIMATIONS DIFFERENTIAL
       $THR FREQ
6411   AUD$DISCRIM NORMAL$MONKEYS
6411   AUD$DISCRIM BRAIN-DAMAGED$MONKEYS
6506   ADJUSTING METHOD$ADJUSTMENT SD DL
6506   EFFECT AURAL$HARMONICS FREQ$DISCRIM
6511   EFFECT VARIABLES DISCRIM
6511   FREQ$DISCRIM CORTICALLY$ABLATED$MONKEYS
6606   APPLICATION EC$MODEL INTERAURAL$JND
6606   AUD$INTEN$PERCEP NEURAL$CODING
6606   DESCRIPTIVE$ANALYSIS DOPPLER$DISCRIM FUNCTION VARIATIONS
       DIMENSION
6606   FREQ$DISCRIM RANDOM-AMPLITUDE$TONES
6606   INSTRUMENTAL$METHOD IMPROVED INTEN$DISCRIM DATA
6606   INTEN$DISCRIM FLUCTUATING$SIGNALS
6606   INTERAURAL$TIME INTENSITY$DIFFERENCES MLD
6606   MASKED$DL PITCH$MEM
6606   PITCH$DISCRIM JITTERED$PULSE$TRAINS
6704   FLUTTER$PERCEP
6704   INTERAURAL$INTENSITY$DL
6706   AMP$DISCRIM NOISE
6706   AUD$INTEN$DISCRIM$SCALE EVIDENCE BINAURAL$INTEN$SUMMATION
6706   FREQ$DISCRIM MEAS AB$AND$ABX$PROCEDURES
6706   FREQ$DISCRIM NOISE
6706   LATERALIZATION INTEN$DISCRIM
6706   MODEL AUD$DISCRIM DETECTION
6706   NUMBER$PULSES REQUIRED MINIMAL$PITCH
6706   PITCH$PERCEP PULSE$PAIRS RANDOM$REPETITION$RATE
6711   FREQUENCY$DL PIGEON CONDITIONED$SUPPRESSION
6713   IMPORTANCE INTENSITY$MODULATION PERCEP$TRILL
6804   PERCEIVING$STEADY$STATE$VOWEL MUSICAL MEANINGLESS
       $SOUNDS
```

6806    ACQUISITION SUCCESSIVE AUD$DISCRIM MONKEYS
6806    APPROACH DL$CONCEPT INFORMATION$THEORY
6806    AUD$PULSED$DOPPLER$DISCRIM
6806    DETECTION RELATIVE$DISCRIM AUD$JITTER
6806    DISCRIM TEMPORAL$INTERVAL JITTERED$AUD$PULSE$TRAINS
6806    DISCRIM AUD$TEMPORAL$DIFFERENCES DOLPHIN HUMAN
6806    EFFECT HARMONIC$COMPONENTS FREQ$DISCRIM
6806    FREQ$DISCRIM MASKING$EFFECTIVENESS
6806    MECHANISMS FREQ$DISCRIM
6806    PERIODICITY$DISCRIM AUD$PULSE$TRAINS
6806    PREDICTION MONAURAL$DETECTION
6806    PT$INTEN$DISCRIM ENERGY$DETECTION
6806    REFERENCE$SIGNAL SIGNAL$QUALITY STUDIES
6811    APPARENT$DURATION AUD$STIMULI
6906    AMP$DISCRIM NOISE PEDESTAL$EXPERIMENTS ADDITIVITY
        MASKING
6906    AUD RANDOM-WALK DISCRIM
6906    CLICK-INTENSITY$DISCRIM BACKGROUND$MASKING$NOISE
6906    EFFECT DURATION AMP$DISCRIM NOISE
6906    EFFECT MASKING$NOISE PULSE$LEVEL JITTER$DETECTION
6906    FLUCTUATIONS AMP REL CLICK-INTENSITY$DISCRIM
6906    FM DL FREQ
6906    FREQ$SELECTIVITY AMP$DISCRIM SIGNALS NOISE
6906    GAP JITTER$DISCRIM
6906    INFLUENCE CONTRALATERAL$NOISE AUD INTEN$DISCRIM
6906    INTEN$DISCRIM RAYLEIGH$NOISE
6906    INTEN$PERCEP PRELIMINARY$THEORY INTEN$RESOLUTION
6906    INTERAURAL$TIME AMP$JNDS
6906    MODULATED$FREQ$DISCRIM REL AGE MUSICAL$TRNG
6906    MONAURAL$DETECTION CONTRALATERAL$CUE ENERGY$DETECTOR
        $PERFORMANCE
6906    PARALLEL$PROCESSING$TECHNIQUES ESTIMATING PITCH$PERIODS
        SP TIME$DO
6906    PERCEIVED$PITCH WHISPERED$VOWELS
6906    PERIODICITY$PITCH INTERRUPTED$WHITE$NOISE ARTIFACT
6906    PERSTIMULATORY$TRACKING PITCH$PERCEP SENSATION$LEVEL
6911    CHANGES MONAURAL$JND PT$STIMULATION$CONTRALATERAL
        $EAR
7004    PHYSIOLOGICAL$DETERMINANTS AUTONOMIC$RESPONSIVITY
        SOUND
7006    AUD$MEM PITCH$DISCRIM
7006    DISCRIM TRAINSIENT$SIGNALS IDENTICAL ENERGY$SPECTRA
7006    EXTENSION NEFF$NEURAL$MODEL DISCRIM COMPLEX$STIMULI
7006    MONAURAL$DETECTION PHASE$DIFFERENCE CLICKS
7006    MONAURAL$DETECTION FILTERING
7006    PERFORMANCE$CHARACTERISTICS HARMONIC$IDENTIFICATION
        $PITCH$EXTRACTI

```
7006   PITCH$PERCEP TWO-FREQ$STIMULI
7006   TIME$DOMAIN
7011   EFFECT INTERVAL$DURATIONS INTERAURAL$LOUDNESS$BALANCING
7011   EFFECT TRNG FREQ$DISCRIM SCH$CHIL
7011   LEARNING-SET$PROCEDURE SOUND$QUALITY$DISCRIM CHINCHILLA
7011   NOISE$EFFECTS SP$DISCRIM
7011   PERCEP$ASYMMETRY DICHOTICALLY$PRESENTED$CLICK-SENTENCE
       $STIMULI
7106   AUD$PERCEP EFFECT STIMULUS$DURATION
7106   DETECTION DURATION$DISCRIM NOISE$INCREMENTS
7106   DISCRIM INTERVAL BRIEF$PULSES
7106   EFFECTS BANDWIDTH-DURATION$CONSTRAINTS FREQ$DISCRIM
7106   MONAURAL$DETECTION CONTRALATERAL$CUE
7106   MONAURAL$DETECTION CONTRALATERAL$CUE SINUSOIDAL$SIGNALS
       CONSTANT
7106   MONAURAL$DETECTION CONTRALATERAL$CUE INTERAURAL$DELAY
       CUE SIGNAL
7106   PERCEP COARTICULATED$NASALITY
7111   FREQUENCY$DISCRIM$THR AUD$CORTEX$ABLATIONS MONKEY
7111   NON-VERBAL$NONMEANINGFUL$STIMULI
7204   OBSERVATIONS ARTIC LABIAL$SENSORY$DEPRIVATIONS
7206   CHANGES FREQ$DISCRIM LEADING$TRAILING$TONES
7206   DISCRIM TEMPORAL$GAPS
7206   DISCRIM INTERAURAL$TIME$INTEN
7206   DURATION$DISCRIM NOISE TONE$BURSTS
7206   FREQ$DISCRIM MLD
7206   FREQ$DISCRIM DOLPHIN
7206   INTEN$DISCRIM PULSED$SINUSOIDS EFFECTS FILTERED$NOISE
7206   INTEN$PERCEP RESOLUTION SMALL-RANGE$IDENTIFICATION
7206   INTEN$PERCEP RESOLUTION ONE-INTERVAL$PARADIGMS
7206   JND SEGMENT$DURATION SP
7206   PT$AUD$THR CARP
7206   TEMPORAL$RESOLUTION TONAL$PULSES
7211   AROUSAL PERSONALITY PITCH$DISCRIM
7211   FACTORS LOUDNESS$DISCRIM SUPRATHR$SIGNAL INCREASING
       $INTENSITY
7211   FREQ$DL DOLPHIN
7211   PROCESSING NON-SYMBOLIC$AUD$INFO
7306   EFFECT INTERAURAL$PHASE FREQ AMPLITUDE$DISCRIM
7306   FREQ DL NARROW$BANDS$NOISE
7306   FREQ DL SHORT-DURATION$TONES
7306   FREQ$DISCRIM PRESENCE$ANOTHER$TONE
7306   INTEN$DISCRIM CLICKS EFFECTS CLICK$BANDWIDTH BACKGROUND
       $NOISE
7306   INTEN$PERCEP RESOLUTION ROVING-LEVEL$DISCRIM
7306   INTERAURAL$TIME$JND SIMULTANEOUS$FUNCTION INTERAURAL
       $TIME
```

7306    PERCEP$CONFUSIONS FOUR-DIMENSIONAL$SOUNDS
7306    PRELIMINARY$RESULTS INTERAURAL$DISCRIM
7306    TEMPORAL$ACUITY FUNCTION FREQ
7311    R$DELAY$EFFECTS DURATION$JUDGMENTS
7404    INTERAURAL$INTENSITY PHASE$ANGLE DISCRIM MONKEYS
7406    AUD$FREQ$DISCRIM VERTEBRATES
7406    DISCRIM INTERAURAL$PHASE$DIFFERENCES
7406    INTEN$DISCRIM RAPID$SEQUENCE TONE$BURSTS
7406    INTEN$DISCRIM NOISE PRESENCE BAND-REJECT$NOISE
7406    INTEN$DISCRIM FREQ$DISCRIM INTERVAL$PARADIGMS
7406    NEURAL$CODING PSYCHOPHYSICAL$DISCRIM$DATA
7406    PT$INTEN$DISCRIM EXPERIMENTS NEAR$MISS WEBERS$LAW
7406    REL CRITICAL$BANDWIDTH FREQ DL
7506    AHUMADA TIME FREQ$ANALYSES AUD$SIGNAL$DETECTION
7506    BODE CNC$DISCRIM SPONDEE$WORDS
7506    DALSTON ACOUSTIC$CHAR ENGLISH$/W,R,L/ CHILD ADULTS
7506    DOOLING AUD$INTENSITY$DISCRIM PARAKEET
7506    ELMASIAN LOUDNESS$ENHANCEMENT
7506    HAFTER DIFFERENCE$THRESHOLDS INTERAURAL$DELAY
7506    JESTEADT DECISION$PROCESSES FREQ$DISCRIM
7506    KAPLAN DISTRACTORS$EXPERIMENT CRITICAL$BAND CONTAMINATED
        $WHITE$NOISE
7506    MACMILLAN PROBE-SIGNAL$INVESTIGATION UNCERTAIN-FREQ
        $DETECTION
7506    MCFADDEN DURATION-INTENSITY$RECIPROCITY EQUAL$LOUDNESS
7506    MOORE INTENSITY$DISCRIM MOISE$BURSTS
7506    PFINGST REACTION-TIME$PROCEDURE MEAS HNG SUPRATHR
        $FUNCTIONS
7506    PFINGST REACTION-TIME$PROCEDURE MEAS HNG THR$FUNCTIONS
7506    POLLACK ID RANDOM$AUD$WAVEFORMS
7506    POLLACK PERCEP COMPLEX$SOUNDS HIDDEN$AUD$FIGURES
7506    RAAB AUD$INTENSITY$DISCRIM BURSTS REPRODUCIBLE$NOISE
7506    RESNICK DISCRIM TIME-REVERSED$CLICK$PAIRS INTENSITY
        $EFFECTS
7506    SINNOTT REGULATION VOICE$AMPLITUDE MONKEY
7506    SMIAROWSKI TEMPORAL$RESOLUTION FORWARD$MASKING SIMULTANEOUS
        $MASKING
7506    SPEAKS INTERAURAL-INTENSIVE$DIFFERENCES DICHOTIC$LISTENING
7506    TAYLOR MONAURAL$DETECTION CONTRALATERAL$CUE MDCC AMPLITUDE
        $DISCRIM
7506    TEAS INTERAURAL$ATTENUATION FREQ GUINEA$PIG CHINCHILLA
        CM$R
7506    THOMPSON UNDERWATER$FREQ$DISCRIM DOLPHIN HUMAN
7506    WATSON DISCRIM TONAL$PATTERNS FREQ TEMPORAL$POSITION
        SILENT$INTERVALS
7506    WIER TEMPORAL$ACUITY FUNCTION FREQUENCY$DIFFERENCE

7511   ALLY INTERFERENCE PITCH$DISCRIM$TASK
7511   ALLY INTERFERENCE PITCH$DISCRIM$TASK
7511   LIEBMAN SISI$SCORES NORMAL$POPULATION
7511   WANG EEG$DESYNCHRONIZATION PITCH$DISCRIM
7511   WANG EEG$DESYNCHRONIZATION PITCH$DISCRIM
7527   DANILOFF CHILDREN'S ARTICULATORY AUD DIFFERENCES VOWEL
       $SOUNDS
7606   BOND IDENTIFICATION VOWELS EXCERPTED /L/ /R/ CONTEXTS
7606   DOMNITZ BINAURAL$DETECTION$MODELS INTERAURAL$TARGET
       $PARAMETERS
7606   EHRET TEMPORAL$AUDITORY$SUMMATION PT WHITE$NOISE HOUSE
       $MOUSE
7606   FADDEN LATERALIZATION HIGH$FREQ BASED ON INTERAURAL
       $TIME$DIFFERENCES
7606   FISH SONAR$TARGET$DISCRIM INSTRUMENTED$HUMAN$DIVERS
7606   GEESA BINAURAL$INTERACTION CAT MAN
7606   GILLIOM GAP$DETECTION TWO-CHANNEL$DETECTION MISSING
       $EVENT
7606   GILLOM CONTRALATERAL$CUES DETECTION SIGNALS UNCERTAIN
       $FREQ
7606   HEBRANK PINNA$DISPARITY$PROCESSING CASE MISTAKEN$ID
7606   HEFFNER PERCEP MISSING$FUNDAMENTAL CATS
7606   HELLMAN GROWTH LOUDNESS
7606   HOOD EYE$COLOR SUSCEPTIBILITY TO TTS
7606   JOHNSTONE TTS SHIFT COCHLEAR$NERVE$FIBERS
7606   LIPPMANN INTENSITY$PERCEP EFFECT PAYOFF$MATRIX ABSOLUTE
       $ID
7606   MASSARO RECOGNITION$MASKING AUD$LATERALIZATION PITCH
       $JUDGEMENTS
7606   MILLER DISCRIM LABELING NOISE-BUZZ$SEQUENCES
7606   MOORE DISCRIM PT$INTENSITIES CALIF$SEA$LION
7606   NORDMARK BINAURAL$TIME$DISCRIM
7606   PATTERSON RESIDUE$PITCH FUNCTION COMPONENT$SPACING
7606   RABINOWITZ INTENSITY$PERCEP DEVIATIONS WEBER,S$LAW
7606   RAJCAN AUD$DISCRIM ONSET-OFFSET$PHASA TONE$BURSTS
7606   RYAN HRING$SENSITIVITY MONGOLIAN$GERBIL
7606   SCHACKNOW NOISE-INTENSITY$DISCRIM BANDWIDTH$CONDITIONS
       MASKER$PRESENT
7606   SCHUSTERMAN CALIF$SEA$LION UNDERWATER$AUD$DETECTION
       RF$SCHEDULES
7606   SHONLE TRILL$THRES REVISITED
7606   SINNOTT SP$SOUND$DISCRIM MONKEYS HUMANS
7606   SMOORENBURG COMBINATION$TONES R NEURONS COCH$NUCLEUS
       CAT
7606   VOGEN COMPARISON RELIABILITY AURALDOME$HEADSET STANDARD
       $HEADSET PT THR

7606    WARD EFFECTIVE$QUIET+MODERATE$TTS IMPLICATIONS NOISE
        $EXPOSURE$STANDARD
7606    WATSON DISCRIM TONAL$PATTERNS ATTENTION LEARNING STIMULUS
        $UNCERTAINTY
7606    WILLIAMS GAP$DETECTION SINGLE-CHANNEL$PROCESS
7606    WOOD DISCRIMINABILITY R$BIAS PHONEME$CATAGORIES DISCRIM
        VOT
7606    ZUREK INTERAURAL$PHASE$DISCRIM COMBINATION$TONES$STIMULI
7621    LEHISTE INFLUENCE FUNDAMENTAL$FREQ$PATTERN PERCEP
        DURATION
7621    STRETTER KIKUYU LABIAL APICAL$STOP$DISCRIMINATION
7703    ANDREWS ASSESSMENT PITCH$DISCRIM CHIL
7706    AHROON SELECTIVE$ATTENTION TWO-CHANNEL$SIMULTANEOUS
        $FREQ$DL
7706    BERLINER INE
7706    BERLINER INTENSITY$PERCEP VII FURTHER DATA ROVING-LEVEL
        $DISCRIM +
7706    BUUNEN PSYCHOPHYS$ELECTROPHYSIO COMBINATION$TONES
        PERCEP PHASE$CHANGES
7706    COLBURN THEORY BINAURAL$INTERACTION AUD-NERVE DETECT
        TONES$IN$NOISE
7706    DIVENYI EAR$DOMINANCE DICHOTIC$CHORD EAR$SUPERIORITY
        FREQUENCY$DISCRIM
7706    DOMNITZ LATERAL$POSITION INTERAURAL$DISCRIM
7706    EFRON EFFECTS SIGNEL$INTENSITY NOISE PITCH$MIXTURE
        DICHOTIC$CHORDS
7706    EHRET POSTNATAL$DEV ACOUS$SYSTEM HOUSE$MOUSE DEV MASKED
        $THR
7706    FASTL DURATION TEMPORAL$MASKING$PATTERNS BROAD-BAND
        $IMPULSES
7706    FETH TWO-TONE$AUDITORY$SPECTRAL$RESOLUTION
7706    GRANTHAM ROLE DYNAMIC$CUES MONAURAL BINAURAL SIGNEL
        $DETECTION
7706    GREEN DETECTION RECOGNITION PURE$TONES NOISE
7706    HALL DETECTION$THRESHOLD TWO-TONE$COMPLEX
7706    HALL SPATIAL$DIFFERENTIATION AUD$SECOND$FILTER ASSESS
        MODEL BAS$MEM
7706    JESTEADT INTENSITY$DISCRIM FREQUENCY SENSATION$LEVEL
7706    JESTEADT COMPARISON MONAURAL BINAURAL,DISCRIM INTENSITY+FREQ
7706    KUHN MODEL INTERAURAL$TIME$DIFFERENCES AZIMUTHAL$PLANE
7706    LIM INTENSITY$PERCEPTION LOUDNESS$COMPARISONS DIFFERENT
        TYPES STIMULI
7706    MOLLER FREQ$SELECTIVITY SINGLE FIBERS R BROADBAND
        STIMULI
7706    MORGAN TEMPORAL$INTEGRATION THR ACOUS$REFLEX
7706    NOORDEN MINIMUM$DIFFERENCES LEVEL FREQ PERCEP$FISSION
        TONE$SEQUENCES

7706    ORR BEHAVIORAL$SYS APPARATUS TONE-DETECTION REACTION-TIMES
        CAT
7706    PISONI IDEN DISCRIM ONSET COMPONENT$TONES VOICING
        $PERCEP STOPS
7706    POLLACK MONAURAL BETWEEN-EAR$TEMPORAL$GAP$DETECTION
7706    REPP MEASURING LATERALITY$EFFECTS DICHOTIC$LISTENING
7706    SHIPP PHYSIOLOGIC$ADJUSTMENTS FREQ$CHANGE TRAINED
        UNTRAINED$VOICES
7706    WIER FREQUENCY$DISCRIM FREQUENCY SENSATION$LEVEL
7706    YENI-KOMSHIAN ID SP$SOUNDS DISPLAYED VIBROTACTILE
        $VOCODER
7706    YUND MODEL RELATIVE$SALIENCE PITCH PURE$TONES PRESENTED
        DICHOTICALLY
7711    ELFNER EFFECT FREQ AURAL$ACUITY LATERALIZATION
7711    HAWKES R$DELAY$EFFECTS CROSS-MODALITY$DURATION$JUDGEMENTS
7711    HUMES THRES OCTAVE$MASKING$TEST PREDICTOR SUSEPTIBILITY
        NOISE-INDUCEHL
7806    BACKUS PRESSURE-FLOW$TECHNIQUE ASSESSING ORAL$PORT
        $SIZE
7806    BERLINER INTENSITY$PERCEPTION FIXED$STANDARD
7806    BURNS CATEGORICAL$PERCEP MELODIC$MUSICAL$INTERVALS
7806    COLLINS TEMPORAL$INTEGRATION TONE$GLIDES
7806    DOOLING AUD$DURATION$DISCRIM PARAKEET
7806    FASTL FREQ$DISCRIM PULSED$VS$MODULATED$TONES
7806    GOLDSTEIN COMPATIBILITY MEAS AURAL$COMBINATION$TONES
7806    GOLDSTEIN ARU
7806    GOLDSTEIN AURAL$PROCESSING PITCH COMPLEX$TONES
7806    GRANTHAM DETECTABILITY INTERAURAL$TEMPORAL$DIFFERENCES
7806    GREY TIMBRE$DISCRIM MUSICAL$PATTERNS
7806    MCFADDEN BINAURAL$DETECTION HIGH$FREQ TIME-DELAYED
        $WAVEFORMS
7806    NELSON FREQ$DISCRIM CHINCHILLA
7806    PENNER POWER$LAW$TRANSFORMATION TIME-INTENSITY$TRADES
        NOISE$BURSTS
7806    POLLACK DECOUPLING AUD$PITCH STIMULUS$FREQ
7806    SCHUSTERMAN UPPER$LIMIT UNDERWATER FREQ$DISCRIM SEA
        $LION
7806    SPARKS INTENSITY$DIFFERENCES BREIF$ADJACENT$TONAL
        $STIMULI
7806    TRAHIOTIS REGRESSION$INTERP TIME-INTENSITY$TRADING
        LATERALITY
7806    WEBER SUPPRESSION CRITICAL$BANDS BAND-LIMITING$EXPERIMENTS
7806    YOST PITCH$DISCRIM BROADBAND$SIGNALS RIPPLED$SPECTRA
7833    GUSSENHOVEN PERCEP PROMINENCE DUTCH$LISTENERS
7833    ROSSI PERCEP FALLING$GLISSANDO PROSODIC$CONTOURS


                              0102


5406    EFFECT ARRIVAL$TIME STEREOPHONIC$LOCALIZATION

5406  EFFECT INTERAURAL$TIME$DIFFERENCES JUDGMENT$SIDEDNESS
5506  AL SINGLE$PAIRED$SOURCES
5506  MONAURAL$DIRECTION$FINDING
5606  EFFECT INTERAURAL$TIME$DIFFERENCES JUDGMENT$SIDEDNESS
5706  AL HIGH-FREQ$TONES
5706  OBJECTIVE$ALLOCATION SOUND-IMAGE BINAURAL$STIMULATION
5806  BINAURAL$LOCALIZATION SPACE-FREQ$EQUIVALENCE
5906  AL CLICKS
5906  LATERALIZATION$THR FUNCTION STIMULUS$DURATION
5906  PI CROSS-EAR$LOCALIZATION$EFFECTS
5906  ROLE INTERAURAL$TIME$INTEN$DIFFERENCES LATERALIZATION
      LOW-FREQ$TON
6006  LATERALIZATION HIGH-FREQ$TONES
6106  LATERALIZATION LOCALIZATION
6106  TIME INTEN LOCALIZATION$TONES
6206  EFFECT MAKING$NOISE LATERALIZATION LOUDNESS CLICKS
6206  EFFECTS UNILATERAL AUD$MASKING AL SPACE
6206  FAILURE LOCALIZE SOURCE$DISTANCE UNFAMILIAR$SOUND
6206  LATERALIZATION ACOUS$TRANSIENTS
6206  MAPPING BINAURAL CLICK LATERALIZATIONS
6211  AL DEPTH
6211  EFFECT DICHOTIC$NOISE AL
6211  TRADING$REL DICHOTIC$TIME INTENSITY$DIFFERENCES AL
6306  INTERPRETATION BUTLER-NAUNTON LOCALIZATION$SHIFTS
6306  MODIFICATION SENSORY$LOCALIZATION CONSEQUENCE OXYGEN
      $INTAKE
6406  ACOUS-IMAGE LATERALIZATION$JUDGMENTS BINAURAL$TONES
6406  ACOUSTIC-IMAGE LATERALIZATION$JUDGMENTS BINAURAL$TRANSIENTS
6406  BINAURAL$LATERALIZATION COPHASIC$ANTIPHASIC$CLICKS
6406  DIRECTIONAL$LOCALIZATION SOUND PLANE-WAVE$SOURCES
6406  LATERALIZING$EFFECTS INTERAURAL$PHASE$DIFFERENCES
6406  ROLE STIMULUS$FREQ DURATION PHENOMENON LOCALIZATION
      $SHIFTS
6506  LATERALIZATION$JUDGMENTS NATURE BINAURAL$ACOUS$IMAGES
6506  LOCALIZATION$AFTEREFFECTS PULSE-TONE PULSE-PULSE STIMULI
6606  END$POINT LATERALIZATION DICHOTIC$CLICKS
6606  LATERALIZATION WEAK$SIGNAL PRESENTED CORRELATED UNCORRELATED
      $NOISE
6606  NOISE$LOCALIZATION UNILATERAL$ATTENUATION
6706  DETECTION LOCALIZATION EXTENSION THEORY$SIGNAL$DETECTABILITY
6706  EFFECT INDUCED$HEAD$MOVEMENT LOCALIZATION SOUNDS
6706  HEAD$MOVEMENTS AL
6711  EFFECTS RHYTHMICALLY$MOVING$AUD$STIMULUS EYE$MOVEMENTS
      ADULTS
6711  ROLE STIMULUS$FREQUENCY LOCALIZATION
6711  UNDERWATER$AL SEA$LION

6806   AL TONAL$STIMULI VERTICAL$PLANE
6806   DIRECTIONAL$HNG SEAL AIR$WATER
6806   FACTORS AL VERTICAL$PLANE
6806   IMPROVEMENT HNG$ABILITY DIRECTIONAL$INFORMATION
6806   LATERAL$LOCALIZATION SP$SIGNALS ANECHOIC$SPACE
6806   LATERALIZATION$THR SIGNAL$IN$NOISE
6806   PERCEP DIRECTION ECHO
6806   PERCEP RANGE SOUND$SOURCE UNKNOWN$STRENGTH
6806   PROXIMITY$IMAGE$EFFECT AL
6806   ROLE PHASE-DIFFERENCE$CUES CUTANEOUS$ANALOG AL
6806   SPECTRAL$CUES MPL
6806   TEMPORAL$INTENSIVE$FACTORS BINAURAL$LATERALIZATION
       AUD$TRANSIENTS
6806   TWO-IMAGE$LATERALIZATION TONES CLICKS
6807   CORRELATION ORIENTED$DEFENSIVE$REFLEXES SOUND
6906   DIRECT$COMPARISON LATERALIZATION DETECTION CONDITIONS
       ANTIPHASIC$M
6906   IMAGE$FUSION BROADENING DISPLACEMENT AL
6906   INTERAURAL$INTENSITY DIFFERENCE INTRACRANIAL$LATERALIZATION
6906   LATERALIZATION DETECTION TONAL$SIGNAL NOISE
6906   ROLE SIGNAL$ONSET AL
6911   MONAURAL$BINAURAL$LOCALIZATION NOISE$BURSTS MEDIAN
       $SAGITTAL$PLANE
6911   UNDERWATER$AL MAN
7004   EFFECT STIMULUS$DURATION AL NOISE$STIMULI
7006   EFFECTS INTERAURAL$FREQ$DIFFERENCES LATERALIZATION
       $FUNCTION
7006   IN-HEAD$LOCALIZATION ACOUS$IMAGES
7011   AL BODY$TILT
7011   AUD$LATERALIZATION BODY$TILT
7011   MONAURAL$AL EFFECTS FEEDBACK INCENTIVE INTERSTIMULUS
       $INTERVAL
7104   MONAURAL$BINAURAL$MINIMUM$AUDIBLE$ANGLES MOVING$SOUND
       $SOURCE
7106   AL LAW FIRST$WAVEFORM MEDIAN$PLANE
7106   DIFFERENCES INTERAURAL$PHASE LEVEL DETECTION LATERALIZATION
7106   DIFFERENCES INTERAURAL$PHASE LEVEL DETECTION LATERALIZATION
7106   EFFECT UNILATERAL$MASKING LATERALIZATION BINAURAL
       $PULSES
7106   LATERALIZATION DETECTION NOISE-MASKED$TONES DURATIONS
7106   LATERALIZATION FILTERED$CLICKS
7106   QUANTITATIVE$EVAL LATERALIZATION$MODEL MASKING-LEVEL
       $DIFFERENCES
7111   CEREBRAL$HEMISPHERE$DOMINANCE$TEST LOCALIZATION$SP
7111   DIRECTIONAL$SENSITIVITY LATERALITY
7206   DIFFERENCES INTERAURAL$PHASE LEVEL DETECTION LATERALIZATION

```
7211    ADAPTATION FUNCTIONAL$LOSS PINNA AL
7211    AL BC EEA$TECHNIQUES
7211    INTERAURAL$INTENSITY$REL MPL
7211    MONAURAL$BINAURAL$AUD$LOCALIZATION NOISE$BURSTS MEDIAN
        $VERTICAL$PL
7211    ROLE PITCH$SENSATION MONAURAL$AL WHITE$NOISE
7211    ROLES PINNA EAM MONAURAL$AL
7306    ACUITY HUMAN AL UNDERWATER
7306    AL HIGH-LOW-FREQ$TRANSIENTS
7306    AL PT
7306    COMPARISON LATERALIZATION MLD MONAURAL$SIGNALS GATED
        $NOISE
7306    DETERMINANTS LOCALIZATION-ADAPTATION$EFFECTS AUD$STIMULI
7306    MONAURAL$BINAURAL$FACETS MPL
7306    PERCEP RANGE SOUND$SOURCE UNKNOWN$DIRECTION
7306    PROBLEM MPL EFFECT PINNAE$CAVITY$OCCLUSION
7306    UNDERWATER AL HUMAN
7311    AL BRAIN-DAMAGED$MONKEYS
7311    CONTROLLED$LATERALIZATION$BC$SOUND
7311    EFFECT HEAD$POSITION AL
7406    AL PAIRED$SOUND$SOURCES RAT SMALL$TIME$DIFFERENCES
7406    AL STRONG$WEAK$SOUNDS
7406    AL$DISTANT$SOUND$SOURCES
7406    DIFFERENCES AL LATERALIZATION
7406    DYNAMIC$THEORY AL
7406    LATERALIZATION BINAURAL$MASKING-LEVEL DIFFERENCE
7406    LATERALIZATION TONAL$STIMULI CAT
7406    PINNA$REFLECTIONS CUES AL
7406    TWO$EARS AL MPL
7503    MOORE AUDITORY$LOCALIZATION INFANTS REINFORCEMENT
        $CONDITIONS
7504    THURLOW LOCALIZATION NOISE OVERLAPPING$TIME
7506    BELENDIUK MONAURAL$LOCALIZATION LOW-PASS$NOISE HORIZONTAL
        $PLANE
7506    LIPORACE LINEAR$ESTIMATION NONSTATIONARY$SIGNALS
7506    MOORE UNDERWATER$LOCALIZATION CALIFORNIA$SEA$LION
7506    MOORE UNDERWATER$LOCALIZATION CLICK PULSED$PT$SIGNALS
        CALIF$SEA$LION
7506    SEARLE BINAURAL$PINNA$DISPARITY AUD$LOCALIZATION$CUE
7511    ALTSHULER STIMULUS$INTENSITY FREQUENCY MEDIAN$PLANE
        LOCALIZATION
7511    ALTSHULER EFFECT STIM$INTENSITY$FREQ MEDIAN$PLANE
        $LOCALIZATION
7511    MCCLCLLAND LOW$FREQ$SOUND$LOCALIZATION KANGAROO$RAT
7511    MCCLELLAND LOW$FREQUENCY$LOCALIZATION KANGAROO$RAT
7511    RUSSEL LOUDNESS$BALANCING COMPLEX$SOUND$LOCALIZATION
```

7511   RUSSELL LOUDNESS$BALANCING COMPLEX$SOUND$LOCALIZATION
7606   ALTES SONAR GENERALIZED$TARGET$DISCRIPTION ANIMAL
       $ECHOLOCATION$SYSTEMS
7606   NUETZEL LATERALIZATION COMPLEX$WAVEFORMS FINE$STRUCTURE
       AMP DURATION
7606   SEARLE MODEL AUDITORY$LOCALIZATION
7611   GATEHOUSE AL MONAURAL$SUBJECTS
7611   RUSSELL LOCALIZATION$RESPONSE$CERTAINTY LISTENING
       $CONDITIONS
7611   RUSSELL EARMUFFS EARPLUGS AZIMUTHAL$CHANGES SPECTRAL
       $PATTERNS THEORIES
7611   RUSSELL ROLE PINNA MONAURAL$PLANE$LOCALIZATION
7706   BUTLER SPECTRAL$CUES LOCATION SOUND MEDIAN$SAGITTAL
       $PLANE
7706   PERROTT BINAURAL$LOCALIZATION MOVING$SOUND$SOURCES
7729   SEITZ CHANGES CLICK$MIGRATION FUNCTION AGE
7806   ALTES ANGLE$ESTIMATION BINAURAL$PROCESSING ANIMAL
       $ECHOLOCATION
7806   AU PROPAGATION DOLPHIN$ECHOLOCATION$SIGNALS
7806   BROWN LOCALIZATION PURE$TONES OLD$WORLD$MONKEYS
7806   SHELTON LOCALIZATION$ACUITY HORIZONTAL$PLANE

## 0103

5406   UTILIZATION INTRATYMPANIC$MUSCLE$REFLEX OBJECTIVE
       $DETERMINATION
6006   POST-TETANIC$POTENTIATION MIDDLE-EAR-MUSCLE AR
6106   METHOD STUDY TYMPANIC$REFLEXES MAN
6106   STUDIES AR CONTRALATERAL$REMOTE$MASKING INDICATOR
       REFLEX$ACTIVITY
6111   COMPARISON ATTENUATION$CHARACTERISTICS ACOUS$REFLEX
       V
6111   PROLONGATION AR
6111   TTS AR
6206   AR MAN
6206   STUDIES AR REFLEX$LATENCY INFERRED REDUCTION TTS IMPULSES
6206   STUDIES AR REDUCTION TTS INTERMITTENT$NOISE REFLEX
       $ACTIVITY
6306   STUDIES AR REFLEX$LATENCY INFERRED REDUCTION TTS IMPULSES
6406   DYNAMICS AR PHENOMENOLOGICAL$ASPECTS
6411   MIDDLE$EAR$MUSCLE ACOUSTIC$REFLEX COCH$SENSITIVITY
6504   EFFECT AR IMPED EARDRUM
6506   BINAURAL$SUMMATION AR
6704   IMPED$STUDIES NORMAL$EARS

6704    REPORT IMPED$STUDIES AR
6706    CONTRALATERAL$MASKING ATTEMPT DETERMINE ROLE$AR
6706    NUMERICAL$MODEL$AR
6711    MIDDLE$EAR$MUSCLE LOW$INTENSITY$SOUNDS
6806    IMPED$EARDRUM MIDDLE-EAR$TRANSMISSION EQUAL$LOUDNESS
6806    REL AR LOUDNESS
6906    CONTRALATERAL REMOTE$MASKING AR
7011    CONDITION AR
7104    ELECTROACOUS$IMPED$BRIDGE STUDIES NORMAL$EARS CHIL
7106    ACOUS STAPEDIAL$REFLEX REL CRITICAL$BANDWIDTH
7106    COMMENTS CONTRALATERAL$REMOTE$MASKING AR
7111    RESPONDENT$CONDITIONING MIDDLE$EAR$REFLEX
7205    IMPED$CONVERSION$TABLE
7206    STUDY AR HUMANS CHARACTERISTICS
7304    AR LOUDNESS$GROWTH PATH$EARS
7306    CRITICAL$BAND ACOUS$STAPEDIUS$REFLEX
7306    LOUDNESS$CHANGES RESULTING ELECTRICALLY$INDUCED$MIDDLE-EAR
        $REFLEX
7306    STAPEDIUS$REFLEX SP$FEATURES
7311    AR LOUDNESS$SHIFTS MASKER
7311    AUD$SENSITIZATION HUMAN$STAPEDIUS$REFLEX
7311    IMPED$ADMITTANCE$BRIDGE MIDDLE$EAR$STUDY
7404    EFFECTS EXTERNAL$EAR$CANAL$PRESSURE MIDDLE-EAR$MUSCLE
        $REFLEX
7404    NOTES ARTIFACT MEAS AR
7406    AR CRITICAL$BANDWIDTH
7417    AR COCH$PATH
7503    BESS ACOUSTIC$IMPEDANCE$MEASUREMENTS CLEFT-PALATE
        $CHIL
7504    WILEY AR+R SUSTAINED$SIGNALS
7506    DANCER HOLOGRAPHIC$INTERFEROMETRY TM$DISPLACEMENTS
        GUINEA$PIG$EARS
7506    MARGOLIS LOUDNESS AR
7511    IWAMOTO ACOUSTIC$REFLEX AIR + BONE-CONDUCTED$WHITE
        $NOISE
7511    IWAMOTO AR AC$BC$WHITE$NOISE
7511    RICHARDS THRESHOLD ACOUSTIC$REFLEX SHORT-DURATION
        BURSTS
7511    RICHARDS THR ACOUS$REFLEX SHORT TONE$BURSTS
7513    SURIA ACOUSTIC$IMPEDANCE AUTISTIC$CHILDREN
7603    SCHWARTZ CRITICAL$BANDWIDTH SENSITIVITY$PREDICTION
        AR
7606    MCPHERSON MIDDLE$EAR$PRESSURE EFFECTS AUD$PERIPHERY
7606    POPELKA ACTIVATING$SIGNAL$BANDWIDTH ACOUSTIC-REFLEX
        $THRESHOLDS
7606    PRICE INTERRUPTING$RECOVERY LOSS COCHLEAR$MICROPHONIC
        $SENSITIVITY

```
7606    SCHARF AR LOUDNESS$SUMMATION CRITICAL$BAND
7606    WOODFORD ACOUS$REFLEX$THR CHINCHILLA STIM$DURATION+FREQ
7611    BLOOD DIMENSIONS ACTIVATING$SIGNELS ACOUSTIC$REFLEX
7611    MACRAE COCHLEAR$EFFECTS TYMPANOMETRY
7703    ABAHAZI ACOUSTIC$REFLEX INFANTS
7704    KARLOVICH ACOUSTIC$REFLEX TTS TEMPORAL$CHAR
7704    MARGOLIS INTERACTIONS TYMPANOMETRIC$VARIABLES
7704    MARGOLIS TYMPANOMETRIC$ASYMMETRY
7704    MCFARLAND MIDDLE$COMPONENTS AER TONE-PIPS
7706    BLOCK STATISTICALLY$BASED$MEASURE ACOUSTIC$REFLEX
        STIMULUS$LOUDNESS
7706    MORGAN TEMPORAL$INTEGRATION THR ACOUS$REFLEX
7713    KEITH ACOUS REFLEX CHILDREN CEREBRAL PALSY
7804    FELDMAN STIM$DURATION STIM$OFF-TIME AUD + AR$THR
7804    HOROVITZ STAPEDIAL$REFLEX ANXIETY DISFLUENT$SPEAKERS
7804    WILEY ACOUSTIC-REFLEX$DYNAMICS PULSED$SIGNALS
7806    WILSON ADAPTATION ACOUSTIC$REFLEX
7806    WILSON THR GROWTH AR
```

## 0104

```
5506    INFLUENCE STIMULUS$DURATION PT$THR RECOVERY$AUD$FATIGUE
5506    PERSTIMULATORY$AUD$FATIGUE CONTINUOUS$INTERRUPTED
        $NOISE
5506    PERSTIMULATORY$FATIGUE MEAS HETEROPHONIC$LOUDNESS
        $BALANCES
5506    SPREAD PERSTIMULATORY$FATIGUE PT
5603    RECOVERY AUD$FATIGUE
5606    ONSET$GROWTH AURAL$HARMONICS OVERLOADED$EAR
5606    TTS INDEX NOISE$SUSCEPTIBILITY
5706    AUD$ADAPTATION
5706    OVERSTIMULATION FATIGUE ONSET$OVERLOAD HUMAN$EAR
5804    CUMULATIVE$AUD$FATIGUE
5806    DEPENDENCE TTS
5806    EXPOSURE$LOUD$SOUNDS
5806    HNG$LEVEL HNG$LOSS THR$SHIFT
5806    INTENSITY DURATION NOISE$EXPOSURE TTS
5806    MONAURAL$TTS MONAURAL$BINAURAL$EXPOSURES
5806    RESIDUAL$EFFECTS LOW$NOISE$LEVELS TTS
5806    TEMPORARY$THR$ELEVATION CONTINUOUS$IMPULSIVE$NOISES
5806    TTS FUNCTION NOISE$EXPOSURE$LEVEL
5806    TTS MASKING NOISE$SPECTRUM$LEVEL
5904    POST-EXPOSURE$RESIDUAL$EFFECTS LOW-LEVEL$NOISE
5906    AUD$ADAPT NOISE
```

5906    EFFECT EARPHONE$CUSHION AUD$THR
5906    NOISE$STRESS LAB$RODENTS EFFECTS CHRONIC$NOISE SEXUAL
        $PERFORMANCE
5906    POSTSTIMULATORY$EFFECTS THR$AUDIBILITY
5906    REL RECOVERY TTS DURATION$EXPOSURE
5906    SUSCEPTIBILITY SEX
5906    TTS INTERMITTENT$EXPOSURE$NOISE
5906    TTS OCTAVE-BAND$NOISE APPLICATIONS DAMAGE-RISK$CRITERIA
6006    INFLUENCE LOUD$CONTRALATERAL$STIMULATION THR PERCEIVED
        $LOUDNESS
6006    LATENT$RESIDUAL$EFFECTS TTS
6006    MEAS PERSTIMULATORY$AUD$ADAPTATION
6006    PROTECTIVE$EFFECT AR IMPULSIVE$NOISES
6006    RECOVERY HIGH$VALUES TTS
6006    TTS CHANGING$NOISE$LEVEL
6104    LOUDNESS$SHIFTS PT CONTRALATERAL$NOISE$STIMULATION
6106    CONTRALATERAL$THR$SHIFT REDUCTION TTS INDICES AR
6106    EFFECT MATCHING$TIME PERSTIMULATORY$ADAPTATION
6106    EXPLORATORY$STUDIES TTS IMPULSES
6106    NONINTERACTION TTS
6106    TTS TONES NOISE$BANDS EQUIVALENT$SPL
6111    TTS AR
6204    RELIABILITY TEMPORAL$COURSE TEMPORARY$CONTRALATERAL
        $THR$SHIFTS
6206    AUD$FATIGUE AUDIO$ANALGESIA
6206    AUD$FATIGUE AUDIO$ANALGESIA
6206    EFFECT TEMPORAL$SPACING TTS IMPULSES
6206    FREE-FIELD THR$SHIFT TTS REDUCTION MEAS EFFICIENCY
6206    GROWTH LOUDNESS REL INTEN$DISCRIM LEVELS AUD$FATIGUE
6206    TTS CHANGING DUTY$CYCLE
6211    AUD$RECOVERY$TIME SHORT$SOUND$STIMULATIONS
6211    THR$AUD$ADAPTATION
6211    TTS HNG$LEVEL INDUSTRIAL$SAMPLES
6304    REL PERSTIMULATORY$ADAPTATION SHORT-TERM$THR$SHIFTING
        $MECHANISMS
6306    CENTRAL$FACTOR PT AUD$FATIGUE
6306    METHODS MEAS RECOVERY SHORT-DURATION$FATIGUE
6306    PREDICTION TTS NOISE INCREASE
6306    TTS PRODUCED LOW-LEVEL$TONES EFFECTS TESTING RECOVERY
6404    EFFECTS REPEATED$EXPOSURE HIGH-INTENSITY$TONES RECOVERY
        AUD$SENSIT
6406    ADAPTATION FATIGUE
6406    EFFECT MONAURAL$FATIGUE PITCH$MATCHING DISCRIM
6406    EFFECT REPEATED$EXPOSURE HIGH-INTENSITY$SOUND
6406    EFFECTS EXTRANEOUS$TASKS AUD$FATIGUE
6406    OBSERVATIONS CENTRAL$FACTOR AUD$FATIGUE

6406    RATE DECAY AUD$SENSATION
6406    TEMPORARY$HNG$LOSSES EXPOSURE PRONOUNCED SINGLE-FREQ
        $COMPONENTS
6411    ABNORMAL$AUD$ADAPTATION AMPLITUDE$MODULATED$TONES
6411    HABITUATION
6506    APPLICATION ADAPTIVE$THR$ELEMENTS RECOGNITION ACOUS-PHONETIC
        $STATE
6506    AUD$FATIGUE INFLUENCE MENTAL$FACTORS
6506    EFFECTS MENTAL$TASKS AUD$FATIGUE
6506    PRELIMINARY$STUDIES TTS ARC-DISCHARGE IMPULSE-NOISE
        $GENERATOR
6506    TTS CHINCHILLA NOISE$EXPOSURE
6506    TTS MONAURAL$BINAURAL$EXPOSURE
6511    PROTECTION IMPULSE$NOISE PRECEDING$NOISE CLICK$STIMULI
6511    REL TTS DIFFERENT$SOURCES
6606    AUD$THR$LOCATION UNCERTAINTY FUNCTION TONE$PARAMETERS
        FATIGUE
6606    MECHANICAL$IMPACT MODEL AUD$EXCITATION FATIGUE
6606    OBSERVATIONS CENTRAL$FACTOR AUD$FATIGUE
6606    RELIABILITY TTS IMPULSE-NOISE$EXPOSURE
6606    TTS HNG EXPOSURE IMPACT/STEADY-STATE$NOISE
6606    TTS MALES FEMALES
6606    USE SL MEAS LOUDNESS TTS
6606    USE SL MEAS$LOUDNESS TTS
6706    CENTRAL$FACTOR AUD$FATIGUE ARTIFACT
6706    EFFECT INTERAURAL$PHASE BINAURAL$EXPOSURES THR$SHIFT
6706    FREQ$DISCRIM NOISE$EXPOSURE
6706    REL AFTEREFFECTS ACOUS$STIMULATION
6711    EFFECT PULSE$DURATION TTS IMPULSE$NOISE
6711    RECOVERY IMPULSE$NOISE ACOUS$TRAUMA
6711    RELATIONSHIP TTS DURATION$NOISE$EXPOSURE
6804    SUPRATHR$AUD$ADAPTATION PATHOLOGICAL$EARS
6806    ADAPTIVE$THR$PROCEDURES BUDTIF
6806    FUNCTIONAL$CHANGES EAR PRODUCED HIGH-INTENSITY$SOUND
6806    IMPULSE$DURATION TTS
6806    MEAS PERSTIMULATORY$LOUDNESS$ADAPTATION
6806    OBSERVATIONS REL LOUDNESS$DISCOMFORT$LEVEL AUD$FATIGUE
        SPL SL
6806    REL THR$SHIFT NOISE HUMAN$EAR
6806    ROLE TONAL$RELEVANCE AUD$FATIGUE
6806    SENSITIZATION AUD$TACTILE$SYSTEMS EXPOSURE INTENSE
        $STIMULATIONS
6806    STUDY PER-AND$POSTSTIMULATORY$FATIGUE PITCH$PERCEP
6806    STUDY TINNITUS INDUCED NOISE
6806    TTS AUD$TASK EXPOSURE
6811    EXPERIMENTAL CENTRAL$FACTORS AUD$FATIGUE

6906 AUD$FATIGUE ARTIC PRELIMINARY$OBSERVATIONS
6906 EFFECTS ATTENTION$STATES AR$ACTIVITY TTS
6906 OBSERVATIONS AUD$FATIGUE VOCAL NONVOCAL SP$ACTIVITIES
6906 RECOVERY TTS FUNCTION TEST EXPOSURE$FREQS
6906 SUPRATHR AUD$ADAPTATION
6906 TTS PULSED MONAURAL ALTERNATE$BINAURAL$EXPOSURE
6911 COMPARISON METHODS MEAS$AUD$ADAPTATION
6911 TTS HIGH$INTENSITY VARIABLE$PEAKED$FARM$MACHINERY
     $NOISE
7004 TTS ROCK-AND-ROLL$MUSICIANS
7006 ADAPTATION LOUDNESS$DECREMENT RECONSIDERATION
7006 ADAPTATION CENTRAL PERIPHERAL
7006 APPLICATION TTS$PARADIGM ASSESSING SOUND$TRANSMISSION
     AUD$SYSTEM
7006 CRITICAL$BAND TTS
7006 FREQ$DISCRIM ADAPTED$EAR
7006 POSTEXPOSURE$RESPONSIVENESS AUD$SYSTEM SENSITIZATION
     DESENSITIZATI
7006 TEMPORARY$CHANGES AUD$SYSTEM EXPOSURE NOISE DAYS
7006 TTS DAMAGE$RISK$CRITERIA INTERMITTENT$NOISE$EXPOSURES
7106 PRELIMINARY$OBSERVATIONS EFFECTS NOISE$EXPOSURE HNG
     INNER$EAR
7106 RECOVERY IMPULSE-NOISE TTS MONKEYS MEN DESCRIPTIVE
     $MODEL
7106 REL TEMPORARY$LOUDNESS$SHIFT TTS
7106 THEORY TTS
7106 TTS PT NOISE ABSENCE AR
7111 TTS ROCK-AND-ROLL$MUSIC
7111 TTS SEX
7111 TTS$RECOVERY IMPULSES STEADY$STATE$NOISE
7204 ADAPTATION$EFFECT
7204 TTS EXPOSURE HIGH-FREQ$NOISE
7204 TTS PROLONGED$EXPOSURE$NOISE
7204 TTS PROLONGED$EXPOSURE$NOISE
7204 TTS REDUCTION FUNCTION CONTRALATERAL$NOISE$LEVEL
7206 AUD$ADAPTATION REL MODEL LOUDNESS
7206 CHANGES TTS HUMMING NONVOCAL$ACTIVITIES
7206 COMPARISON OBJECTIVE THR-SHIFT$METHODS MEAS REAL-EAR
     $ATTENUATION
7206 FUNCTIONAL$CHANGES EAR PRODUCED HIGH-INTENSITY$SOUND
7206 INFLUENCE BINAURAL$INTERACTION MEAS PERSTIMULATORY
     $LOUDNESS$ADAPTA
7206 MECHANICAL$IMPACT FATIGUE REL NONLINEAR$COMBINATION
     $TONES COCH
7206 MONAURAL$PERSTIMULATORY$LOUDNESS$ADAPTATION
7206 TEMPORARY$HNG$LOSS NOISE VIBRATION

7206    TTS CHINCHILLA ELECTROPHYSIOLOGICAL$CORRELATES
7206    TTS HNG EXPOSURE NOISE$SPECTRA
7206    TTS RECOVERY$PATTERNS ROCK$ROLL$MUSIC
7211    ADAPTATION LOUDNESS$RECRUITMENT
7211    INFLUENCE AR TTS CONTINUOUS$PT
7304    COMBINED$EFFECTS RECOVERY$PERIOD STIMULUS$INTENSITY
        HUMAN
7304    DECAY$TTS NOISE
7304    SPREAD-OF-MASKING$EFFECTS PURE$TONE SP$STIMULI
7304    THR$SHIFTS EXPOSURE$NOISE CHINCHILLAS NOISE-INDUCED
        $HNG$LOSSES
7304    TTS PERMENENT$THR$SHIFTS NINE-DAY$EXPOSURES$NOISE
7306    EFFECTS INTENSE$AUD$STIMULATION HNG$LOSSES INNER$EAR
        $CHANGES MONKE
7306    MONAURAL$LOUDNESS$ADAPTATION
7306    PERSTIMULATORY$LOUDNESS$ADAPTATION
7306    SUPRATHR$LOUDNESS$ADAPTATION
7306    SUSCEPTIBILITY DAMAGE IMPULSE$NOISE CHINCHILLA MAN
        MONKEY
7306    THR$ADAPTATION NORMAL$LISTENERS
7317    ADAPTATION FATIGUE OPERATIONAL$DEFINITIONS
7403    TTS TOY$CAP$GUN
7404    SPECTRAL$TEMPORAL$PARAMETERS CONTRALATERAL$SIGNALS
        TTS
7406    AUDIOMETRIC$HISTOLOGICAL$CORRELATES EXPOSURE
7406    HNG$LOSS CONTINUOUS$EXPOSURE STEADY-STATE$BROAD-BAND
        $NOISE
7406    PERSTIMULATORY$LOUDNESS$ADAPTATION COCH$DAMAGE MASKED
        $NORMAL$LISTE
7406    SPECIES$DIFFERENCES COCH$FATIGUE ACOUS OUTER$MIDDLE
        $EARS GUINEA$PI
7511    WEILER DICHOTIC$HETEROPHONIC$MEASUREMENT ADAPTATION
7511    WEILER DICHOTIC$HETEROPHONIC$MEAS PERSTIMULATORY$ADAPTATION
7511    YOUNG LOUDNESS$RECRUITMENT FATIGUED$EAR
7511    YOUNG TYPES LOUDNESS$RECRUITMENT
7606    DRESCHER EFFECT TEMP COCHLEAR$R EXPOSURE NOISE
7606    IRWIN TEMPORAL$SUMMATION DECAY HEARING
7606    MARGOLIS MONAURAL$LOUDNESS$ADAPTION LOW$SL NORMAL
        $IMPAIRED
7606    MARGOLIS MONAURAL$LOUDNESS$ADAPT LOW$SL NORMAL + IMPAIRED
        $EARS
7606    PARKER INFLUENCE AUDITORY$FATIGUE MASKED$PURE-TONE
        $THRESHOLDS
7606    WARD TTS NEIGHBORHOOD$AIRCRAFT$NOISE
7704    KARLOVICH ACOUSTIC$REFLEX TTS TEMPORAL$CHAR
7706    HETU TEMPORAL$DISTRIBUTION SOUND$ENERGY TTS NOISE
        $EXPOSURES

7806    BERGER NOISE$INDUCED PTS
7806    BLAKESLEE THR$SHIFT CHINCHILLAS EXPOSED IMPULSE$NOISE
7806    BURDICK THRESHOLD$SHIFTS CHINCHILLAS EXPOSED OCTAVE
        $BANDS
7806    HAYASHI PSYCHOLOGICAL$ASSESSMENT AIRCRAFT$NOISE$INDEX
7806    RYAN NOISE-INDUCED$THR$SHIFT COCH$PATH GERBIL
7806    TOBIAS ESTIMATING$PERFORMANCE HEARING$PROTECTORS


## 0105

5406    COCH$FUNCTION
5406    CORTICAL$TEST AUD$FUNCTION EXPERIMENTALLY$DEAFENED
        $CATS
5406    EXPLORATION COCH$POTENTIALS GUINEA$PIG MICROELECTRODE
5406    NEURAL$R CLICKS ANALYSIS MASKED$UNMASKED$INTENSITY
        $FUNCTIONS
5406    VARIATION SPL GUINEA$PIGS$EARS ABNORMAL$EARDRUMS
5506    HUMAN$SKIN$PERCEP TRAVELING$WAVES COCH
5506    MUSICIAN GUINEA$PIG
5506    PARADOXICAL$DIRECTION WAVE$TRAVEL COCH$PARTITION
5706    ELECTROPHYSIOLOGICAL$EVIDENCE AUD$SENSITIZATION
5706    FLUID$MOTION COCH$MODEL
5706    FUSION$SOUNDS SENSE$ORGANS
5706    NEURAL$VOLLEYS SIMILARITY SENSATIONS TONES SKIN$VIBRATIONS
5706    OBSERVATIONS MODELS BASILAR$PAPILLA FROG$EAR
5706    R ELECTRICAL$MODEL COCH$PARTITION POSITIONS$EXCITATION
5806    CHANGES COCH$ENDOLYMPHATIC$OXYGEN$AVAILABILITY AP
        CM ASPHYXIA HYPO
5806    EFFECTS LOCALIZED$HYPOXIA ELECTROPHYSIOLOGICAL$ACTIVITY
        COCH$GUINE
5806    ENDOLYMPHATIC$OXYGEN$TENSION COCH$GUINEA$PIG
5806    HARMONIC$DISTORTION COCH$MODELS
5806    LOCALIZATION$AURAL$HARMONICS BASILAR$MEMBRANE$GUINEA
        $PIGS
5806    MEDIAL$GENICULATE$BODY
5806    PITCH BINAURAL$INTERACTIONS
5906    ACTION MIDDLE$EAR$MUSCLES CATS
5906    LATENCY ACTION$POTENTIALS COCH$GUINEA$PIG
5906    NEURAL$FUNNELING SKIN INNER$OUTER$HAIR$CELLS COCH
5906    NOISE$STRESS LAB$RODENTS BEHAVIORAL$ENDOCRINE$R
5906    R AUD$CORTEX REPETITIVE$ACOUS$STIMULI
5906    REPRODUCTIVE$FUNCTION GUINEA$PIGS
5906    SYNCHRONISM NEURAL$DISCHARGES DEMULTIPLICATION PITCH
        $PERCEP SKIN H

5906    TONOTOPIC$ORGANIZATION CAT$AUD$CORTEX COMPLEX$STIMULI
6006    DIMENSIONAL$ANALYSIS COCH$MODELS
6006    MODEL CROSS$SECTION COCH
6006    R COCH$MODELS APERIODIC$SIGNALS RANDOM$NOISES
6006    SHEARING$MOTION SCALA$MEDIA COCH$MODELS
6106    ACOUS$TRAUMA GUINEA$PIG
6106    COCHLEAR$MODEL NERVE$SUPPLY
6106    CRITICAL$BANDWIDTH FREQ$COORDINATES BASILAR$MEMBRANE
6106    EFFECT ANOXIA COCH$POTENTIALS
6106    FACTOR$ANALYSIS COCH$INJURIES CHANGES ELECTROPHYSIOLOGICAL
        $POTENTI
6106    MECHANISM MIDDLE$EAR
6106    NETWORK$MODEL MIDDLE$EAR
6106    STUDIES ENDOLYMPHATIC$DC$POTENTIAL GUINEA$PIG$COCH
6206    ADVANCES NEUROPHYSIOLOGY NEUROANATOMY COCH
6206    ANALYSIS MIDDLE-EAR$FUNCTION INPUT$IMPED
6206    AUD$EVOKED$POTENTIALS COCH CORTEX INFLUENCED ACTIVATION
        EFFERENT
6206    BASILAR$MEMBRANE
6206    CENTRIFUGAL$INHIBITION AFFERENT$SECONDARY$NEURONS
        COCH$NUCLEUS SOU
6206    CHANGES COCH$MICROPHONIC GUINEA$PIG PRODUCED MECHANICAL
        $FACTORS
6206    COCH$POTENTIALS RHESUS$SQUIRREL$MONKEY
6206    COCH$R ACOUS$TRANSIENTS INTERPRETATION wHOLE-NERVE
        ACTION$POTENTIA
6206    COMPRESSIONAL$BC COCH$MODELS
6206    COMPUTATIONAL$MODEL BASILAR-MEMBRANE$DISPLACEMENT
6206    EVIDENCE LATERAL-LINE$ORGAN R NEAR-FIELD SOUND$DISPLACEMENT
        $SOURCE
6206    FUNCTIONAL$IMPLICATIONS NATURE SUBMICROSCOPE$STRUCTURE
        TECTORIAL
6206    INHIBITORY$MECHANISM VESTIBULAR$SYSTEM MAN COMPARISON
        HNG
6206    INNER$EAR R HIGH-LEVEL$SOUNDS
6206    INNER$EAR
6206    MEAS SIZE DC$POTENTIALS MICROPHONICS COCH
6206    MINIMUM PHASE R BASILAR$MEMBRANE
6206    MORPHOLOGICAL$BASIS DIRECTIONAL$SENSITIVITY
6206    NERUAL$MECHANISMS PERIPHERAL$AUD$SYS CENTRAL$AUD$SYSTEM
        MONKEY
6206    NERVOUS$DISCHARGES END$ORGANS VIBRATORY$STIMULATION
        SKIN
6206    OLIVO-COCH$BUNDLE
6206    OUTER$HAIR$CELLS ORGAN$CORTI
6206    PROPERTIES EIGHTH$NERVE ACTION$POTENTIAL

6206    R AUD$NERVE REPETITIVE$ACOUS$STIMULI
6206    RATE$FUNCTION AUD$NERVE R NOISE$BURSTS EFFECT CHANGES
6206    STRUCTURE FUNCTION SENSORY$HAIRS INNER$EAR
6211    VERTICAL$ORGANIZATION AUD$CORTEX CAT
6306    ANALYSIS MIDDLE-EAR$FUNCTION GUINEA$PIGS$EAR
6306    MEDIAL$SUPERIOR-OLIVARY-UNIT R$PATTERNS MONAURAL$BINAURAL
        $CLICKS
6306    MODIFICATION SENSORY$LOCALIZATION CONSEQUENCE OXYGEN
        $INTAKE
6306    NONLINEARITY MIDDLE$EAR SOURCE SUBHARMONICS
6306    POST-MORTEM ACOUS$IMPED HUMAN$EARS
6306    R ACOUS$STIMULI SINGLE$UNITS EIGHTH$NERVE BULLFROG
6306    R COCH$POTENTIALS CHANGES HYDROSTATIC$PRESSURE
6306    STUDIES ARTIFICIAL$NEURONS BINAURAL TEMPORAL$RESOLUTION
        CLICKS
6306    SUMMATING$POTENTIAL COCH GUINEA$PIG
6306    TRANSFER$FUNCTION MIDDLE$EAR
6406    CHANGES COCH-MICROPHONIC$POTENTIAL RESECTION EFFERENT
        $COCH$FIBERS
6406    EXPERIMENT COCH$SUMMATION
6406    LATERAL$LINE VIBRATION$RECEPTOR
6406    MEAS DISPLACEMENTS NONLINEARITIES GUINEA-PIG$TYMPANUM
6406    MODEL NEURAL$INHIBITION MAMMALIAN$COCH
6406    R ACOUS$STIMULI SINGLE$UNITS EIGHTH$NERVE GREEN$FROG
6411    AMPLITUDE$CHANGES EVOKED$POTENTIALS INFERIOR$COLLICULUS
        ACOUSTIC
6411    DAMAGE EIGHTH$CRANIAL$NERVE CAT
6506    BINAURAL$INTERACTION ACCESSORY$SUPERIOR-OLIVARY$NUCLEUS
        CAT
6506    DISTORTION$PROCESSES COCH-MICROPHONIC$R ABNORMAL$PHYSIOLOGICAL
        $CON
6506    EXPERIMENTAL$OBSERVATIONS DC$RESTING$POTENTIAL GUINEA-PIG
        $COCH
6506    INFLUENCES NEURAL$ACTIVITY BINAURAL$ACOUS$IMAGES
6506    NEUROPHYSIOLOGICAL$EVIDENCE STEVENS$POWER$FUNCTION
        MAN
6506    ROLE PINNA HNG
6506    SENSORY$SYSTEM INTERNAL$NOISE
6506    STIMULUS$CORRELATES WAVE$ACTIVITY SUPERIOR-OLIVARY
        $COMPLEX CAT
6511    COCH$POTENTIALS RAT
6511    COMPARISON SINGLE$UNIT$RESPONSES AUD$NERVE GSR$THR
        MICE
6511    STRUCTURE FUNCTION LIZARD$EAR
6606    BEHAVIORAL PINNA-REFLEX THR RAT AUDIOMETRIC TTS COVARIATIONS
6606    EFFECTS CALCIUM SOUND-EVOKED COCH$POTENTIALS GUINEA
        $PIG

6606    EFFERENT$INHIBITION AUD-NERVE$R DEPENDENCE ACOUS-STIMULUS
        $PARAMETE
6606    INPUT-OUTPUT$CHARACTERISTICS LATERAL-LINE SENSE$ORGAN
        XENOPUS$LAEV
6606    INTERACTIONS SYNCHRONOUS NEURAL$R PAIRED$ACOUS$SIGNALS
6606    MEAS STAPEDIAL-FOOTPLATE$DISPLACEMENTS SOUND$TRANSMISSION
        MIDDLE$E
6606    MEMBRANE$RESISTANCE ENDOLYMPHATIC$WALLS FIRST$TURN
        $COCH GUINEA$PIG
6606    ORIGIN SUMMATING$POTENTIAL
6606    PERIPHERAL$ORIGIN AUD$R RECORDED EIGHTH$NERVE BULLFROG
6606    REEXAMINATION COCH$MODEL
6606    SUBHARMONIC$COMPONENTS COCH-MICROPHONIC$POTENTIALS
6606    SUPERIOR-OLIVARY$R$PATTERNS MONAURAL$BINAURAL$CLICKS
6706    ACTIVATION AUD$CORTEX CLICKS BILATERAL$LESIONS BRACHIUM
        $INFERIOR$C
6706    DISPLACEMENT$MODEL TECTORIAL$MEMBRANE RETICULAR$LAMINA
6706    DYNAMIC$R MIDDLE-EAR$STRUCTURES
6706    EFFERENT$INHIBITION COCH REL HAIR-CELL$DC$ACTIVITY
        STUDY
6706    ENCODING STIMULUS$FREQ INTEN CAT SUPERIOR$OLIVE$S-SEGMENT
        $CELLS
6706    MECHANISTIC$ASPECTS HNG
6706    MIDDLE-EAR$CHARACTERISTICS ANESTHETIZED$CATS
6706    POSTSYNAPTIC$ACTIVITY CROSSED$OLIVOCOCH$FIBERS CAT
6706    PROPERTIES SOUND$TRANSMISSION MIDDLE$OUTER$EARS CATS
6706    SHAPES TUNING$CURVES SINGLE$AUD-NERVE$FIBERS
6711    CORRELATION$STUDIES FREQUENCY$RESOLUTION COCHLEA
6711    HNG ARBOREAL$EDENTATES COCHLEA$MICROPHONICS
6711    NEURAL$SENSITIVITY TRANSIENT$SOUND$BURSTS
6804    AMPLITUDE$DISTRIBUTIONS CM ACOUS$SINUSOIDS NOISE
6804    COMPARATIVE$MEAS COCH$APPARATUS
6804    EFFECTS CEREBROSPINAL$FLUID$PRESSURE CM$R
6806    APICAL$COCH$R PULSE$TRAINS
6806    DISTORTION COMPENSATING CONDENSER-EARPHONE PHYSIOLOGOCAL
        $STUDIES
6806    DISTORTION COMPENSATING CONDENSER-EARPHONE DRIVER
        PHYSIOLOGICAL$ST
6806    EFFECT SODIUM$DEFICIENCY COCH$POTENTIALS
6806    EFFECT TETRODOTOXIN PROCAINE COCH$POTENTIALS
6806    EFFECTS TONAL$INTERACTIONS COCH$MICROPHONIC
6806    LONGITUDINAL$DISTRIBUTION COCH$MICROPHONICS COCH$DUCT
        GUINEA$PIG
6806    MODEL NONLINEAR$CHARACTERISTICS COCH$POTENTIALS
6806    NEGATIVE$POTENTIAL ORGAN$CORTI
6806    RATE$VS$LEVEL$FUNCTIONS AUD-NERVE$FIBERS CATS TONE-BURST
        $STIMULI

6806  REPRESENTATION BINAURAL$STIMULI   SINGLE$UNITS PRIMARY
      $AUD$CORTEX
6806  SINGLE-UNIT$ACTIVITY PRIMARY$AUD$CORTEX UNANESTHETIZED
      $CATS
6806  STUDIES TWO-TONE$INTERACTION GUINEA$PIG$MICROPHONIC
6806  SUBMICROSCOPIC$DISPLACEMENT$AMPLITUDES TYMPANIC$MEMBRANE
      CAT MEAS
6806  TWO-TONE$DISTORTION$PRODUCTS NONLINEAR$MODEL$BASILAR
      $MEMBRANE
6806  TWO-TONE$INHIBITION AUD-NERVE$FIBERS
6807  MORPHOLOGICAL$CHANGES BRAIN SOUND$STIMULUS
6807  STRUCTURAL$ORG CORTICAL$REPRESENTATION ANALYSORS$MAN
6807  STUDY FUNCTION MANS$ACOUS$ANALYZOR
6811  ANALYSIS SINGLE$UNIT$RESPONSE$AREAS COCHLEAR$NERVE
6811  COCHLEA$MICROPHONICS$POTENTIAL BASAL$THIRD$TURNS RAT
      $COCHLEA
6811  NEURAL$RESPONSES SOUND CRICKET
6811  NON-LINEAR$BEHAVIOR INNER$EAR SENSATION$RAREFACTION
      $CLICKS
6811  RELATIONSHIP TEMPERATURE COCHLEAR$RESPONSE POIKILOTHERM
6811  STEREOTAXIC$INSTRUMENT ACOUSTIC$STUDIES RAT
6811  VOCAL$SPECTRA COCHLEAR$SENSITIVITY GERBIL
6904  REL AUDIOMETRY CM
6904  RELEASE$MASKING STUDYING HAIR$CELL$FUNCTION
6906  ALTERATION AFFERENT TONE-EVOKED$ACTIVITY NEURONS COCH
      $NUCLEUS
6906  CAT$SUPERIOR$OLIVE$S-SEGMENT$CELL$DISCHARGE
6906  COCH$HAIR-CELL$DAMAGE GUINEA$PIGS EXPOSURE IMPULSE
      $NOISE
6906  COCH$R BITONAL$STIMULI FUNCTION EFFERENTS
6906  COMBINATION$TONE MICROPHONIC$POTENTIALS
6906  COMMENTS DIFFERENTIAL-ELECTRODE$TECHNIQUE
6906  DEPENDENCE COCH$MICROPHONICS SUMMATING$POTENTIAL ENDOCOCH
      $POTENTIA
6906  DISTRIBUTION$PATTERN COCH$COMBINATION$TONES
6906  DISTRIBUTION$PATTERN COCH$HARMONICS
6906  EXPLANATION SYNCHRONY AUD$NERVE IMPULSES COMBINATION
      $TONES
6906  PROBLEMS MEAS COCH$DISTORTION
6906  PROPERTIES SUMMATING$POTENTIAL GUINEA$PIG COCH
6906  R SINGLE$AUD$UNITS EIGHTH$NERVE LEOPARD$FROG
6906  STIMULUS-R REL AUD-NOISE$FIBERS TWO-TONE$STIMULI
6906  TIME-DOMAIN$MEAS COCH$NONLINEARITIES COMBINATION$CLICK
      $STIMULI
6906  TRAVELING-WAVE$VELOCITY HUMAN COCH
6906  UNIT$R CAT COCH$NUCLEUS AMPLITUDE-MODULATED$STIMULI

6906   WAVEFORM$PRESERVATION COCH
6911   LATERAL$LINE$SENSITIVITY GOLDFISH
6911   TECHNIQUE WIDE$APPROACH$MEDULLA AUD$BULLAE CAT
7004   ORGANIZATION AUD$BEHAVIOR
7004   RELEASED$INFANTILE$ORONEUROMOTOR$ACTIVITY
7006   AUD-NERVE$FIBER$R TONE$BURSTS
7006   BEHAVIORAL$INVEST EFFECTS SECTIONING CROSSED$OLIVOCOCH
       $BUNDLE
7006   COCH$INNERVATION SIGNAL$PROCESSING REL AUD$TIME-INTENSITY
       $EFFECTS
7006   COMMENT WAVEFORM$PRESERVATION COCH
7006   DEGREES FREEDOM COCH$PATTERNS
7006   EFFECT CALCIUM$DEFICIENCY COCH$POTENTIALS
7006   EFFECTS ELECTRIC$STIMULATION CROSSED$OLIVOCOCH$BUNDLE
       AUD-NERVE$FI
7006   EFFECTS ELECTRICAL$CURRENT COCH$PARTITION DISCHARGES
       AUD-NERVE$FIB
7006   MAGNITUDE COCH$MICROPHONICS COMPONENTS BROAD-BAND
       $NOISE
7006   MEAS COCH$POTENTIALS GUINEA$PIG SPL EARDRUM COCH$MICROPHONIC
7006   MECHANICS GUNIEA$PIG$COCH
7006   MECHANISM PROD COCH$MICROPHONICS
7006   MODEL TWO-TONE$INHIBITION COCH-NERVE$FIBERS
7006   NONLINEARITIES COCH$HYDRODYNAMICS
7006   ON$OFF$R MEAS COCH$GUINEA$PIG
7006   PATTERN STAPEDIAL$VIBRATION
7006   PERIPHERAL$INHIBITION AUD$FIBERS FROG
7006   PERIPHERAL$ACTIVATION OLIVOCOCH$BUNDLE$ENDINGS
7006   POSTEXPOSURE$RESPONSIVENESS AUD$SYSTEM
7006   R NEURONS COCH$NUCLEI VARIATIONS NOISE$BANDWIDTH TONE-NOISE
       $COMBIN
7006   ROLE HEAT PROD ULTRASONIC$FOCAL$LESIONS
7006   STIMULATION VESTIBULAR$APPARATUS GUINEA$PIG STATIC
       $PRESSURE$CHANGE
7006   STUDY SINGLE$UNITS COCH$NUCLEUS CHINCHILLA
7006   VARIATIONS EFFECTS ELECTRIC$STIMULATION CROSSED$OLIVOCOCH
       $BUNDLE C
7011   COCH$NEURAL$ACTIVITY AUD$SYSTEM RACOON
7011   CONVOLUTIONAL$ORG LATERAL$SUPERIOR$OLIVARY$NUCLEI
7011   CORTICAL$AUDIOMETRY GUINEA$PIGS
7011   OSSICULAR$CHAIN$GRAFTING SOUND$CONDITIONED$CATS
7011   SENSITIVITY RAT$EAR CM
7104   CORTICAL$R
7104   NEUROPHYSIOLOGICAL$FEATURE$DETECTORS SP$PERCEP DISCUSSION
7106   COMMENT EXPLANATION SYNCHRONY AUD-NERVE$IMPULSES COMBINATION
       $TONES

7106  COMMENTS CORRESPONDENCE COCH$MICROPHONICS SENSITIVITY
7106  CORRESPONDENCE COCH$MICROPHONIC SENSITIVITY BEHAVIORAL
      $THR CAT
7106  CORTICAL$R AWAKE$CAT NARROW-BAND$FM$NOISE
7106  DETERMINATION MICROPHONIC$GENERATOR$TRANSFER$CHARACTERISTICS
7106  EFFECTS ELECTRICAL$STIMULATION CROSSED$OLIVOCOCH$BUNDLE
      COCH$POTEN
7106  ERROR HELMHOLTZ$CALCULATION DISPLACEMENT TYMPANIC
      $MEMBRANE
7106  INHIBITION AUD$NERVE
7106  INTRACOCH$ELECTRODES GUINEA$PIG
7106  INTRACOCH$POTENTIAL RECORDED MICROPIPETS CORRELATIONS
7106  INTRACOCH$POTENTIAL RECORDED MICROPIPET R COCH$SCALAE
      TONES
7106  INTRACOCH$POTENTIAL RECORDED MICROPIPET REL COCH$MICROPHONIC
      $POTEN
7106  LIMITATIONS COCH-MICROPHONIC$MEAS
7106  MICROPIPET$LOCATION
7106  OBSERVATIONS VIBRATION BASILAR$MEMBRANE SQUIRREL$MONKEY
7106  OLIVARY$R DICHOTIC$STIMULI
7106  R NEURONS COCH$NUCLEUS TONE-INTENSITY INCREMENTS
7106  STAPES$VELOCITY
7106  STUDY INFLUENCE OLIVOCOCH$BUNDLE R TONE$PULSES
7106  SUGGESTIONS BASILAR$MEMBRANE$DISPLACEMENT SIGNAL$AUDIBILITY
7106  TEMPORAL$POSITION DISCHARGES SINGLE$AUD$NERVE$FIBERS
      CYCLE SINE-WA
7106  TRANSFORM BASILAR$MEMBRANE
7106  TRAVEL$TIME COCH DETERMINATION COCH-MICROPHONIC$DATA
7106  VIBRATORY$PATTERN ROUND$WINDOW CAT
7111  FIELD$POTENTIAL$STUDY INHIBITION CAT SUPERIOR$OLIVARY
      $COMPLEX
7111  INTRACOCHLEAR$PRESSURE$VARIATION ANOXEMIA GUINEA$PIG
7111  NEURONAL$ACTIVITY DIFFERENT$LEVELS$AUD$SYSTEM
7206  COCH$MICROPHONE$POTENTIAL STAPES$VELOCITY
7206  COCH$RESONANCE PHASE-REVERSAL$SIGNALS
7206  COCH-MICROPHONIC MIDDLE-EAR$PRESSURE$CHANGES NITROUS-OXIDE
7206  COMMENT INTRACOCH$POTENTIAL RECORDED MICROPIPETS REL
7206  CROSSED$OLIVOCOCH$BUNDLE GUINEA$PIG$COCH
7206  DERIVATIVE$REL STAPES$MOVEMENT COCH$MICROPHONIC
7206  EARPHONE$COUPLING$SYSTEM PHYSIOLOGICAL$STUDIES
7206  ELECTROPHYSIOLOGICAL$STUDIES SPATIAL$DISTRIBUTION
7206  ENHANCEMENT MECHANOSENSITIVITY HAIR$CELLS LATERAL-LINE
      $ORGANS
7206  FRACTIONAL$DISTORTION$PAIRS COCH
7206  HYBRID-COMPUTER$MODEL COCH$PARTITION
7206  INFLUENCE DC$POLARIZATION COCH$PARTITION SUMMATING
      $POTENTIALS

7206   LATENCY WHOLE-NERVE$ACTION$POTENTIALS INFLUENCE HAIR-CELL
       $NORMALCY
7206   MAGNETICALLY$COUPLED$STIMULATION OSSICULAR$CHAIN MEAS
       KANGAROO$RAT
7206   MODELING SIMULATION COCH$POTENTIALS GUINEA$PIG
7206   NETWORK$REPRESENTATION EXTERNAL$EAR
7206   OXYGEN$AVAILABILITY TUNNEL$OF$CORTI MEAS MICROELECTRODE
7206   POTASSIUM$IONS
7206   R$PATTERNS SINGLE$COCH$NERVE$FIBERS CLICK$STIMULI
       DESCRIPTIONS CAT
7206   SIGNIFICANCE RESISTANCE$MEAS SCALA$MEDIA
7206   SOIND-INDUCED$ELECTRICAL$IMPED$CHANGES GUINEA$PIG
       $COCH
7206   TYMPANIC$MEMBRANE$VIBRATIONS CATS TIME-AVERAGED$HOLOGRAPHY
7206   TYMPANIC-MEMBRANE$VIBRATIONS HUMAN$CADAVER$EARS
7211   COMPUTER-GENERATED$DISPLAY COCH$TRAVELING$WAVES
7211   EFFECTS INTRACOCH$PRESSURE$CHANGES COCH$POTENTIALS
       GUINEA$PIGS
7304   REFLEX$CONTRACTION MIDDLE-EAR$MUSCLES STIMULATION
       $LARYNGEAL$NERVES
7306   ACOUS$BEHAVIOR OUTER$EAR GUINEA$PIG INFLUENCE MIDDLE
       $EAR
7306   AUD$NERVE$DISCHARGES
7306   COMPARISON SINGLE-AND-DOUBLE-CHAMBER$MODELS$COCH
7306   COMPUTER$SIMULATION GENERATION DISTRIBUTION COCH$POTENTIALS
7306   ELECTRIC$NETWORK$EFFECTS COCH
7306   INTEGRABLE$MODEL BASILAR$MEMBRANE
7306   MECHANISM SHORT-TERM$POSTSTIMULATORY$DEPRESSION COCH
       $MICROPHONIC
7306   NERVE-FIBER$DISTRIBUTION COCH BAT
7306   PRECEDENCE$EFFECTS AUD$CELLS LONG$CHARACTERISTIC$DELAYS
7306   QUANTITATIVE$STUDY COCH$POTENTIALS SCALA$MEDIA GUINEA
       $PIG
7306   RECOVERY DETECTION$PROBABILITY SOUND$EXPOSURE COMPARISON
       PHYSIOLOG
7306   RECOVERY SOUND$EXPOSURE AUD-NERVE$FIBERS
7306   SYSTEM NONLINEAR$DIFFERENTIAL$EQUATIONS MODEL BASILAR-MEMBRANE
       $MOT
7306   THEORY$BINAURAL$INTERACTION AUD-NERVE$DATA GENERAL
       $STRATEGY
7306   TRANSMISSION RADIAL$SHEAR$FORCES COCH$HAIR$CELLS
7311   COCH$EXCITATION FAINT$AUD$SIGNALS
7311   COMPUTER-AVERAGED$PT$R AUD$NERVE WAKING$SQUIRREL$MONKEY
7311   ORGANIZATION INFERIOR$COLLICULUS$CHINCHILLA
7311   REL CORTICAL$R ACOUS$STIMULI SPL SL
7311   SPACE-TIME$REFLECTION WHOLE-NERVE$AP COCH

| | |
|---|---|
| 7404 | ELECTRIC$RESPONSES$AUD |
| 7406 | AUDIOMETRIC HISTOLOGICAL$EFFECTS |
| 7406 | BASILAR$MEMBRANES TUNING$CURVES GUINEA$PIG |
| 7406 | BEHAVIOR BASILAR$MEMBRANE PT$EXCITATION |
| 7406 | COCH$MECHANICS NONLINEARITIES COCH$POTENTIALS |
| 7406 | COCH$PARTITION$STIFFNESS COMPOSITE$BEAM$MODEL |
| 7406 | CODING SOUNDS VARYING$SPECTRUM COCH$NUCLEUS |
| 7406 | DEPENDENCE MIDDLE-EAR$PARAMETERS BODY$WEIGHT GUINEA $PIG |
| 7406 | ELECTRICAL$POTENTIALS FLUID$BOUNDARIES ORGAN$CORTI |
| 7406 | EVIDENCE MOSSBAUER$EXPERIMENTS NONLINEAR$VIBRATION COCH |
| 7406 | INTRACELLULAR$R ACOUS$CLICKS INNER$EAR ALLIGATOR$LIZARD |
| 7406 | INVEST SOURCES WHOLE-NERVE$ACTION$POTENTIALS RECORDED PLACES GUINE |
| 7406 | LOSS$RECOVERY$PROCESSES LEVEL COCH$MICROPHONIC INTERMITTENT $STIMUL |
| 7406 | MEAS GUINEA$PIG MIDDLE-EAR$TRANSFER$CHARACTERISTIC |
| 7406 | MIDDLE-EAR$FUNCTION GUINEA$PIG |
| 7406 | MODEL MECHANICAL$TO$NEURAL$TRANSDUCTION AUD$RECEPTOR |
| 7406 | PERIPHERAL$AUD$FUNCTION PLATYPUS |
| 7406 | R$PATTERNS COCH$NUCLEUS$NEURONS EXCERPTS$SUSTAINED $VOWELS |
| 7406 | STIFFNESS REISSNERS$MEMBRANE |
| 7406 | TAILS TUNING$CURVES AUD-NERVE$FIBERS |
| 7406 | TRANSFORMATION$FUNCTION EXTERNAL$EAR R IMPULSIVE$STIMULATION |
| 7406 | TYMPANIC$MUSCLE$EFFECTS MIDDLE-EAR$TRANSFER$CHARACTERISTICS |
| 7412 | ANATOMY PHYSIOLOGY BIOCHEM AUD$PROCESSING |
| 7506 | ABBAGNARA MEASUREMENTS DIFFRACTION INTERAURAL$DELAY HUMAN$HEAD |
| 7506 | BOER SYNTHETIC$WHOLE-NERVE$ACTION$POTENTIALS CAT |
| 7506 | BURKHARD ANTHROPOMETRIC$MANIKIN ACOUSTIC$RESEARCH |
| 7506 | CHADWICK MECHANICAL$COCHLEAR$MODEL |
| 7506 | FLAMMINO NEURAL$R INFERIOR$COLLICULUS ALBINO$RAT BINAURAL $STIMULI |
| 7506 | HOLLIEN EXTERNAL$AUDITORY$MEATUS AUDITORY$SENSITIVITY $UNDERWATER |
| 7506 | KUHN FRONT$CAVITY$RESONANCE SP$PERCEPTION |
| 7506 | PFEIFFER COCHLEAR$NERVE FIBER$R COCHLEAR$PARTITION |
| 7506 | SEARLE BINAURAL$PINNA$DISPARITY AUD$LOCALIZATION$CUE |
| 7506 | WILSON BASILAR$MEMBRANE MID-EAR$VIBRATION GUINEA$PIG CAPACITIVE$PROBE |
| 7511 | NUNLEY STIMULATION CHINCHILLA'S$OSSICULAR$CHAIN ELECTRODE |
| 7511 | NUNLEY STIMULATION CHINCHILLA$OSSICULAR$CHAIN IMPLANTED $ELECTRODE |
| 7512 | BRUGGE MECHANISMS CODING$INFORMATION AUD$SYSTEM |

7512   PISONI MECHANISMS AUD$DISCRIM CODING LINGUISTIC$INFO
7606   ABBAS
7606   BOSTON AC$DC$COMPONENTS LATERAL$LINE MICRIPHONIC$POTENTIALS
7606   DRAGSTEN INTERFEROMETER VIBRATION$MEAS AUD$ORGANS
7606   DRESCHER EFFECT TEMP COCHLEAR$R EXPOSURE NOISE
7606   DUIFHUIS COCHLEAR$NONLINEARITY SECOND$FILTER
7606   FLOTTORP MECHANICAL$IMPED HUMAN$HEADBONES
7606   HOOD EYE$COLOR SUSCEPTIBILITY TO TTS
7606   JOHNSTONE TTS SHIFT COCHLEAR$NERVE$FIBERS
7606   KHANNA MECHANICAL$PARAMETERS HNG BONE$CONDUCTION
7606   MOORE R COCHLEAR-NUCLEUS$NEURONS SYNTHETIC$SP
7606   OZDAMAR INPUT-OUTPUT$FUNCTIONS COCHLEAR$ACTION$POTENTIALS
7606   REINIS ACUTE$CHANGES ANIMAL$INNER$EARS SIMULATED$SONIC
       $BOOMS
7606   ROBLES TRANSIENT$R BASILAR$MEM SQUIRREL$MONKEYS MOSSBAUER
       $EFFECT
7606   SMOORENBURG COMBINATION$TONES R NEURONS COCH$NUCLEUS
       CAT
7606   SOKOLICH R$POLARITIES COCHLEAR$HAIR$CELLS
7606   YATES LOCALIZED$COCHLEAR$MICROPHONICS SPIRAL$LAMINA
7606   ZWEIG COCHLEAR$COMPROMISE
7611   GUELKE TRANSMISSION$LINE$THEORY COCHLEAR$MECHANICS
7611   JETER WAVEFORM$PATTERNS REFLEX VOLUNTARY$CONTRACTION
       MIDDLE$EAR$MUSCLE
7611   MITCHELL FREQUENCY$SPECIFIC N
7611   RUBINSTEIN INFLUENCE EFFERENT$FIBERS COCHLEAR$ELECTRICAL
       $ACTIVITY
7611   RUSSELL ROLE PINNA MONAURAL$PLANE$LOCALIZATION
7611   WALLOCH ACOUSTIC$TRAUMA GUINEA$PIGS
7622   CELESIA AUD$CORTICAL$AREAS MAN, ORGANIZATION
7632   CAMPAIN GROSS$CONFIGURATIONS AUDITORY$CORTEX
7706   ALLEN COCHLEAR$MICROMECHANICS MECHANISM TRANSFORMING
       $TUNING COCHLEA
7706   ALLEN TWO-DIMENSIONAL$COCHLEAR$FLUID$MODEL
7706   COLBURN THEORY BINAURAL$INTERACTION AUD-NERVE DETECT
       TONES$IN$NOISE
7706   COOPER SYNTACTIC$BLOCKING PHONOLOGICAL$RULES SP$PRODUCTION
7706   GANS OLIVOCOCHLEAR STIMULATION COCHLEAR$SUMMATING
       $POTENTIAL
7706   HALL SPATIAL$DIFFERENTIATION AUD$SECOND$FILTER ASSESS
       MODEL BAS$MEM
7706   HALL TWO-TONE$SUPPRESSION NONLINEAR$MODEL BASILAR
       $MEMBRANE
7706   KRUGER MIDDLE$EAR$TRANSMISSION CATS EXPERIMENTALLY
       $INDUCED$TM$PERFS
7706   MEHRGARDT TRANSFORMATION$CHAR  EXTERNAL$HUMAN EAR

7706    MOLLER FREQ$SELECTIVITY SINGLE FIBERS R BROADBAND
        STIMULI
7706    TROTT EFFECTIVE$ACOUSTIC$CENTER
7708    MONNIN SUPERVISED$EXPERIENCE SCHOOLS
7732    FERRARO BRACHIUM INFERIOR$COLLICULUS HUMAN$AUD$PATHWAYS
7732    FERRARO LATERAL$LEMNISCUS HUMAN$AUD$PATHWAYS
7732    GATES CEREBRAL$HEMISPHERES MUSIC
7732    MINCKLER HUMAN$AUD$PATHWAYS
7732    PIROZZOLO HEMISPHERIC$SPECIALIZATION READING WORD
        $RECOGNITION
7806    ABBAS EFFECTS FREQ TWO-TONE$SUPPRESSION
7806    ALDER APPROACH GUINEA$PIG AUDITORY$NERVE
7806    BACKUS PRESSURE-FLOW$TECHNIQUE ASSESSING ORAL$PORT
        $SIZE
7806    BOER COCHLEAR$ENCODING REVERSE-CORRELATION$TECHNIQUE
7806    BUUNEN RESPONSES FIBERS CAT$AUDITORY$NERVE DIFFERENCE
        $TONE
7806    COLBURN THEORY BINAURAL$INTERACTION AUD-NERVE$DATA
7806    CROW PHASE$LOCKING MEDULLARY$NEURONS BINAURAL$PHENOMENA
7806    EHRET STIFFNESS$GRADIENT BASILAR$MEMBRANE FREQUENCY
        $ANALYSIS COCHLEA
7806    FAY CODING SINGLE$AUD-NERVE$FIBERS GOLDFISH
7806    FRY ACOUSTICAL$PROPERTIES HUMAN$SKULL
7806    FUNNELL MODELING CAT$EARDRUM FINITE-ELEMENT$METHOD
7806    GOSS ULTRASONIC$PROPERTIES MAMMALIAN$TISSUES
7806    JAVEL TWO-TONE$SUPPRESSION AUD$NERVE CAT
7806    KEMP STIMULATED$ACOUSTIC$EMISSIONS HUMAN$AUDITORY.SYSTEM
7806    LIBERMAN AUD-NERVE$R CATS RAISED LOW-NOISE$CHAMBER
7806    MORGAN ME$MUSCLE$CONTRACTION THR PT
7806    PRICE AP LOW$INTENSITIES
7806    RHODE OBSERVATIONS COCH$MECHANICS
7806    SAMBUR REDUCING BUZZ LPC$SYNTHESIS
7806    SCHMIEDT CM$TUNING$CURVES GERBIL
7806    SONDHI COMPUTING$MOTION TWO-DIMENSIONAL$COCH$MODEL
7806    STERN THEORY BINAURAL$INTERACTION BASED AUD-NERVE
        DATA
7806    VIERGEVER BASILAR$MEMBRANE$MOTION SPIRAL-SHAPED$COCHLEA


                              0106


5406    LAB$EVAL FIELD$MEAS LOUDNESS TRUCK$EXHAUST$NOISE
5407    EFFECTS HIGH$INTENSITY$NOISE MAN BIBLIOGRAPHY
5506    COMPARISONS PT NOISE$BANDS STIMULI EAR$PROTECTOR$ATTENUATION
        $MEAS

5506    DESIGN TESTING EARMUFFS
5506    SEMIPLASTIC$EARPLUGS
5506    SUBJECTIVE$MEAS LINEARITY EAR$DEFENDERS
5516    PRESCH$HNG$CONSERVATION
5603    OHIO$COUNTY$FAIR$HNG$SURVEY
5606    CRITERIA OFFICE$QUIETING QUESTIONNAIRE$RATING$STUDIES
5606    NOISE$BANDS PT STIMULI MEAS ACOUS$ATTENUATION EAR
        $PROTECTORS
5615    INDUSTRIAL$A
5706    HNG NAVAL$AIRCRAFT$MAINTENANCE$PERSONNEL
5706    HNG$PROTECTION
5803    OHIO$HNG$CRUISER
5817    HNG$CONSERVATION
5906    NOISE$MEAS ROCKET$ENGINES NOZZLE$PRESSURE$RATIOS
5906    SCALING$HUMANS$REACTIONS SOUND AIRCRAFT
6003    PRESCH$HNG$CONSERVATION STATEWIDE
6006    VALUE EAR$DEFENDERS MENTAL$WORK INTERMITTENT$NOISE
6006    VARIATION EAR$PROTECTOR$ATTENUATION MEAS METHODS
6206    DAMAGE-RISK$CRITERIA LINE$SPECTRA
6206    EAR$PROTECTORS
6206    IMPLICATIONS DAMAGE-RISK$CRITERIA
6306    EXPERIMENTAL$STUDY NOISE$REDUCTION CENTRIFUGAL$BLOWERS
6306    USE AR MEAS EAR-PROTECTOR$ATTENUATION HIGH$LEVEL$SOUND
6506    HNG$LOSS$TREND$CURVES DAMAGE-RISK$CRITERION DIESEL-ENGINEROOM
        $PERS
6506    STUDY NOISE HNG JUTE$WEAVING
6706    DAMAGE-RISK$CRITERION IMPULSIVE$NOISE TOYS
6803    ASPECT STATE$PUBLIC$SCH HNG$CONSERVATION$PROGRAM
6804    COCKPIT$NOISE$INTENSITY
6804    CROP-DUSTING$AIRCRAFT
6806    HNG$HAZARD SMALL-BORE$WEAPON
6806    PT THIRD-OCTAVE$OCTAVE-BAND$ATTENUATION EAR$PROTECTORS
6904    HNG$STUDIES TELEPHONE$OPERATING$PERSONNEL
6906    ROCK-AND-ROLL$MUSIC DAMAGE-RISK$CRITERIA
6907    ARCHITECTURAL$DESIGN NOISE$CONTROL
6907    CARS TRUCKS TRACTORS NOISE$SOURCES
6907    CITY$PLANNING NOISE
6907    COMMUNITY$NOISE
6907    CONTROL AIRCRAFT$NOISE SOURCE
6907    EFFECTS NOISE PSYCHOLOGICAL$STATE
6907    EFFECTS NOISE PHYSIOLOGICAL$STATE
6907    EFFECTS NOISE COMMUNITY$BEHAVIOR
6907    GENERAL$AIRCRAFT$NOISE
6907    METHODS SCALES NOISE$MEAS
6907    NOISE$CONTROL PROPAGANDA$EDUC
6907    NOISE$CONTROL LAWS REGULATIONS

| | |
|---|---|
| 6907 | NOISE$EXPOSURE DAMAGE$RISK$CRITERIA |
| 6907 | SONIC$BOOM COMMUNITY$STUDY |
| 6907 | SONIC$BOOM$OVERPRESSURE SST$OPERATION |
| 6917 | DENTISTRY ACOUS$TRAUMA |
| 7006 | DAMAGE$RISK$CRITERIA |
| 7006 | EFFECT AMBIENT-NOISE$LEVEL THR$SHIFT MEAS EAR-PROTECTOR $ATTENUATIO |
| 7011 | EFFECTS INCUBATOR$NOISE HUMAN$HNG |
| 7306 | DAMAGE-RISK$CRITERIA TRADING$RELATION INTENSITY |
| 7306 | DBA$ATTENUATION EAR$PROTECTORS |
| 7506 | BERGLUND SCALING$LOUDNESS NOISINESS ANNOYANCE AIRCRAFT $NOISE |
| 7506 | LEE NOMOGRAM ESTIMATING NOISE$PROPAGATION URBAN$AREAS |
| 7604 | YATES DAMAGE$RISK EVAL EFFECTS DBA$NOISE |
| 7606 | BOER HNG$PROTECTOR$RATING |
| 7606 | CHANAUD POROUS$BLADES FAN$NOISE |
| 7606 | DALLOS COMPOUND$ACTION$POTENTIAL TUNING$CURVES |
| 7606 | HARRIS DAMAGE$RISK HABITABILITY$CRITERIA PURE-TONE $PULSE$TRAINS |
| 7606 | REINIS ACUTE$CHANGES ANIMAL$INNER$EARS SIMULATED$SONIC $BOOMS |
| 7606 | WARD EFFECTIVE$QUIET+MODERATE$TTS IMPLICATIONS NOISE $EXPOSURE$STANDARD |
| 7606 | WARD TTS NEIGHBORHOOD$AIRCRAFT$NOISE |
| 7706 | BRAMMER MONITORING SOUND$PRESSURES APPLICATION NOISE $EXPOSURE |
| 7706 | COLWILL SURFACE-WAVE$SIMULATOR STUDY JET-NOISE$SOURCES |
| 7706 | HODGSON SURFACE$ACOUSTICAL$INTENSITY$METHOD NOISE $POWER MACHINE |
| 7706 | JOHNSON MEASUREMENT CONTINUOUS$SOUND$EXPOSURE |
| 7804 | FELDMAN STIM$DURATION STIM$OFF-TIME AUD + AR$THR |
| 7806 | AKAY REVIEW IMPACT$NOISE |
| 7806 | FIDELL URBAN$NOISE$SURVEY |
| 7806 | HAYASHI PSYCHOLOGICAL$ASSESSMENT AIRCRAFT$NOISE$INDEX |
| 7806 | ROCHE LONGITUDINAL$STUDY HEARING$CHIL NOISE$EXPOSURE |
| 7806 | SCHULTZ SYNTHESIS SOCIAL$SURVEYS NOISE$ANNOYANCE |
| 7806 | TOBIAS ESTIMATING$PERFORMANCE HEARING$PROTECTORS |
| 7806 | UNGAR ESTIMATION PERCENTAGE OVEREXPOSED$WORKERS |

## 0107

| | |
|---|---|
| 5406 | ANESTHESIA HNG |
| 5406 | AUD$SENSITIZATION |
| 5406 | EARPHONE$R EARS COUPLERS |

| | |
|---|---|
| 5406 | NOTE AUDIBILITY INTENSE$ULTRASONIC$SOUND |
| 5419 | HNG CHIL |
| 5506 | AUD$THR CAT |
| 5506 | MEAS HNG$ACUITY SUBMARINERS$NOISE$LEVELS |
| 5506 | SOUND$LEVEL$IDENTIFICATION INTERTRIAL$STIMULUS$VARIATIONS |
| 5515 | BISENSORY$PERCEP |
| 5603 | OHIO$COUNTY$FAIR$HNG$SURVEY |
| 5606 | EARPHONE PROBE$TUBE$MICROPHONY AUDIOMETRIC$ZERO |
| 5703 | RECOGNITION INTELLIGIBILITY$TEST$MATERIALS |
| 5703 | ZERO$HNG$LOSS |
| 5706 | ACOUS$IRRITATION$THR RINGBILLED$GULLS |
| 5706 | ACOUS$IRRITATION$THR PEKING$DUCKS DOMESTIC$WILD$FOWL |
| 5706 | ATTENUATION$EAR$PROTECTORS LOUDNESS$BALANCE THR$METHODS |
| 5706 | THR THERMAL$NOISE FUNCTION DURATION INTERRUPTION$RATE |
| 5706 | THR$HNG EQUAL-LOUDNESS$REL PT LOUDNESS$FUNCTION |
| 5706 | UNDERWATER$HNG$THR |
| 5804 | SWITCHING$TRANSIENTS THR$DETERMINATION |
| 5806 | COMPARISON HNG$THR AIR$WATER |
| 5806 | EFFECT PRACTICE MOTIVATION THR$AUDIBILITY |
| 5806 | LAB$STANDARD$NORMAL$HNG |
| 5806 | PROPAGATION$VELOCITY SOUND HUMAN$SKULL |
| 5806 | THR$HNG RINGBILLED$GULL |
| 5815 | INVESTIGATION BINAURAL$HNG |
| 5904 | REL NORMAL$HNG PT SP |
| 5905 | INTERNATIONAL$AUDIOMETRIC$ZERO |
| 5906 | AGE SEX$DIFFERENCES PT$THR |
| 5906 | EXPERIMENTS BC$THR FREE$FIELD |
| 5906 | REL HNG$THR DURATION TONE$PULSES |
| 6004 | FACTORS THR SHORT$TONES |
| 6006 | AIR$DAMPED ARTIFICIAL$MASTOID |
| 6011 | HNG SNAKES |
| 6104 | HNG$THR RANDOM$NOISE |
| 6106 | HNG$THR PERIODIC$TONE$PULSES |
| 6106 | PRACTICE$EFFECT AUD$THR |
| 6106 | SENSITIVITY WATER-IMMERSED$EAR HIGH-LOW$LEVEL$TONES |
| 6107 | INTERNATIONAL$AUDIO$ZERO |
| 6111 | HNG$BAT COCH$POTENTIALS |
| 6204 | PT$AUDIOMETRY SINGLE$THR$CROSSING |
| 6206 | INTERAURAL$PHASE ABSOLUTE$THR TONE |
| 6206 | INTERAURAL$PHASE ABSOLUTE$THR TONE |
| 6206 | PT$LOUDNESS REL |
| 6206 | THR$AUDIBILITY SHORT$PULSES |
| 6206 | UNDERWATER HNG$THR |
| 6211 | EFFECT RADIATION AUD$THR RAT |
| 6306 | EFFECT CIRCUMAURAL$EARPHONES EARPHONE$CUSHIONS AUD $THR |

| | |
|---|---|
| 6306 | POST-MORTEM ACOUS$IMPED HUMAN$EARS |
| 6306 | SENSORY$THR R$BIAS |
| 6306 | TONAL$THR SHORT-DURATION$STIMULI REL SUBJECT HNG$LEVEL |
| 6315 | PT$AC$THR CHIL |
| 6403 | AGE NORMAL$HNG |
| 6404 | AUD$BEHAVIOR HUMAN$NEONATE |
| 6404 | PT$AUD$FEEDBACK |
| 6404 | RACE$DIFFERENCE AUD$SENSITIVITY |
| 6404 | SENSITIVITY ACUITY |
| 6406 | EFFECT AUD$DEPRIVATION |
| 6406 | EFFECT AUD$DEPRIVATION |
| 6406 | EFFECT CIRCUMAURAL$EARPHONES AUD$THR |
| 6406 | EFFECTS HEAD AIR-LEAKAGE SIDETONE MONAURAL-TELEPHONE $SPEAKING |
| 6406 | EFFECTS HEAD AIR-LEAKAGE SIDETONE MONAURAL-TELEPHONE $SPEAKING |
| 6406 | INTERNATIONAL$AUDIO$ZERO |
| 6411 | ALERTED$EFFECTIVE$THR AUD$VIGILANCE |
| 6411 | AUDITORY$RESPONSES LIZARD |
| 6503 | NORMAL$EARS |
| 6503 | QUANTIFYING LOMBARD$EFFECT |
| 6506 | PT$ACUITY INTELLIGIBILITY EVERYDAY$SP |
| 6506 | THR$AUD MONKEY |
| 6511 | AUD$BEHAVIOR HUMAN$NEONATE METHODOLOGIC$PROBLEMS DESIGN |
| 6511 | AUD$THR BAT |
| 6511 | AUD$THR RACOON |
| 6515 | ISO$AUDIOMETRIC$ZERO |
| 6604 | EFFECTS LOW$FREQ$TONES AUD$THR |
| 6605 | INCONSISTENCY AUDIOMETRIC$ZERO$REFERENCE |
| 6606 | AUD$THR$LOCATION UNCERTAINTY FUNCTION TONE$PARAMETERS FATIGUE |
| 6606 | EARCANAL$PRESSURE FREE$SOUND$FIELD |
| 6606 | EARCANAL$PRESSURE FREE$FIELD |
| 6606 | EARPHONE SOUND-FIELD$THR SPL SPONDEE$WORDS |
| 6606 | EFFECT SIGNAL$DURATION AUD$SENSITIVITY HUMANS MONKEYS |
| 6606 | INTEGRATION ACOUS$POWER THR NORMAL$HNG |
| 6606 | NORMAL$HNG$THR DETERMINED MANUAL$TECHNIQUES SELF-RECORDING TECHNIQ |
| 6606 | NORMAL$THR$HNG PT EARPHONE$LISTENING SELF-RECORDING $AUDIOMETRIC$TE |
| 6606 | TOLERABLE$LIMIT$LOUDNESS CLINICAL$PHYSIOLOGICAL$SIGNIFICANCE |
| 6703 | ARTIFACT MEAS TEMPORAL$SUMMATION AUD$THR |
| 6704 | MEAS INTERPRETATION HNG$THR$LEVELS |
| 6704 | METHODOLOGY DIGIT$MEM$TESTING COLLEGE$STUDENTS |
| 6704 | REL HNG REACTION$TIME AGE |
| 6704 | VARIABILITY OCCLUDED$BC$THR |

6706    ACCUMULATION$THEORY BINAURAL-MASKED$THR
6706    AUD$SENSITIZATION
6706    EFFECTS VIBRATOR$TYPES PLACEMENT BC$THR$MEAS
6706    UNDERWATER HNG$THR MAN
6711    CONDITIONAL$SUPPRESSION DETERMINATION$AUD$SENSITIVITY
        PIGEONS
6711    HIGH$FREQUENCY$AUD
6711    HNG CHINCHILLA
6804    INDEX$FREQ$SENSITIVITY
6806    INTERNATIONAL$STANDARD$REFERENCE$ZERO
6806    PROBE-SIGNAL$METHOD
6806    REL ABSOLUTE$THR DURATION-OF-TONE$PULSES PORPOISE
6806    SOUND$PRESSURE EXTERNAL-EAR$REPLICA HUMAN$EARS POINT
        $SOURCE
6806    SPECIFICATION NORMAL$BC$THR
6806    TRANSFORMATION SPL FREE$FIELD EARDRUM HORIZONTAL$PLANE
6806    VARIABLES SOUND$PRESSURE EAR$CANAL AUDIOMETRIC$EARPHONE
6811    AUD$R GOLDFISH
6811    AUD$RESPONSES SHREWS PRIMATES
6811    COMPARISON BC$THRESHOLDS CRANIAL$LOCATIONS
6811    SKULL$VIBRATIONS$INFLUENCES OCCLUSION$EFFECT BC
6904    EFFECT MEDIAN$FREQ$LEVELS ROUGHNESS JITTERED$STIMULI
6904    EFFECT MEDIAN$FREQ$LEVELS ROUGHNESS JITTERED$STIMULI
6906    AUD$SENSITIZATION
6906    AUD$THR STROBOSCOPIC$VISUAL$STIMULATION
6906    CONTEXT SEQUENCE$EFFECTS ADAPTIVE$THR$PROCEDURE
6906    EFFECT AIR$BUBBLES EAM UNDERWATER HNG$THR
6906    HNG$THR EAR-CANAL$PRESSURE ACOUS$FIELDS
6906    PRACTICE$EFFECTS SIGNAL$DETECTION AUD$VIGILANCE$TASK
6906    UNDERWATER HNG$THR MAN FUNCTION WATER$DEPTH
6911    AUD$THR MONKEY CLOSED$SYSTEM$HELMET
6911    BEHAVIORAL$AUDIOGRAM GOLDFISH
6911    HNG PRIMITIVE$MAMMALS TREE$SHREW
6911    HNG PRIMITIVE$MAMMALS OPOSSUM
6911    SHOCK-AVOIDANCE$TECHNIQUE A$THR MONKEY
6915    AUD$BEHAVIORAL$R HNG$INF
7006    AUD$THR VISUAL$STIMULATION FUNCTION SIGNAL$BANDWIDTH
7006    AUDIBILITY$CURVE CHINCHILLA
7006    AUDIOMETER$EARPHONE$MOUNTING IMPROVE INTERSUBJECT
        $RELIABILITY
7006    LOW-FREQ$AUD$CHARACTERISTICS SPECIES$DEPENDENCE
7006    PT$AUD$BEHAVIORAL$THR LEMURS
7011    EARPHONE$CUSHIONS STANDARD$UNIT
7011    MEAS GENERAL$MOTOR$ACTIVITY REL ACOUS$STIMULATED$HUMAN
        $NEONATES
7011    PERCEP ACOUS$STIMULI$NEAR$THR

```
7103   OBSERVATIONS REL THR$PT THR$SP
7104   EXPERIMENTAL$STUDIES UNCOMFORTABLE$LOUDNESS$LEVEL
7104   R HOFMANN
7106   AUD$THR SHORT$DURATION PULSES
7106   AUD$THR FUNCTION SIGNAL$DURATION SIGNAL$FILTERING
7106   BEHAVIORAL$THR CAT
7106   LEMUR HNG
7111   BEHAVIORAL$THR INTERAURAL$PHASE$DIFFERENCES
7111   EFFECT JAW$POSITION HNG BONE$CONDUCTION
7111   EFFECT OCCLUDING$DEVICES BC$THR SPLS OCCLUDED$MEATUS
7111   EFFECT OCCLUDER$CAVITY$SIZE RESTRICTION$SKULL$VIBRATION
7111   EFFECTS SIZE AUD$CAPACITIES GOLDFISH
7111   NON-VERBAL$NONMEANINGFUL$STIMULI
7111   STABILITY NARROW-BAND$NOISE$THR VISUAL$STIMULATION
7204   ACOUS$STIMULUS$DURATION REL BEHAVIORAL$R NEWBORN$INF
7204   EFFECTS BODY$POSITION AUD$SYSTEM
7204   EFFECTS PHYSIOLOGICAL$NOISE AUD$THR
7206   ANESTHESIA CATS
7206   AUD$THR GOLDFISH
7206   AUD$THR DOLPHIN
7206   AUD$THR KILLER$WHALE
7206   EARPHONE$COUPLING$SYSTEM PHYSIOLOGICAL$STUDIES
7206   PT$AUD$THR CARP
7211   AUD$SENSITIVITY TURKEY
7211   EFFECT CLICK$INTENSITY RW$POTENTIALS CAT
7211   EFFECT MARIHUANA AUD$THR
7211   THEORETICAL$INVEST COCH$EFFECTS IMPED
7211   ULTRASONIC$SIGNALLING MICE
7311   EFFECT MASTOID$PLACEMENT BONE$OSCILLATOR THR$ACUITY
7311   PT$AUDIOMETRY NOISE-BARRIER$HEADSETS
7311   REL LEVELS PT SP AR LOUDNESS$DISCOMFORT
7404   BODY$ACOUS$IMMITANCE EAR
7406   AUD$SENSITIVITY SEA$LION AIRBORNE$SOUND
7406   CHINCHILLA
7406   HUMAN AUD$THR DEEP$SATURATION$HELIUM-OXYGEN$DIVES
7406   LOUDNESS$DISCOMFORT$LEVEL EARPHONE FREE$FIELD EFFECTS
7406   PT$THR MONKEY
7406   PT$THR MONKEY
7406   THR$AUDIBILITY LOW-FREQ$PT
7414   RIGHT$EAR$ADVANTAGE SP$PRESENTED$MONAURALLY
7503   WATROUS AUDITORY$RESPONSES INFANTS
7506   CLACK SUBJECTIVE$TONES TONE-ON-TONE$MASKING
7506   HAFTER DIFFERENCE$THRESHOLDS INTERAURAL$DELAY
7506   HELLMAN RELATION LOUDNESS$FUNCTION INTENSITY$CHARACTERISTICS
7506   MOORE INTENSITY$DISCRIM MOISE$BURSTS
7506   ROSENTHAL SP$RECEPTION LOW-FREQ$SP$ENERGY
```

7506   TYSZKA INTERAURAL$PHASE AMPLITUDE$RELATIONSHIPS BC
       $SIGNELS
7506   WEBER NONMONOTONIC$BEHAVIOR CUBIC$DISTORTION$PRODUCTS
       HUMAN$EAR
7506   WILSON SYSTEMATIC$ERROR REVERSE$CORRELATION
7511   LIEBMAN SISI$SCORES NORMAL-HEARING
7513   LABELLE COMP SIMPLE SENTENCES CHILDREN
7526   BARON SEMANTIC$FEATURES RETREVIAL$SPEED
7526   FRASER MOTHERS$SP CHILD
7526   STINSON EFFECTS RATE WORD$BOUNDRY$AMBIGUITY RECALL
7526   WERTSCH INFLUENCE PERCEP SPEAKER RECOGNITION$MEMORY
7533   GILBERT DISCRIM NASALIZED NON-NASALIZED VOWELS CHILDREN
7604   DIRKS BONE$CONDUCTION$THR NORMAL$LISTENERS
7604   DIRKS PSYCHOMETRIC$FUNCTIONS LOUDNESS$DISCOMFORT MCL
7604   SORENSON BINAURAL$MASKING BC$NOISE
7606   FLOTTORP MECHANICAL$IMPED HUMAN$HEADBONES
7606   HOUTGAST SUBHARMONIC$PITCHES PT LOW$S/N$RATIO
7606   MICHAEL CALIBRATION$DATA CIRCUMAURAL$HEADSET HNG$TESTING
7606   PARKER INFLUENCE AUDITORY$FATIGUE MASKED$PURE-TONE
       $THRESHOLDS
7606   PRICE AGE FACTOR SUSCEPTIBILITY HNG$LOSS YOUNG VERSUS
       ADULT$EARS
7611   WEATHERTON EAR$COUPLER$EFFECTS HNG$SENSITIVITY HIGH
       $FREQUENCY
7627   CARPENTER DEV ACOUS$CUE$DISCRIM CHILDREN
7704   BILLINGS CALIBRATION$FORCE FOR BONE$VIBRATORS
7706   JOHNSON MEASUREMENT CONTINUOUS$SOUND$EXPOSURE
7706   KALIKOW SP$INTELL SENTENCE$MATERIALS CONTROLLED$WORD
       $PREDICTABILITY
7706   MICHAEL REAL-EAR$COMPARISONS EARPHONE METEL$OUTER
       $SHELL PLASTIC SHELL
7711   TILLIS AUDIOMETRIC$SCREENONG$CRITERIA FIRLD$STUDY
7713   STOVALL AUD$ASSEMBLY$ABILITY CHILDREN MILD SEVERE
       $MISARTIC
7729   SEITZ CHANGES CLICK$MIGRATION FUNCTION AGE
7729   TYLER ACTION$POTENTIALS R LOW$FREQ$STIMULI
7803    BARRY ABSOLUTE$THR FM$SIGNALS RATE PATTERN PERCENTAGE
       $MODULATION
7806   MORGAN ME$MUSCLE$CONTRACTION THR PT
7806   ROCHE LONGITUDINAL$STUDY HEARING$CHIL NOISE$EXPOSURE
7806   SIMON COMFORTABLE$LISTENING$LEVELS SP$EXPERIMENTS
7827   BLACHE CLINICAL$PROTOTYPE AUD$MEMORY$SPAN
7833   GANDOUR DIMENSIONS TONES MULTIDIMENSIONAL$SCALING


                              0108


5406   ACOUS COMM

5506    ARTIC$SCORES REVERBERANT$ROOMS POLYCYLINDRICAL$DIFFUSERS
5515    ACOUS$ENGINEERING
5906    SYNCHRONIZATION MUSIC JUXTAPOSITION DUAL—CHANNEL$TAPES
6106    PHASOR$ANALYSIS STEREOPHONIC$PHENOMENA
6206    SPACE—TIME$CORRELATION SPHERICAL$CIRCULAR$NOISE$FIELDS
6306    PHYSICS$STUDENTS STUDY ACOUS
6306    SIREN$EXPERIMENTS NONCIRCULAR$HOLES NONCIRCULAR$NOZZLE
6506    RESONANCE—ABSORPTION CROSS$SECTION PIPE$ORGAN
6606    SONAR$ECHO
6606    TABLE INTENSITY$INCREMENTS
6704    INTERAURAL$INTENSITY TIME$DIFFERENCES ANECHOIC$REVERBERANT
        $ROOMS
6806    PROPERTIES LONGITUDINAL$SHEAR$WAVES STUDY COMPUTER
        $SIMULATIONS
6816    ACOUS$DESIGN CLASSROOMS$DEAF
6911    BEHAVIORAL$BIOACOUS
7106    HEAD—RELATED TWO—CHANNEL STEREOPHONY LOUDSPEAKER$REPROD
7306    NUMBER NONREVERBERANT$IMPULSES
7406    AMBIENT$NOISE$FIELD EDGE$EFFECTS PRODUCT$ARRAY$PROCESSING
7406    LOG$SPECTRA GAUSSIAN$SIGNALS
7506    ABBAGNARA MEASUREMENTS DIFFRACTION INTERAURAL$DELAY
        HUMAN$HEAD
7506    ANDERSON ACOUSTIC$SIGNAL$PROCESSING
7506    BENDER INTERNAL—COMBUSTION$ENGINES$INTAKE EXHAUST
        $SYSTEM$NOISE
7506    BERANEK ACOUSTICS CONCERT$HALL
7506    BERMAN BOUNDED$SPACE
7506    BLUMENTHAL AIRCRAFT$COMMUNITY$NOISE$RESEARCH
7506    BURGESS DIGITAL$SPECTRUM$ANALYSIS PERIODIC$SIGNELS
7506    CHANAUD AERODYNAMIC$NOISE MOTOR$VEHICLES
7506    DEUTSCH
7506    DUMNITZ HEADPHONES$MONITORING$SYSTEM BINAURAL$EXPERIMENTS
7506    FINCK ORB—WEB ACOUSTIC$DETECTOR
7506    HILLQUIST MOTOR$VEHICLE$NOISE$SPECTRA CHARACTERISTICS
7506    HOLMES LOW—FREQUENCY$PHASE$DISTORTION SP$RECORDINGS
7506    LAUCHLE RADIATION SOUND LOUDSPEAKER CIRCULAR$BAFFLE
7506    LEASURE TIRE—ROAD$NOISE
7506    LIPORACE LINEAR$ESTIMATION NONSTATIONARY$SIGNALS
7506    MCDONALD ASYMPTOTIC$FREQUENCY$SPREAD SURFACE—SCATTER
        $CHANNELS
7506    OSMAN DETECTION MONAURAL$SIGNAL NOISE$CORRELATION
        FREQ
7506    SCHROEDER DIFFUSE$SOUND$REFLECTION MAXIMUM—LENGTH
        $SEQUENCES
7506    SCHULTZ MEASUREMENT ACOUSTIC$INTENSITY SOUND$FIELD
7506    VAN ZYL EVAL INTENSITY$METHOD SOUND—POWER$DETERMINATION

```
7506   VER LOW-NOISE$CHAMBERS AUDITORY$RESEARCH
7506   YEGNANARAYANA INTELLIGIBILITY SP NONEXPOTENTIAL$DECAY
       $CONDITIONS
7606   BIES IMPEDANCE-TUBE$CALIBRATION REVERBERANT$ROOM SOUND
       $POWER TONES
7606   FISH SONAR$TARGET$DISCRIM INSTRUMENTED$HUMAN$DIVERS
7606   GALAITSIS PREDICTION NOISE$DISTRIBUTION FREE-FIELD
       $MEASUREMENTS
7606   ISHIZAKI SOUND-VELOCITY$MEAS PULSE-SUPERPOSITION$METHOD
7606   KILLION NOISE EARS MICROPHONES
7606   SCHULTZ ALTERNATIVE$TEST$METHOD EVALUATING$NOISE
7706   BERANEK NOTEBOOKS SABINE
7706   COLWILL SURFACE-WAVE$SIMULATOR STUDY JET-NOISE$SOURCES
7706   COOK HISTORY AMERICAN$ACOUSTICS
7706   DAVIS PSYCHOLOGICAL PHYSIOLOGICAL$ACOUSTICS
7706   DUNENS IMPULSIVE$SOUND-LEVEL R$STATISTICS REVERBERANT
       $ENCLOSURE
7706   FAHY MEAS INTENSITY CROSS-SPECTRAL$DENSITY MICROPHONE
       $SIGNALS
7706   HILLIARD ELECTROACOUSTICS$
7706   HODGSON SURFACE$ACOUSTICAL$INTENSITY$METHOD NOISE
       $POWER MACHINE
7706   IVEY ACOUSTICAL$SCALE$MODEL ATTENUATION WIDE$BARRIERS
7706   KUHN ACOUS$PRESSURE$FIELD ALONGSIDE MANIKINS$HEAD
       WITH VIEW TOWARDS IN
7706   MANGIANTE ACTIVE SOUND$ABSORPTION
7706   MILLER ACOUSTIC$MEASUREMENTS INSTRUMENTATION
7706   MORELAND MEASUREMENT SOUND$ABSORPTION ROOMS
7706   NILSSON ACOUSTICAL$PROPERTIES FLOATING-FLOOR$CONSTRUCTION
7706   PATTERSON STIMULUS$VARIABILITY AUDITORY$FILTER$SHAPE
7706   PIERCY REVIEW NOISE$PROPAGATION ATMOSPHERE
7706   SHANKLAND ARCHITECTURAL$ACOUSTICS AMERICA
7806   FRY ACOUSTICAL$PROPERTIES HUMAN$SKULL
7806   KOIDAN ACOUSTICAL$PROPERTIES NBS ANECHOIC$CHAMBER
7806   LEGGAT AEROACOUSTIC$MECHANISM ROTOR-VORTEX$INTERACTIONS
7806   MEHL ANALYSIS RESONANCE STANDING-WAVE$MEASUREMENTS
```

## 0109

```
5403   AUDIBILITY-RECOGNITION$SOUND$PRESSURE$FUNCTIONS VOICED
       $COGNATES
5403   SIGNAL$RECEPTION INTELLIGIBILITY SIDE-TONE
5403   VISUAL$COMPONENTS ORAL$SYMBOLS SP$COMPREHENSION LISTENERS
5406   EXPERIMENTS SP$RECOGNITION ONE$TWO$EARS
```

```
5406   FACTORS MULTICHANNEL$LISTENING
5406   R OVERLAPPING$MESSAGES
5410   PERCEP PHONETIC$VARIABLES
5506   ADDITION CHERRYS$FINDINGS SWITCHING$SP TWO$EARS
5506   RELATIVE$INTELLIGIBILITY SP RECORDED$SIMULTANEOUSLY
       $EAR$MOUTH
5509   RELATIVE$INTELLIGIBILITY LANG$GRPS
5603   FACTORIAL$ANALYSIS SP$PERCEP
5606   DUAL$MESSAGES
5606   EFFECT ATTENUATING$ONE$CHANNEL DICHOTIC$CIRCUIT WORD
       $RECEPTION
5606   HUMAN$CROSS-CORRELATOR TECHNIQUE MEAS PARAMETERS SP
       $PERCEP
5606   NOISE$DURATION CUE DISTINGUISHING FRICATIVE$AFFRICATE
       $STOP$CONSONA
5609   LISTENING SP$SOUNDS
5703   AUD$COMPREHENSION REL LISTENING$RATE VERBAL$REDUNDANCY
5703   AUD$COMPREHENSION HIGH-SPEED$MESSAGES
5703   PERCEP$RECOGNITION WORDS
5706   ANALYSIS MULTIPLE$RECEIVER$CORRELATION$SYSTEM
5706   RESEARCH SP$PERCEP
5716   RECOGNITION MAGNITUDES INTERPHONEMIC$TRANSITIONAL
       $INFLUENCE
5806   AUTOMATIC$RECOGNITION PHONETIC$PATTERNS SP
5806   CONFIDENCE$RATINGS MESSAGE$RECEPTION ROC
5806   LIMITS SP$COMM$IN$NOISE
5814   EFFECT LISTENERS$ANTICIPATION INTELLIGIBILITY
5814   EXPERIMENTS PERCEP$STRESS
5814   PERCEP COMPOUND$CONSONANTS
5819   RELATIVE$CONTRIBUTION AUD$TACTILE$CUES SP
5904   FACTORS SPONDEE$THR NORMAL-HNG
5904   FREQ$BANDS INTELLIGIBILITY$TESTING
5904   TRANSITION RELEASE PERCEP$CUES FINAL$PLOSIVES
5906   MULTIPLE$OBSERVERS MESSAGE$RECEPTION RATING$SCALES
5906   REPROD IDENTIFICATION ELEMENTS AUD$DISPLAYS
5906   SYNTHESIS PERCEP NASAL$CONSONANTS
6004   FACTORIAL$STUDY SP$PERCEP
6006   ANALYSIS INCORRECT$R UNKNOWN$MESSAGE$SET
6006   CONFIDENCE$RATINGS SECOND-CHOICE$R CONFUSION$MATRICES
6006   MODEL SP$RECOGNITION
6006   SP$PROCESSING SELECTIVE$AMPLITUDE$SAMPLING$SYSTEM
6006   SPOKEN$DIGITS$RECOGNITION TIME-FREQ$PATTERN$MATCHING
6006   STUDY COCKTAIL$PARTY$PROBLEM
6014   CONSONANT$CONFUSIONS CONSTANT-RATIO$RULE
6014   PERCEP CONSONANT$VOICING NOISE
6014   PERCEP CONSONANT$VOICING NOISE
```

6014 PERCEP ENG$STOPS ENG$SPEAKERS FOREIGN$SPEAKERS
6014 PERCEP UNRELEASED$VOICELESS$PLOSIVES ENG
6014 TIME$FACTORS PERCEP DOUBLE$CONSONANT
6103 WORD$CUE$REMOVAL ADAPTATION ADJACENCY
6104 INTRINSIC$CUES CONSONANT$PERCEP
6106 INFORMATION MULTIDIMENSIONAL$SP$MESSAGES
6106 NOISE-BAND$MASKING APPLICATION PREDICTION SP$INTELLIGIBILITY
6106 PERCEP SOUNDS CHANGING$RESONANT$FREQ
6106 VOWEL$RECOGNITION
6106 VOWEL$RECOGNITION MULTIPLE$DISCRIMINANT$FUNCTION
6109 AURAL$RECEPTION SENTENCES DIFFERENT$LENGTHS
6114 CONTINUITY$SP$UTTERANCE DETERMINANTS SIGNIFICANCE
6114 EFFECT SUCCEEDING$VOWEL CONSONANT$RECOGNITION NOISE
6114 LISTENER$COMPREHENSION SPEAKERS STATUS$GRPS
6204 SP$RECEPTION ALTERING$SIGNAL
6206 AUD$ACUITY PERCEP$SP
6206 COMPARISON ROC MESSAGES EAR EYE
6206 COMPARISON ROC MESSAGES EAR EYE
6206 SPOKEN$DIGIT$RECOGNITION VOWEL-CONSONANT$SEGMENTATION
6206 STUDY TIME$CUES SP$PERCEP
6211 REL FREQ$DISCRIM SP$PERCEP
6214 CHOICE STRATEGIES IDENTIFICATION SPOKEN$WORDS NOISE
6214 INCORRECT$R UNKNOWN$MESSAGES WORD$FREQ
6304 EFFECTS PRETRNG SOUND$DISCRIM$LEARNING
6306 ARTIC$INDEX AVERAGE$CURVE-FITTING$METHODS PREDICTING
     $SP$INTERFEREN
6306 DIMENSIONS CONSONANT$PERCEP
6306 PHYSICAL$MEAS SP-INTERFERING NAVY$NOISES
6306 SIGNAL CONTEXT COMPONENTS WORD-RECOGNITION$BEHAVIOR
6306 WORD-FREQ EFFECT ERRORS SP$PERCEP
6314 EFFECTS SEMANTIC$GRAMMATICAL$CONTEXT PROD PERCEP SP
6314 R$TIMES KNOWN$MESSAGE-SETS NOISE
6406 CONSISTENCY IDENTIFICATION CONSONANTS HEAR-IN-NOISE
6406 PERCEP RETENTION VERBAL$INFORMATION AUD$SHADOWING
6406 PERCEPTUAL$BASES SPEAKER$IDENTITY
6411 BINAURAL$HNG INTELLIGIBILITY
6411 INFLUENCE CONSONANTS DISCRIM NOISE
6414 EXPERIMENTS PERCEP RESONANT$CONSONANTS
6414 INTERACTION SOURCES VERBAL$CONTEXT WORD$IDENTIFICATION
6414 INTERACTION AUD$VISUAL$INFORMATION$SOURCES WORD$IDENTIFICATION
6504 EFFECT CONTEXT AURAL$PERCEP WORDS
6504 METHOD MEAS SP$IDENTIFICATION
6511 AUD$CONFUSION ALPHABET$LETTERS
6514 EXPERIMENTS PERCEP GEMINATE$CONSONANTS ARABIC
6514 VARIABILITY VOWEL$PERCEP
6604 AUD$RECOGNITION NOUNS

6606   PERCEP SEGMENTS VCCV$UTTERANCES
6606   PERCEP SEGMENTS ENGLISH-SPOKEN CV$SYLLABLES
6610   PERCEP FOREIGN$ACCENT JAPANESE$ENG AMERICAN$BRITISH
       $JAPANESE$LISTE
6614   EFFECT CONTEXT PROD HOSTILE$ASSOCIATES AMBIGUOUS$VERBAL
       $STIMULI
6614   NAMING$SEQUENTIALLY$PRESENTED$LETTERS$WORDS
6614   WORD$IDENTIFICATION
6704   HELD$POSITION$IDENTIFICATION
6704   SYNTHETIC$SENTENCE$IDENTIFICATION ROC
6704   TEMPORAL$ORDERING SP$IDENTIFICATION
6706   AUD$SEARCH EMBEDDED$SYLLABLES MEANINGFUL$SENTENCES
6706   PHONEME$GROUPING SP$RECOGNITION
6706   ROLE FORMANT$TRANSITIONS VOWEL$RECOGNITIONS
6706   TRANSITIONS AMERICAN$ENGLISH$S CUES IDENTIFY ADJACENT
       $STOP$CONSONA
6714   ATTENTION SIMULTANEOUS$TRANSLATION
6714   AURAL$PERCEP SENTENCES SYNTACTIC$STRUCTURES LENGTHS
6714   EFFECT NOISE$SPECTRA IDENTIFICATION$CONSONANTS
6714   PHONEME$CATEGORIZATION SYNTHETIC$VOCALIC$STIMULI FOREIGN
       $SPEAKERS
6804   PHONETIC$DISTORTIONS SERIAL$TRANSMISSION SHORT$SP
       $SAMPLES
6804   R MULTIPLE-CHOICE$INTELLIGIBILITY$TESTS
6806   AUD$PRESENTATIONS SP
6806   EFFECT PITCH$AVERAGING QUALITY NATURAL$VOWELS
6810   EXPERIMENTAL$STUDY ASSESS EFFECTS LEVELS$MISPRONUNCIATION
       COMPREHE
6811   UNDERWATER SRT DISCRIM
6814   PERCEP STOP$CONSONANTS SYNTHETIC$CV$SYLLABLES
6814   PERCEP$CATEGORIZATION SYNTHETIC$VOWELS TOOL DIALECTOLOGY
       TYPOLOGY
6814   PERCEP$TIMING NATURAL$SP COMPENSATION SYLLABLE
6814   PERCEP$VERBAL$DISCRIM ELABORATED$RESTRICTED$CODE$USERS
6814   PHONEMIC$INTERFERENCE PERCEP$PHENOMENON
6903   VISION AUD SP$RECEP
6903   VISION AUD SP$RECEP
6904   APPLICATIONS ULTRASOUND SP$RESEARCH
6904   INTERACTION AUDITION VISION RECOGNITION ORAL$SP
6904   MASKING$EFFECTS SP$COMPETING$MESSAGES
6906   COMPARISON ROC$CURVES INTERVAL$RATING$SCALE$PROCEDURES
6906   COMPARISON ROC$CURVES INTERVAL$RATING$SCALE$PROCEDURES
6906   EFFECT ACOUS$CUES FRICATIVES PERCEP$CONFUSIONS PRESCH
       $CHIL
6906   EFFECT CIRCUMAURAL$EARPHONE$CUSHIONS THR$SENSITIVITY
       SP

6906    FEATURES PERCEP CONSONANTS
6906    MULTIPLE$RATINGS SOUND$STIMULI
6906    PERCEP$PHYSICAL$SPACE VOWELS
6909    WORD$LISTS LOADED$PASSAGE DISTANT$VOWEL$ASSIMILATIONS
6911    COMPARISON SENTENCE$CONTINUOUS$DISCOURSE$INTELLIGIBILITY
6911    COMPARISON METHODS SP$INTERFERENCE ARTIC$INDEX
6911    CONTRALATERAL$SHIFT CEREBRAL$DOMINANCE NONVERBAL$SOUNDS
        SP$PERCEP
6911    EFFECT CONSONANT$DISCRIM LOW-FREQ$PASSBAND HIGH-FREQ
        $PASSBAND
6914    CROSSLANG$STUDY VOWEL$PERCEP
6920    RESEARCH SLOW-PLAYED$SP LISTENER$TRNG CONSONANT$ERRORS
7004    DISTRACTING$PROPERTIES COMPETING$SP
7004    PERCEP SIMULTANEOUS$DICHOTIC$MONOTIC$MONOSYLLABLES
7004    ROLE$PRACTICE OBSERVATION$PRACTICE SP$DISCRIM$LEARNING
7004    VOWEL$RECOGNITION FUNCTION TEMPORAL$SEGMENTATIONS
7006    COMMENTS SP$RECOGNITION STUDIES
7006    COOPERATION LISTENER COMPUTER RECOGNITION$TASK EFFECTS
7006    EVAL SP$RECOGNITION$WORK
7006    HEMISPHERIC$SPECIALIZATION SP$PERCEP
7006    PACED$RECOGNITION WORDS MASKED WHITE$NOISE
7006    TEMPORAL$ORDER PERCEP VOWELS
7011    COMPARISON SP$RECEPTION MONOTIC$DICHOTIC$LISTENING
7011    EAR$PREFERENCE LANG$SOUNDS UNILATERAL$BRAIN$FUNCTION
7012    AUD$VERBAL$RECOGNITION ADULTS LISTENING$CONDITIONS
7014    FRICATIVE$PLOSIVE$PERCEP$IDENTIFICATION FUNCTION PHONETIC
        $CONTEXT
7014    PERCEP$STUDY AMERICAN$ENG$DIPHTHONGS
7014    PHONEME$REPETITION STRUCTURE$LANG
7017    CHIL$COMPREHENSION INTELLIGIBLE$UNINTELLIGIBLE$SP
7103    PHONETIC$CONTEXTS SP-SOUND$RECOGNITION PROD$PRACTICE
7104    ECHO-REACTION APPROACH SEMANTIC$RESOLUTION
7104    PERCEP$SIMILARITIES MINIMAL$PHONEMIC$DIFFERENCES
7104    RELATIVE$CONTRIBUTION VISUAL$AUD$COMPONENTS SP SP
        $INTELLIGIBILITY
7106    EAR$PREFERENCE DICHOTICALLY$PRESENTED VERBAL$STIMULI
        FUNCTION
7106    PERCEP SYNTHESIZED$ISOLATED$VOWELS WORDS FUNCTION
        FUND$FREQ
7106    PERCEP$STUCTURE AMERICAN$ENG$VOWELS
7106    PHONOLOGICAL$OPPOSITIONS CHIL PERCEP$STUDY
7111    AURAL$IDENTIFICATION CHIL$VOICES
7111    REACTION$TIME AUDITORY$IDENTIFICATION SEGMENTS SYLLABLES
7111    RECOGNITION SP$MODULATED$NOISE
7114    METHODOLOGY EXPERIMENTS PERCEP SYNTHETIC$VOWELS
7114    OBSERVATIONS METATHEORY SP$PERCEP

| | |
|---|---|
| 7114 | PERCEP$PARAMETERS CONSONANT$S |
| 7114 | PERCEPTUAL$REALITY PHONEME HI$CHIL |
| 7204 | INDIVIDUAL$CONSISTENCY HNG$SP LISTENING$CONDITIONS |
| 7204 | INDIVIDUAL$CONSISTENCY HNG$SP LISTENING$CONDITIONS |
| 7204 | INFLUENCE LINGUISTIC$SITUATIONAL$VARIABLES PHONEMIC $ACCURACY |
| 7204 | PERCEP COARTICULATION ENG$VCV$SYLLABLES |
| 7204 | PERCEP VOWEL$PHONEMES FORT$ERIE$ONTARIO BUFFALO$NEW $YORK APPLICATI |
| 7204 | PERCEP$EFFECTS FORWARD$COARTICULATION |
| 7204 | SP$PERCEP SPECTRAL$TRANSFORMATIONS PHONETIC$CHARACTERISTICS |
| 7206 | COOPERATION LISTENER COMPUTER RECOGNITION$TASK EFFECTS |
| 7206 | EFFECT INTERAURAL$SWITCHING RECOGNITION SP |
| 7206 | PERCEP TEMPORAL$PHENOMENA SP |
| 7206 | PERCEP$STRUCTURE PREVOCALIC$ENG$CONSONANTS |
| 7210 | CHIL$DEPENDENCE VISUAL$CONTEXT SENTENCE$COMPREHENSION |
| 7211 | MINIMAL-CONTRASTS$CLOSED-R$SP$TEST |
| 7212 | HEARD$VIEWED VERBAL$MATERIALS |
| 7214 | DIRECT$MAGNITUDE$SCALING$METHOD INVEST MODES SP$PERCEP |
| 7304 | DEVELOPMENTAL COMPARISON VOWELS$CONSONANTS DICHOTIC $LISTENING |
| 7304 | PERCEP SYLLABLES REMEMBERING$PHONEMES |
| 7304 | SPEAKING$RATE EFFECTS CHIL$COMPREHENSION NORMAL$SP |
| 7306 | ANOMALOUS$LOUDNESS$FUNCTION SP |
| 7306 | DICHOTIC$SP$PERCEP INTERPRETATION RIGHT-EAR$ADVANTAGES |
| 7306 | INTERNAL$PROCESSES SP$PERCEP |
| 7306 | PERCEP DICHOTICALLY$PRESENTED$VOWELS |
| 7311 | EFFECT CATEGORY$SET AUD$WORD$RECOGNITION |
| 7314 | AUD$LINGUISTIC$PROCESSES PERCEP INTONATION$CONTOURS |
| 7314 | EFFECT FORWARD$BACKWARD$COARTIC IDENTIFICATION SP |
| 7314 | PERCEP PROD CORRELATIONS VOICING INITIAL$STOP |
| 7314 | PERCEP SUB-PHONEMIC$PHONETIC$DIFFERENCES |
| 7404 | AUD$VISUAL$CONTRIBUTIONS PERCEP ENG$CONSONANTS |
| 7404 | PERCEP DURATIONS$SILENT$INTERVAL NONSP$STIMULI MOTOR $THERAPY SP$PE |
| 7406 | AUD$FEEDBACK REGULATION$VOICE |
| 7406 | BILATERAL$COMPONENT SP$PERCEP |
| 7406 | CATEGORICAL$NONCATEGORICAL$MODES SP$PERCEP VOICING $CONTINUUM |
| 7406 | CUES SYLLABLE$JUNCTURE$PERCEP ENG |
| 7406 | PERCEP$STRUCTURE PREVOCALIC$ENG$CONSONANTS SENTENTIALLY $EMBEDDED |
| 7406 | PRIMARY$AUD$STREAM$SEGREGATION REPEATED$CV$SEQUENCES |
| 7406 | RECEPTION CONSONANTS CLASSROOM MONAURAL$BINAURAL$LISTENING NOISE |
| 7406 | RECEPTION CONSONANTS CLASSROOM MONAURAL$BINAURAL$LISTENING NOISE |

7406    ROLE FORMANT$TRANSITIONS VOICED-VOICELESS$DISTINCTION
        STOPS
7410    INFLUENCE FACTORS IDENTIFICATION$VOWELS TEMPORAL$CUES
7413    EFFECT NOISE ACOUS$PARAMETER$SP
7414    CONSONANT$GRPS FUNCTION UNITS WORD$PROD
7414    ORTHOGRAPHY PERCEP STOPS$AFTER$PHONEME$S
7414    R$STRATEGIES SENTENCE$COMPREHENSION
7414    R$STRATEGIES SENTENCE$COMPREHENSION
7504    EILERS FRICATIVE$DISCRIMINATION INFANCY
7504    EISELE INFANT$SUCKING$R CHANGES SPL AUDITORY$STIMULI
7504    PANAGOS SP$COMPREHENSION DEVIENT+NORMAL$SPEAKING$CHILD
7504    RAPHAEL VOWEL+NASAL$DURATION WORD-FINAL$STOP SPECTROGRAPHIC+PERC
7504    RAPHAEL VOWEL + NASAL$DURATION VOICING STOP SPECTROGRAPHIC
        + PERCEP
7504    WALDEN DIMENSIONS CONSONANT$PERCEP NORMAL+HI
7504    WINGFIELD ACOUS$REDUNDENCY TIME-COMPRESSED$SP
7504    ZLATIN VOICING$CONTRAST PERCEP STOP$CONSONANTS
7506    AGRAWAL EFFECT VOICED$PARAMETERS INTELLIGIBILITY PB
        $WORDS
7506    BODE CNC$DISCRIM SPONDEE$WORDS
7506    BORDELON PRESERVATION INFO MATRIX$FILTERING SIGNAL
7506    BURDICK SP$PERCEPTION CHINCHILLA DISCRIM
7506    COLE PERCEP VOICING ENGLISH$AFFRICATES+FRICATIVES
7506    GLAVE EFFORT$DEPENDENCE SP$LOUDNESS ACOUSTICAL$CUES
7506    GUPTA PERCEPTION HINDU$CONSONANTS CLIPPED$SP
7506    HOLMES LOW-FREQUENCY$PHASE$DISTORTION SP$RECORDINGS
7506    LARIVIERE VOCALIC$TRANSITIONS PERCEP VOICELESS$INITIAL
        $STOPS
7506    MCFADDEN DURATION-INTENSITY$RECIPROCITY EQUAL$LOUDNESS
7506    NACHSHON STIMULUS$FAMILIARITY EAR$SUPERIORITY DICHOTIC
        $LISTENING
7506    PATISAUL TIME-FREQ$RESOLUTION SP$ANALYSIS+SYNTHESIS
7506    PORTER EFFECT DELAYED$CHANNEL PERCEP DICHOTICALLY
        $PRESENTED$SP+NONSP
7506    REPP DICHOTIC$MASKING CONSONANTS VOWELS
7506    ROSENTHAL SP$RECEPTION LOW-FREQ$SP$ENERGY
7506    YEGNANARAYANA INTELLIGIBILITY S P NONEXPOTENTIAL$DECAY
        $CONDITIONS
7511    *ICKS INTERFERENCE NONSYMBOLIC$AUD$INFO
7511    KEMPTON USE MICRO-KINESIC$SIGNELS SP$UNDERSTANDING
7511    KEMPTON MICRO-KINESIC$SIGNALS SP$UNDERSTANDING
7511    MASTERSON PSYCHOACOUS$PROCESSING DICHOTIC$SENTENCES
        PRE-SCH$CHILD
7521    COOPER ARTIC$EFFECTS SP$PERCEP
7521    CUTTING PERCEP STOP-LIQUID$CLUSTERS PHONOLOGICAL$FUSION
7521    SEMILOFF-ZELASKO ACOUSTIC-PERCEP$STUDY MODERN$HEBREW

```
7526    BEVER DETECTION NONLINGUISTIC$STIMULUS
7526    BEVER PROJECTION$MECHANISMS READING
7526    FISHER OBJECT IMAGE OBJECT
7526    GARCIA AMBIGUITY PERCEP$PROCESSES
7526    JAMES BLACK$CHILD$PERCEP BLACK$ENGLISH
7526    LEONARD CHILD$JUDGEMENTS LINGUISTIC$FEATURES
7526    WEIST PARENT SIBLING COMP CHILD$SP
7533    SAVITT COGNATE$RECOGNITION DIALECTS
7533    WANGLER VOWEL$PERCEP GERMAN
7603    BEASLEY CHILDREN'S$PERCEP TIME-COMPRESSED$SP SP$DISCRIM
7604    BARAN PHONOLOGICAL$RULES BLACK$ENGLISH DISCRIM WORD
        $PAIRS
7604    BEITER EAR$ADVANTAGE LAG$EFFECT DICHOTIC$LISTENING
7604    BRENNAN WORD$LENGTH VISUAL$COMPLEXITY VERBAL$REACTION
        $TIMES
7604    DANHAUER INDSCAL CONSONANTS VISUAL-TACTILE INPUTS
7604    MILLER CATEGORICAL$SP$DISCRIM INFANTS
7604    RAFFIN TIME-INTENSITY$TRADE SP SP-STENGER$EFFECT
7606    BOND IDENTIFICATION VOWELS EXCERPTED /L/ /R/ CONTEXTS
7606    CORLISS METHOD ESTIMATING AUDIBILITY EFFECTIVE$LOUDNESS
        SIRENS SP AUTO
7606    OHALA COMMENTS TEMPORAL$INTERACTIONS WITHIN PHRASE+SENTENCE
        $CONTEXT
7606    PARSONS SEPARATION SP INTERFERING$SP HARMONIC$SELECTION
7606    PORTER PRACTICE PERCEP DICHOTICALLY$PRESENTED$SYLLABLES
7606    SCOTT TEMPORAL$FACTORS VOWEL$PERCEP
7606    STRANGE CONSONANT$ENVIRONMENT VOWEL$ID
7606    VERBRUGGE WHAT INFO ENABLES LISTENER TO MAP TALKERS
        VOWEL$SPACE
7611    REINSCHE DISCRIM TIME-COMPRESSED$CNC$MONOSYLLABLES
        NORMAL$LISTENERS
7620    WHEELER CHILD$SOCIAL$PERCEP CHILD$SPEAKERS
7621    COOPER ARTIC$EFFECTS SP$PERCEP
7621    DOHERTY EVAL ACOUSTIC$PARAMETERS SPAEKER$IDENTIFICATION
7621    MILLER SELECTIVE$TUNING FEATURES$DETECTORS SP
7621    OSTREICHER COARTIC IDENTIFICATION DELETED$CONSONANT
        $VOWEL
7621    PURCELL PITCH$PEAK$LOCATION PERCEP SERBO-CROATIAN
        $WORD$TONE
7621    VANVALIN PERCIEVED$DISTANCE VOWEL$STIMULI
7623    EILERS ROLE SP$DISCRIM DEVELOPMENTAL$SOUND$SUBSTITUTIONS
7629    PRIDEAUX RECOGNITION AMBIGUITY
7632    BOND INPUT$UNITS SP$PERCEP
7632    CATLIN MONAURAL$RIGHT-EAR$ADVANTAGE TARGET-IDENTFICATION
7632    DONNENFELD EFFECTS EXPECTANCY ORDER$OF$REPORT AUD
        $ASYMMETRIES
```

```
7632    WARREN EEG$ALPHA WORD$PROCESSING RECALL
7633    BENGUEREL PERCEP COARTIC$LIP$ROUNDING
7704    CULLINAN PERCEP TEMPORAL$ORDER VOWELS CV$SYLLABLES
7704    EILERS DEV$CHANGES SP$DISCRIM INFANTS
7704    KONKLE INTELLIGIBILITY TIME-ALTERED$SP CHRONOLOGICAL
        $AGING
7704    MILLER NONINDEPENDENCE FEATURE$PROCESSING INITIAL
        $CONSONANTS
7704    MORSE OVERT+COVERT$ASPECTS ADULT$SP$PERCEP
7704    OHDE ORDER$EFFECT ACOUSTIC$SEGMENTS STOP+VOWEL$IDENTIFICATION
7704    SPRING DISCRIM LINGUISTIC$STRESS INFANCY
7706    BLUMSTEIN PROPERY$DETECTORS SP$PRODUCTION
7706    CARNEY NONCATEGORICAL$PERCEPTION STOP$CONSONANTS DIFFERING
        VOT
7706    EILERS CONTEXT-SENSITIVE$PERCEPTION CONSONANTS INFANTS
7706    KALIKOW SP$INTELL SENTENCE$MATERIALS CONTROLLED$WORD
        $PREDICTABILITY
7706    KLATT REVIEW ARPA SP$UNDERSTANDING$PROJECT
7706    MILLER PROPERTIES FEATURE$DETECTORS VOT
7706    PARKER DISTINCTIVE$FEATURES ACOUSTIC$CUES
7706    PISONI IDEN DISCRIM ONSET COMPONENT$TONES VOICING
        $PERCEP STOPS
7706    POWERS INTELLIGIBILITY TEMPORALLY$INTERRUPTED$SP INTERVENING
        $NOISE
7706    REMINGTON PROCESSING PHONEMES SP SPEED-ACCURACY STUDY
7711    FAGER PRESENTATION$MODACLITY PRONOUNCEABILITY FREE
        $RECALL$TRIGRAMS
7721    BOND PERCEP ANTICIPATORY$COARTIC CONSONANTS
7721    DEBROCK ACOUSTIC$CORRELATE FORCE ARTIC
7721    JANSON ASYMMETRY VOWEL$CONFUSION$MATRICES
7721    MAJEWSKI ACOUSTIC$COMPARISONS AMERICAN$ENGLISH POLISH
7721    WILSON INDSCAL$ANALYSIS VOWELS
7723    FOWLES COMPETENCE TALENT VERBAL$RIDDLE$COMPREHENSION
7732    HEILMAN EAR$ASYMMETRIES SELECTIVE$ATTENTIONAL
7732    MORAIS LISTENING SP RETAINING$MUSIC RIGHT-EAR$ADVANTAGE
7732    PIROZZOLO HEMISPHERIC$SPECIALIZATION READING WORD
        $RECOGNITION
7732    WINGFIELD PERCEP ALTERNATED$SP
7732    WOLF PROCESSING FUNDAMENTAL$FREQ DICHOTIC$MATCHING
        $TASK
7804    DOWNS PROCESSING$DEMANDS AUD$LEARNING DEGRADED$LISTENING
7806    AINSWORTH PERCEP SP FORMANTS OPPOSITE$EARS
7806    BRADY RANGE$EFFECT PERCEP VOICING
7806    COLE PERCEP PHONETIC$FEATURES FLUENT$SP
7806    DEFILIPPO TRAINING EVALUATING RECEPTION ONGOING$SP
7806    KEATING TRANSITION$LENGTH PERCEP STOP$CONSONANTS
```

7806    KUHL SP$PERCEP CHINCHILLA VOT$STIMULI
7806    MERMELSTEIN DIFFERENCE$LIMENS FORMANT$FREQ VOWELS
7806    NABELEK PRECEDENCE$EFFECT WORD$ID HI$SUBJECTS
7806    NAKATANI PROSODIC$CUES WORD$PERCEP
7806    POLS IDENTIFICATION DELETED$CONSONANTS
7806    SIMON COMFORTABLE$LISTENING$LEVELS SP$EXPERIMENTS
7806    SIMON SELECTIVE$ANCHORING ADAPTATION PHONETIC$CONTINUA
7806    STEVENS CUES PLACE$ARTICULATION STOP$CONSONANTS
7806    WALTZMAN SP$INTERFERENCE$LEVEL PREDICTOR COMM NOISE
7806    WATANABE  R CATS$COLLICULAR NEURON SP
7806    WILLIAMS DISCRIM YOUNG$INFANTS VOICED$STOP
7821    BENSON ACOUSTIC$SIMILARITY DICHOTIC$LISTENING
7821    ODEN INTEGRATION PLACE + VOICING$INFO IDEN SYN$STOP
7821    PARNELL SPEAKER$AGE PERCEPTUAL$CUE$DISTRIBUTION
7821    ROSSI PERCEPTION INTENSITY$GLIDES VOWELS
7826    MEHLER SENTENCE$PERCEPTION
7826    RAZEL CHILDREN'S$SENTENCE$COMPREHENSION
7827     NELSON COMPREHENSION STANDARD$ENGLISH SPEAKING$RATES
        BLACK$ENGLISH
7829    MANZER INTENSITY$PRESENTATION$LEVELS DICHOTIC$LISTENING
7833    GUSSENHOVEN PERCEP PROMINENCE DUTCH$LISTENERS


                            0110


5406    NOTE ACOUS$ATTENUATION EARS
5406    OBSERVATION TARTINI$PITCH
5506    THEORY$PITCHES
5606    COMMENT DIPLACUSIS AUD$THEORY
5606    IMPLICATION AUD$THEORY UNITARY$PITCH$PERCEP DIPLACUSIS
5606    NEUROLOGICAL$THEORY BEAT$TONES
5706    MECHANISM BINAURAL$FUSION HNG$SP
5806    FUNNELING NERVOUS$SYSTEM ROLE LOUDNESS SENSATION$INTENSITY
        SKIN
5906    MECHANISMS BINAURAL$FUSION
6006    HYPOTHESIS HYDRAULIC$FUNCTIONING COCH MASKING
6006    THEORY TEMPORAL$AUD$SUMMATION
6011    NYSTAGMUS$AUDIOCINETIQUE
6206    BC REVIEW CONTRIBUTIONS BEKESY
6206    DEV TRAVELING—WAVE$THEORIES
6206    MODIFIED$PLACE$CONCEPT
6206    TIME$FREQ$ANALYSIS PARTITION COCH$MODELS
6206    VARIATION THEME BEKESY MODEL BINAURAL$INTERACTION
6306    DIPLACUSIS AUD$THEORY
6306    HNG$THEORIES COMPLEX$SOUNDS

6306    NEUROLOGICAL$THEORY BEAT$TONES
6406    DETECTION MARKOVIAN$SEQUENCES SIGNALS
6406    OHMS$ACOUS$LAW SHORT-TERM$AUD$MEM
6406    REL SP-INTERFERENCE$CONTOURS IDEALIZED ARTIC$INDEX
        $CONTOURS
6604    ELEMENTS ACOUS$PHONETIC$THEORY
6604    GLOSSARY$TERMS PHYSIOLOGICAL$ACOUS$PHONETIC$THEORIES
6706    ACCUMULATION$THEORY BINAURAL-MASKED$THR
6706    DETECTION LOCALIZATION EXTENSION THEORY$SIGNAL$DETECTABILITY
6711    AUD TACTUAL$RIVALRY VERIFICATION$GRADIENT BRAIN$BLOOD
        SHIFT$THEORY
6806    BROWNIAN$MOTION COCH$PARTITION
6806    EXTERNAL-EAR$ACOUS$MODELS SIMPLE$GEOMETRY
6806    MATHEMATICAL$ELECTRICAL$MODELS AUD$DETECTION
6906    CONSONANCE$THEORY CONSONANCE DYADS
7007    ACOUS$ANALOGUE$STUDIES
7206    BANDPASS$NOISE$STIMULATION SIMULATED$BASILAR$MEMBRANE
7206    BOUNDARY$CONDITIONS RESULTS PETERSON-BOGERT$COCH$MODEL
7206    BOUNDARY$CONDITIONS RESULTS PETERSON-BOGERT$COCH$MODEL
7406    COCH$WAVES INTERACTION THEORY EXPERIMENTS
7406    HIGH-LEVEL$INTERRUPT$THEORY
7406    PSYCHOPHYSICAL$VERIFICATION PREDICTED$INTERAURAL$DIFFERENCES
7406    SIMPLE$SHORT-WAVE$COCH$MODEL RANKE
7506    OSMAN DETECTION MONAURAL$SIGNAL NOISE$CORRELATION
        FREQ
7606    DUIFHUIS COCHLEAR$NONLINEARITY SECOND$FILTER
7606    HEBRANK PINNA$DISPARITY$PROCESSING CASE MISTAKEN$ID
7606    SEARLE MODEL AUDITORY$LOCALIZATION
7611    GUELKE TRANSMISSION$LINE$THEORY COCHLEAR$MECHANICS
7706    ALLEN TWO-DIMENSIONAL$COCHLEAR$FLUID$MODEL
7706    BILSEN PITCH NOISE$SIGNELS EVIDENCE CENTRAL$SPECTRUM
7706    PIERCE UNCERTAINTY CONCERNING DIRECT USE TIME$INFO
        HRG PLACE$CUES
7806    COLBURN THEORY BINAURAL$INTERACTION AUD-NERVE$DATA
7806    RHODE OBSERVATIONS COCH$MECHANICS
7806    SONDHI COMPUTING$MOTION TWO-DIMENSIONAL$COCH$MODEL
7806    STERN THEORY BINAURAL$INTERACTION BASED AUD-NERVE
        DATA


                         0111


5406    ANESTHESIA HNG
5406    CORTICAL$TEST AUD$FUNCTION EXPERIMENTALLY$DEAFENED
        $CATS

| | |
|---|---|
| 5406 | EXPLORATION COCH$POTENTIALS GUINEA$PIG MICROELECTRODE |
| 5406 | VARIATION SPL GUINEA$PIG$EARS ABNORMAL$EARDRUMS |
| 5506 | AUD$THR CAT |
| 5506 | MUSICIAN GUINEA$PIG |
| 5513 | PSYCHOLOGICAL$REL ONE'S$OWN$VOICE |
| 5515 | BISENSORY$PERCEP |
| 5515 | SOUND$PERCEP BREATH$CONTROL |
| 5606 | LEARNING FACTOR PREFERENCES HIFI$REPRODUCING$SYSTEMS |
| 5606 | SOURCE RECEIVER$BEHAVIOR CRITERION |
| 5706 | ACOUS$IRRITATION$THR PEKING$DUCKS DOMESTIC$WILD$FOWL |
| 5706 | ACOUS$IRRITATION$THR RINGBILLED$GULLS |
| 5706 | LEARNING FACTOR PREFERENCES HIFI$REPRODUCING$SYSTEMS |
| 5706 | OBSERVATIONS MODELS BASILAR$PAPILLA FROG$EAR |
| 5806 | EFFECTS LOCALIZED$HYPOXIA ELECTROPHYSIOLOGICAL$ACTIVITY COCH$GUINE |
| 5806 | ENDOLYMPHATIC$OXYGEN$TENSION COCH$GUINEA$PIG |
| 5806 | LOCALIZATION$AURAL$HARMONICS BASILAR$MEMBRANE$GUINEA $PIGS |
| 5806 | THR$HNG RINGBILLED$GULL |
| 5906 | ACTION MIDDLE$EAR$MUSCLES CATS |
| 5906 | BINAURAL$COMM$SYSTEMS |
| 5906 | HYDROSTATIC$BALANCING$MECHANISM |
| 5906 | LATENCY ACTION$POTENTIALS COCH$GUINEA$PIG |
| 5906 | REPRODUCTIVE$FUNCTION GUINEA$PIGS |
| 5914 | QUANTIFICATION PHONIC$INTERFERENCE |
| 6006 | DETERMINATION ABSOLUTE-INTENSITY$THR FREQ-DIFFERENCE $THR CATS |
| 6011 | HNG SNAKES |
| 6106 | ACOUS$TRAUMA GUINEA$PIG |
| 6106 | STUDIES ENDOLYMPHATIC$DC$POTENTIAL GUINEA$PIG$COCH |
| 6111 | EFFECT STIMULUS$RISE$TIME EVOKED$R CEREBRAL$CORTEX $CAT |
| 6111 | HNG$BAT COCH$POTENTIALS |
| 6206 | CHANGES COCH$MICROPHONIC GUINEA$PIG PRODUCED MECHANICAL $FACTORS |
| 6206 | COCH$POTENTIALS RHESUS$SQUIRREL$MONKEY |
| 6211 | EFFECT RADIATION AUD$THR RAT |
| 6211 | VERTICAL$ORGANIZATION AUD$CORTEX CAT |
| 6304 | HNG MICE GSR$AUDIOMETRY |
| 6306 | ANALYSIS MIDDLE-EAR$FUNCTION GUINEA$PIG$EAR |
| 6306 | MASKING TONES NOISE CAT |
| 6306 | R ACOUS$STIMULI SINGLE$UNITS EIGHTH$NERVE BULLFROG |
| 6306 | SUMMATING$POTENTIAL COCH GUINEA$PIG |
| 6404 | PT$AUD$FEEDBACK |
| 6404 | SENSITIVITY ACUITY |
| 6406 | EFFECT AUD$DEPRIVATION |

6406    EFFECT AUD$DEPRIVATION
6406    MEAS DISPLACEMENTS NONLINEARITIES GUINEA-PIG$TYMPANUM
6406    R ACOUS$STIMULI SINGLE$UNITS EIGHTH$NERVE GREEN$FROG
6406    SONIC-PULSE$COMPRESSION BATS PEOPLE
6406    SONIC-PULSE$COMPRESSION BATS
6410    FACTORS ERRORS AUDITION FOREIGN$STUDENTS
6411    AUD$DISCRIM NORMAL$MONKEYS
6411    AUD$DISCRIM BRAIN-DAMAGED$MONKEYS
6411    AUD$DISCRIM BRAIN-DAMAGED$MONKEYS
6411    AUDITORY$RESPONSES LIZARD
6411    DAMAGE EIGHTH$CRANIAL$NERVE CAT
6506    BINAURAL$INTERACTION ACCESSORY$SUPERIOR-OLIVARY$NUCLEUS
        CAT
6506    EXPERIMENTS FOUR-EARED$MAN
6506    EXPERIMENTAL$OBSERVATIONS DC$RESTING$POTENTIAL GUINEA-PIG
        $COCH
6506    STIMULUS$CORRELATES WAVE$ACTIVITY SUPERIOR-OLIVARY
        $COMPLEX CAT
6506    THR$AUD MONKEY
6506    TTS CHINCHILLA NOISE$EXPOSURE
6511    AUD$THR BAT
6511    AUD$THR RACOON
6511    COCH$POTENTIALS RAT
6511    COMPARISON SINGLE$UNIT$RESPONSES AUD$NERVE GSR$THR
        MICE
6511    ECHOLOCATION$SIGNALS BAT
6511    FREQ$DISCRIM CORTICALLY$ABLATED$MONKEYS
6511    STRUCTURE FUNCTION LIZARD$EAR
6511    UNANESTHETIZED$CATS AUD$EVOKED$POTENTIALS TEST$CAGE
        $ACOUS STUDY
6604    EFFECTS PT$SYNCHRONOUS$DAF KEYTAPPING PROGRAMMED$VISUAL
        $STIMULUS
6604    KEYTAPPING DAF
6606    BEHAVIORAL PINNA-REFLEX THR RAT AUDIOMETRIC TTS COVARIATIONS
6606    EFFECT SIGNAL$DURATION AUD$SENSITIVITY HUMANS MONKEYS
6606    EFFECTS CALCIUM SOUND-EVOKED COCH$POTENTIALS GUINEA
        $PIG
6606    INPUT-OUTPUT$CHARACTERISTICS LATERAL-LINE SENSE$ORGAN
        XENOPUS$LAEV
6606    MEMBRANE$RESISTANCE ENDOLYMPHATIC$WALLS FIRST$TURN
        $COCH GUINEA$PIG
6606    PERIPHERAL$ORIGIN AUD$R RECORDED EIGHTH$NERVE BULLFROG
6606    VOCAL$R BULLFROG NATURAL$SYNTHETIC$MATING$CALLS
6704    TONE$
6706    ENCODING STIMULUS$FREQ INTEN CAT SUPERIOR$OLIVE$S-SEGMENT
        $CELLS

6706    INTEGRATION ENERGY REPEATED$TONE$PULSES MAN GOLDFISH
6706    MIDDLE-EAR$CHARACTERISTICS ANESTHETIZED$CATS
6706    POSTSYNAPTIC$ACTIVITY CROSSED$OLIVOCOCH$FIBERS CAT
6706    PROPERTIES SOUND$TRANSMISSION MIDDLE$OUTER$EARS CATS
6711    CONDITIONAL$SUPPRESSION DETERMINATION$AUD$SENSITIVITY
        PIGEONS
6711    FREQUENCY$DL PIGEON CONDITIONED$SUPPRESSION
6711    HNG CHINCHILLA
6711    UNDERWATER$AL SEA$LION
6804    HNG MICE GSR$AUDIOMETRY MAGNITUDE UNCONDITIONED$GSR
        FUNCTION
6804    HNG$MICE GSR$AUDIOMETRY MAGNITUDE UNCONDITIONED$GSR
6806    ACQUISITION SUCCESSIVE AUD$DISCRIM MONKEYS
6806    LONGITUDINAL$DISTRIBUTION COCH$MICROPHONICS COCH$DUCT
        GUINEA$PIG
6806    MASKED$TONAL$THR PORPOISE
6806    RATE$VS$LEVEL$FUNCTIONS AUD-NERVE$FIBERS CATS TONE-BURST
        $STIMULI
6806    REL ABSOLUTE$THR DURATION-OF-TONE$PULSES PORPOISE
6806    REL ABSOLUTE$THR DURATION-OF-TONE$PULSES PORPOISE
6806    SINGLE-UNIT$ACTIVITY PRIMARY$AUD$CORTEX UNANESTHETIZED
        $CATS
6806    STUDIES TWO-TONE$INTERACTION GUINEA$PIG$MICROPHONIC
6806    SUBMICROSCOPIC$DISPLACEMENT$AMPLITUDES TYMPANIC$MEMBRANE
        CAT MEAS
6811    AUD$R GOLDFISH
6811    AUD$RESPONSES SHREWS PRIMATES
6811    COCHLEA$MICROPHONICS$POTENTIAL BASAL$THIRD$TURNS RAT
        $COCHLEA
6811    NEURAL$RESPONSES SOUND CRICKET
6811    STEREOTAXIC$INSTRUMENT ACOUSTIC$STUDIES RAT
6811    VOCAL$SPECTRA COCHLEAR$SENSITIVITY GERBIL
6906    COCH$HAIR-CELL$DAMAGE GUINEA$PIGS EXPOSURE IMPULSE
        $NOISE
6906    PROPERTIES SUMMATING$POTENTIAL GUINEA$PIG COCH
6906    R SINGLE$AUD$UNITS EIGHTH$NERVE LEOPARD$FROG
6906    TEMPORAL$SUMMATION ACOUS$SIGNALS CHINCHILLA
6911    AUD$EVOKED$R MICE BRAIN$WEIGHTS
6911    AUD$THR MONKEY CLOSED$SYSTEM$HELMET
6911    BEHAVIORAL$AUDIOGRAM GOLDFISH
6911    EVOKED$R AUD$CORTEX MONKEY
6911    HNG PRIMITIVE$MAMMALS TREE$SHREW
6911    HNG PRIMITIVE$MAMMALS OPOSSUM
6911    LATERAL$LINE$SENSITIVITY GOLDFISH
6911    SHOCK-AVOIDANCE$TECHNIQUE A$THR MONKEY
6911    TECHNIQUE WIDE$APPROACH$MEDULLA AUD$BULLAE CAT

7006    AUDIBILITY$CURVE CHINCHILLA
7006    CAT
7006    LOW-FREQ$AUD$CHARACTERISTICS SPECIES$DEPENDENCE
7006    MEAS COCH$POTENTIALS GUINEA$PIG SPL EARDRUM COCH$MICROPHONIC
7006    MECHANICS GUNIEA$PIG$COCH
7006    ON$OFF$R MEAS COCH$GUINEA$PIG
7006    PERIPHERAL$INHIBITION AUD$FIBERS FROG
7006    PT$AUD$BEHAVIORAL$THR LEMURS
7006    STIMULATION VESTIBULAR$APPARATUS GUINEA$PIG STATIC
        $PRESSURE$CHANGE
7006    STUDY SINGLE$UNITS COCH$NUCLEUS CHINCHILLA
7006    VARIATIONS EFFECTS ELECTRIC$STIMULATION CROSSED$OLIVOCOCH
        $BUNDLE C
7011    AUD$COMPARISONS STETHOSCOPES
7011    COCH$NEURAL$ACTIVITY AUD$SYSTEM RACOON
7011    CORTICAL$AUDIOMETRY GUINEA$PIGS
7011    LEARNING-SET$PROCEDURE SOUND$QUALITY$DISCRIM CHINCHILLA
7011    OSSICULAR$CHAIN$GRAFTING SOUND$CONDITIONED$CATS
7011    SENSITIVITY RAT$EAR CM
7106    AUD$MASKING PT PORPOISE
7106    BEHAVIORAL$THR CAT
7106    CHINCHILLA
7106    CORRESPONDENCE COCH$MICROPHONIC SENSITIVITY BEHAVIORAL
        $THR CAT
7106    INTRACOCH$ELECTRODES GUINEA$PIG
7106    LEMUR HNG
7106    OBSERVATIONS VIBRATION BASILAR$MEMBRANE SQUIRREL$MONKEY
7106    VIBRATORY$PATTERN ROUND$WINDOW CAT
7111    ECHO$RANGING$SIGNALS SONAR SEA$LION
7111    EFFECTS SIZE AUD$CAPACITIES GOLDFISH
7111    FIELD$POTENTIALS$STUDY INHIBITION CAT SUPERIOR$OLIVARY
        $COMPLEX
7111    FREQUENCY$DISCRIM$THR AUD$CORTEX$ABLATIONS MONKEY
7111    INTRACOCHLEAR$PRESSURE$VARIATION ANOXEMIA GUINEA$PIG
7205    SURVEY HAE$PROCEDURES
7206    ANESTHESIA CATS
7206    AUD$THR KILLER$WHALE
7206    AUD$THR DOLPHIN
7206    AUD$THR GOLDFISH
7206    CROSSED$OLIVOCOCH$BUNDLE GUINEA$PIG$COCH
7206    FREQ$DISCRIM DOLPHIN
7206    MAGNETICALLY$COUPLED$STIMULATION OSSICULAR$CHAIN MEAS
        KANGAROO$RAT
7206    MODELING SIMULATION COCH$POTENTIALS GUINEA$PIG
7206    PT$AUD$THR CARP
7206    PT$AUD$THR CARP

7206    R$PATTERNS SINGLE$COCH$NERVE$FIBERS CLICK$STIMULI
        DESCRIPTIONS CAT
7206    SOIND-INDUCED$ELECTRICAL$IMPED$CHANGES GUINEA$PIG
        $COCH
7206    T1S CHINCHILLA ELECTROPHYSIOLOGICAL$CORRELATES
7206    TYMPANIC$MEMBRANE$VIBRATIONS CATS TIME-AVERAGED$HOLOGRAPHY
7211    AUD$SENSITIVITY TURKEY
7211    EFFECT CLICK$INTENSITY RW$POTENTIALS CAT
7211    EFFECTS INTRACOCH$PRESSURE$CHANGES COCH$POTENTIALS
        GUINEA$PIGS
7211    FREQ$DL DOLPHIN
7211    ULTRASONIC$SIGNALLING MICE
7304    ThR$SHIFTS EXPOSURE$NOISE CHINCHILLAS NOISE-INDUCED
        $HNG$LOSSES
7306    ACOUS$BEHAVIOR OUTER$EAR GUINEA$PIG INFLUENCE MIDDLE
        $EAR
7306    EVOKED$R$AUDIBILITY$CURVE CHINCHILLA
7306    EVOKED$R$AUDIBILITY$CURVE CHINCHILLA
7306    NERVE-FIBER$DISTRIBUTION COCH BAT
7306    QUANTITATIVE$STUDY COCH$POTENTIALS SCALA$MEDIA GUINEA
        $PIG
7311    AL BRAIN-DAMAGED$MONKEYS
7311    COMPUTER-AVERAGED$PT$R AUD$NERVE WAKINGS$SQUIRREL$MONKEY
7311    ORGANIZATION INFERIOR$COLLICULUS$CHINCHILLA
7404    EFFECTS LOW-PASS$FILTERING RATE$LEARNING$RETRIEVAL
        $MEMORY SP$STIMU
7404    INTERAURAL$INTENSITY PHASE$ANGLE DISCRIM MONKEYS
7406    AUD$FREQ$DISCRIM VERTEBRATES
7406    AUD$SENSITIVITY SEA$LION AIRBORNE$SOUND
7406    BASILAR$MEMBRANES TUNING$CURVES GUINEA$PIG
7406    BILATERAL$HNG$ASYMMETRY
7406    CHINCHILLA
7406    CHINCHILLA
7406    DEPENDENCE MIDDLE-EAR$PARAMETERS BODY$WEIGHT GUINEA
        $PIG
7406    DETECTION BINAURALLY$MASKED$TONES CAT
7406    EFFECTS INTENSE$AUD$STIMULATION HNG$LOSSES INNER$EAR
        $CHANGES CHINC
7406    INTRACELLULAR$R ACOUS$CLICKS INNER$EAR ALLIGATOR$LIZARD
7406    INVEST SOURCES WHOLE-NERVE$ACTION$POTENTIALS RECORDED
        PLACES GUINE
7406    MEAS GUINEA$PIG MIDDLE-EAR$TRANSFER$CHARACTERISTIC
7406    MIDDLE-EAR$FUNCTION GUINEA$PIG
7406    PERIPHERAL$AUD$FUNCTION PLATYPUS
7406    PT$THR MONKEY
7406    PT$THR MONKEY

7406    SPECIES$DIFFERENCES COCH$FATIGUE ACOUS OUTER$MIDDLE
        $EARS GUINEA$PI
7412    AUD$PROCESSES
7504    GOLDENBERG AVERAGE$EP CATS LESIONS$AUDITORY$PATHWAY
7506    ALTES MECHANISM AURAL$PULSE$COMPRESSION MAMMALS
7506    BERANEK CHANGING$ROLE "EXPERT"
7506    BILSEN R SINGLE$UNITS COCHLEAR$NUCLEUS CAT COSINE
        $NOISE
7506    BILSEN R SINGLE$UNITS COCHLEAR$NUCLEUS CAT COSINE
        $NOISE
7506    BOER SYNTHETIC$WHOLE-NERVE$ACTION$POTENTIALS CAT
7506    BURDICK SP$PERCEPTION CHINCHILLA DISCRIM
7506    BURKHARD ANTHROPOMETRIC$MANIKIN ACOUSTIC$RESEARCH
7506    CHADWICK MECHANICAL$COCHLEAR$MODEL
7506    DANCER HOLOGRAPHIC$INTERFEROMETRY TM$DISPLACEMENTS
        GUINEA$PIG$EARS
7506    DOOLING AUD$INTENSITY$DISCRIM PARAKEET
7506    FLAMMINO NEURAL$R INFERIOR$COLLICULUS ALBINO$RAT BINAURAL
        $STIMULI
7506    GREEN GOLD PUMPREY REVISITED
7506    KELLY HRG$THR HORN$SHARK
7506    MAESTRELLO MECHANISMS NOISE$GENERATION RADIATION SUBSONIC
        $JET
7506    MOORE UNDERWATER$LOCALIZATION CALIFORNIA$SEA$LION
7506    MOORE UNDERWATER$LOCALIZATION CLICK PULSED$PT$SIGNALS
        CALIF$SEA$LION
7506    SEARLE BINAURAL$PINNA$DISPARITY AUD$LOCALIZATION$CUE
7506    SEATON COMPARISON CRITICAL$RATIOS CRITICAL$BANDS MONAURAL
        CHINCHILLA
7506    SPEAKS INTERAURAL-INTENSIVE$DIFFERENCES DICHOTIC$LISTENING
7506    TEAS INTERAURAL$ATTENUATION FREQ GUINEA$PIG CHINCHILLA
        CM$R
7506    TERHUNE MASKED$HEARING$THRESHOLDS SINGED$SEALS
7506    THOMPSON UNDERWATER$FREQ$DISCRIM DOLPHIN HUMAN
7506    WILSON BASILAR$MEMBRANE MID-EAR$VIBRATION GUINEA$PIG
        CAPACITIVE$PROBE
7511    MCCLCLLAND LOW$FREQ$SOUND$LOCALIZATION KANGAROO$RAT
7511    MCCLELLAND LOW$FREQUENCY$LOCALIZATION KANGAROO$RAT
7511    NUNLEY STIMULATION CHINCHILLA'S$OSSICULAR$CHAIN ELECTRODE
7511    NUNLEY STIMULATION CHINCHILLA$OSSICULAR$CHAIN IMPLANTED
        $ELECTRODE
7511    PETERSON NOISE CARDIOVASCULAR$FUNCTIONS RHEDUS$MONKEYS
7511    PETERSON NOISE CARDIOVASCULAR$FUNCTIONS MONKEYS
7532    PORTER DEV$CHANGES DICHOTIC$RIGHT-EAR$ADVANTAGE
7532    SATZ DEV$PARAMETERS EAR$ASYMMETRY
7606    ALTES SONAR GENERALIZED$TARGET$DISCRIPTION ANIMAL
        $ECHOLOCATION$SYSTEMS

7606 BROWN COMFORTABLE$EFFORT$LEVEL
7606 EGGERMONT AP TONE$BURSTS HUMAN + GUINEA$PIG$COCHLEA
7606 EHRET TEMPORAL$AUDITORY$SUMMATION PT WHITE$NOISE HOUSE
     $MOUSE
7606 FROST TACTILE$LOCALIZATION SOUNDS
7606 GEESA BINAURAL$INTERACTION CAT MAN
7606 GREENWOOD TWO-TONE$SUPPRESS COMB-TONE$DRIVE COCH$NUCLEUS
     CAT
7606 HEFFNER PERCEP MISSING$FUNDAMENTAL CATS
7606 MCGEE PSYCHOPHYSICAL$TUNING$CURVES CHINCHILLAS
7606 MOORE DISCRIM PT$INTENSITIES CALIF$SEA$LION
7606 PICKLES AUDITORY-NERVE-FIBER$BANDWIDTHS CRITICAL$BANDWIDTHS
     CAT
7606 REINIS ACUTE$CHANGES ANIMAL$INNER$EARS SIMULATED$SONIC
     $BOOMS
7606 ROBLES TRANSIENT$R BASILAR$MEM SQUIRREL$MONKEYS MOSSBAUER
     $EFFECT
7606 RYAN HRING$SENSITIVITY MONGOLIAN$GERBIL
7606 SCHACHT BIOCHEMISTRY NEOMYCIN$OTOTOXICITY
7606 SCHUSTERMAN CALIF$SEA$LION UNDERWATER$AUD$DETECTION
     RF$SCHEDULES
7606 SINNOTT SP$SOUND$DISCRIM MONKEYS HUMANS
7606 SMOORENBURG COMBINATION$TONES R NEURONS COCH$NUCLEUS
     CAT
7606 WOODFORD ACOUS$REFLEX$THR CHINCHILLA STIM$DURATION+FREQ
7611 MEIKLE PREVENTION SPONTANEOUS$MIDDLE$EAR$MUSCLE$ACTIVITY
     GUINEA$PIG
7611 NELSON AUTOMATED$CONDITIONED$AVOIDANCE$AUDIOMETRY
     CHINCHILLA
7611 TANIGUCHI ACOUSTIC$FAR-FIELD$RESPONSE KANAMYCIN-TREATED
     $GUINEA$PIG
7611 WALLOCH ACOUSTIC$TRAUMA GUINEA$PIGS
7621 STRETTER KIKUYU LABIAL APICAL$STOP$DISCRIMINATION
7706 ANDO EFFECTS NOISE SLEEP BABIES
7706 CORNILLON SIMPLE$MODEL SIMULATING TRAFFIC$NOISE$SPECTRA
7706 EHRET POSTNATAL$DEV ACOUS$SYSTEM HOUSE$MOUSE DEV MASKED
     $THR
7706 GEISLER ALTERNATING$ELECTRICAL-RESISTANCE$CHANGES
     GUINEA-PIG$COCHLEA
7706 KRUGER MIDDLE$EAR$TRANSMISSION CATS EXPERIMENTALLY
     $INDUCED$TM$PERFS
7706 NAKATANI COMPUTER-AIDED$SIGNAL$HANDLING SP$RESEARCH
7706 ORR BEHAVIORAL$SYS APPARATUS TONE-DETECTION REACTION-TIMES
     CAT
7706 SCHMIEDT SOUND-TRANSMISSION CM$CHAR MONGOLIAN$GERBIL
     GUINEA$PIG

7706  YENI-KOMSHIAN ID SP$SOUNDS DISPLAYED VIBROTACTILE
      $VOCODER
7806  ALDER APPROACH GUINEA$PIG AUDITORY$NERVE
7806  ALTES ANGLE$ESTIMATION BINAURAL$PROCESSING ANIMAL
      $ECHOLOCATION
7806  ALTES FOURIER-MELLIN MAMMALIAN$HRG
7806  AU PROPAGATION DOLPHIN$ECHOLOCATION$SIGNALS
7806  BLAUERT GROUP$DELAY$DISTORTIONS ELECTROACOUSTICAL
      $SYSTEMS
7806  BROWN LOCALIZATION PURE$TONES OLD$WORLD$MONKEYS
7806  BURKICK THRESHOLD$SHIFTS CHINCHILLAS ESPOSED OCTAVE
      $BANDS
7806  BUUNEN RESPONSES FIBERS CAT$AUDITORY$NERVE DIFFERENCE
      $TONE
7806  DOOLING AUD$DURATION$DISCRIM PARAKEET
7806  FAY CODING SINGLE$AUD-NERVE$FIBERS GOLDFISH
7806  FOSTER AUD$R CATS PULSED$ULTRASOUND
7806  GOSS ULTRASONIC$PROPERTIES MAMMALIAN$TISSUES
7806  JACKSON ACOUSTIC$INPUT$IMPEDANCE DOG$LUNGS
7806  JAVEL TWO-TONE$SUPPRESSION AUD$NERVE CAT
7806  KRUGER TM$PERFORATIONS CATS CONFIGURATIONS$LOSSES
7806  KUHL SP$PERCEP CHINCHILLA VOT$STIMULI
7806  LIBERMAN AUD-NERVE$R CATS RAISED LOW-NOISE$CHAMBER
7806  NELSON FREQ$DISCRIM CHINCHILLA
7806  NIELSON MONKEY TTS LOW-PITCH$NOISE
7806  PRICE AP LOW$INTENSITIES
7806  PROSEN KANAMYMYCIN-INDUCED HL GUINEA$PIG
7806  RYAN NOISE-INDUCED$THR$SHIFT COCH$PATH GERBIL
7806  SCHMIEDT CM$TUNING$CURVES GERBIL
7806  SCHULTZ SYNTHESIS SOCIAL$SURVEYS NOISE$ANNOYANCE
7806  SCHUSTERMAN UPPER$LIMIT UNDERWATER FREQ$DISCRIM SEA
      $LION
7806  THR$SHIFT CHINCHILLAS EXPOSED IMPULSE$NOISE
7806  WATANABE  R CATS$COLLICULAR NEURON SP


## 0112


5406  HISTORICAL$NOTE THERMAL$MASKING$NOISE PT$PITCH$CHANGES
5406  MASKING$SP NOISE$BURSTS
5506  INDEPENDENCE MASKING$AUDIOGRAM PERSTIMULATORY$FATIGUE
      AUD$STIMULUS
5603  MASKING IMPAIRED$EARS NOISE
5706  DOWNWARD$SPREAD$MASKING
5706  MASKING$SP LINE-SPECTRUM$INTERFERENCE

5706    PHYSIOLOGICAL$EVIDENCE MASKING$LOW$FREQ
5706    REMOTE$MASKING
5806    INTENSIVE$DETERMINANTS REMOTE$MASKING
5806    MASKING ENG$WORDS PROLONGED$VOWEL$SOUNDS
5906    ADDITIVITY TYPES MASKING
5906    BACKWARD$MASKING
5906    LAMBDA$LOUDNESS$FUNCTION MASKING LOUDNESS MULTICOMPONENT
        $TONES
5906    MASKED$THR OCTAVE$BAND$NOISE
5906    MASKING TONES NOISE$BANDS
5906    MASKING$PATTERNS TONES
5906    OBSERVATIONS SIGNALS NOISE
5906    PT$MASKING
5906    RESIDUAL$MASKING LOW$FREQ
6006    MONAURAL$TEMPORAL$MASKING INVEST BINAURAL$INTERACTION
6006    NOTE EQUALIZATION CANCELLATION$THEORY BINAURAL$MASKING
        $LEVEL
6006    STUDY COCKTAIL$PARTY$PROBLEM
6010    USE FAST-LIMITING IMPROVE INTELLIGIBILITY SP$IN$NOISE
6104    DIFFERENTIAL$SENSITIVITY MASKED$THR
6104    SP$NOISE
6106    AUD$MASKING CRITICAL$BAND
6106    AUD$THR$SHIFTS SIMULTANEOUSLY$CONTRALATERAL$STIMULI
6106    CHANGES MASKING TIME
6106    FORWARD$BACKWARD$MASKING ACOUS$CLICKS
6106    LOUDNESS$SUMMATION MASKING
6106    LOUDNESS$FUNCTION MASKING$NOISE
6106    MASKING PULSED$TONES NOISE$BANDS
6206    BACKWARD$MASKING MONOTIC DICHOTIC
6206    BACKWARD$FORWARD$MASKING PROBE$TONES FREQ
6206    EFFECT NOISE ONE$EAR MASKED$THR TONE OTHER
6206    MASKING INTERAURAL$PHASE
6206    WIDTH CRITICAL$BANDS
6211    MASKING PT SP
6211    MASKING$EFFICIENCY WIDE$BAND$NARROW$BAND$NOISE
6306    AUD$UNMASKING
6306    EFFECT NOISE DEPENDENCE CORRELATION DETECTION MEAS
6306    EFFECT VARYING INTERAURAL$NOISE$CORRELATION DETECTABILITY
        TONAL$SI
6306    EQUALIZATION CANCELLATION$THEORY BINAURAL$MASKING
        $LEVEL$DIFFERENCE
6306    MASKING TONES NOISE CAT
6306    PHYSICAL$MEAS SP-INTERFERING NAVY$NOISES
6306    SIGNAL-PLUS-NOISE$INPUTS
6306    TEMPORAL$MASKING CLICKS NOISE$BURSTS
6306    THR$MECHANISM MASKING$NOISE

6314    R$TIMES KNOWN$MESSAGE-SETS NOISE
6404    GENERALIZED$SP$INTERFERENCE$NOISE$CONTOURS
6406    BACKWARD$MASKING DURATIONS MASKING$STIMULUS
6406    BACKWARD$MASKING TONES NARROW-BAND$NOISE
6406    BINAURAL$MASKING-LEVEL$DOFFERENCES HIGH$FREQ
6406    LOUDNESS$FUNCTION
6406    LOUDNESS$FUNCTION PRESENCE MASKING$NOISE
6406    MASKER$LEVEL NOISE-SIGNAL$DETECTION
6406    MASKING$NOISE
6406    NOTE BINAURAL$MASKING-LEVEL$DIFFERENCES HIGH$FREQ
6406    NOTE BINAURAL$MASKING-LEVEL DIFFERENCES FUNCTION INTERAURAL
        $CORREL
6406    TEMPORAL$SUMMATION BACKWARD$MASKING
6411    INTERACTION FORWARD$BACKWARD$MASKING
6506    AUD$MASKING RAT
6506    CHANGES SIMULTANEOUS$MASKED$THR BRIEF$TONES
6506    DEMONSTRATION MASKING-LEVEL$DIFFERENCES BINAURAL$BEATS
6506    EFFECT MASKING PITCH PERIODIC$PULSES
6506    MASKING TWO$TONES
6506    MASKING-LEVEL$DIFFERENCES FUNCTION INTERAURAL$DISPARITIES
        INTENSIT
6506    RELEASE$MASKING SP
6506    SHIFTS AC$THR PRODUCED PULSED CONTINUOUS CONTRALATERAL
        $MASKING
6506    TEMPORAL$EFFECTS SIMULTANEOUS$MASKING WHITE-NOISE
        $BURSTS
6506    TIME-INTENSITY$REL BINAURAL$UNMASKING
6506    USE NOISE ELIMINATE$ONE$EAR MASKING$EXPERIMENTS
6511    EFFECT CENTRAL$MASKING THR$SP
6606    BINAURAL$MASKING SP PERIODICALLY$MODULATED$NOISE
6606    BINAURAL$UNMASKING COMPLEX$SIGNALS
6606    INTERAURAL$PHASE$EFFECTS MASKING SIGNALS$DIFFERENT
        $DURATIONS
6606    INTERAURAL$PHASE EFFECTS MASKING$SIGNALS DURATIONS
6606    MASKING DISCRIM
6606    MASKING DISCRIM
6606    MASKING DISCRIM
6606    MASKING$SP AIRCRAFT$NOISE
6606    MASKING-LEVEL$DIFFERENCES CONTINUOUS$MASKING$NOISE
        BURST$MASKING$N
6606    PHYSIOLOGICAL$CORRELATE TONAL$MASKING
6606    POWER-GROUP TRANSFORMATIONS GLAKE MASKING RECRUITMENT
6606    REMOTE$MASKING ABSENCE INTRA-AURAL$MUSCLES
6606    RESULTS BINAURAL$UNMASKING EC$MODEL
6606    SHIFTS AUD$THR PRODUCED IPSILATERAL$CONTRALATERAL
        $MASKERS

6606    SPECTRUM$WIDTH BINAURAL$RELEASE$MASKING
6706    ADDITIVITY MASKING
6706    AURAL$HARMONICS MASKING
6706    BINAURAL$RELEASE$MASKING$SP GAIN$INTELLIGIBILITY
6706    DETECTION IN-PHASE$SIGNAL UNCERTAINTY INTERAURAL$PHASE
        MASKING$NOI
6706    EXPLANATION MASKING-LEVEL$DIFFERENCES INTERAURAL$INTENSIVE
        $DISPARI
6706    FREQ$SELECTIVITY EAR FORWARD$MASKING
6706    MASKER$LEVEL SINUSOIDAL-SIGNAL$DETECTION
6706    MASKING WHITE$NOISE PT$FM$TONE NARROW-BAND$NOISE
6706    OBSERVATIONS CONTRALATERAL$REMOTE$MASKING
6706    PREDICTING BINAURAL$GAIN$INTELLIGIBILITY RELEASE$MASKING
        $SP
6706    RELEASE MASKING SP INTERAURAL$TIME$DELAY
6804    UNMASKING PT SPONDEES INTERAURAL$PHASE$TIME$DISPARITIES
6804    UNMASKING PT SPONDEES INTERAURAL$PHASE$TIME$DISPARITIES
6806    AURAL$HARMONICS TIME-INTENSITY$REL TONE-ON-TONE$MASKING
        $TECHNIQUE
6806    EFFECT MASKER$SPECTRUM$LEVEL MASKING-LEVEL$DIFFERENCES
        LOW$FREQ
6806    EFFECTS INTERAURAL$TIME$DELAYS MASKING TWO$COMPETING
        $SIGNALS
6806    FREQ$DISTRIBUTION CENTRAL$MASKING
6806    MASKED$TONAL$THR PORPOISE
6806    MASKING-LEVEL$DIFFERENCES INTERAURAL$DISPARITIES MASKER
        $INTENSITY
6806    MONAURAL$LOUDNESS$FUNCTION MASKING
6806    MONAURAL$TEMPORAL$MASKING TRANSIENTS
6806    RESULTS BINAURAL$UNMASKING EC$MODEL NOISE$BANDWIDTH
        INTERAURAL$PHA
6806    SHIFTS MASKING TIME
6806    SINE$COSINE$MASKING
6904    RELEASE$MASKING STUDYING HAIR$CELL$FUNCTION
6906    AUD$TEMPORAL$MASKING PERCEP$ORDER
6906    BINAURAL$MASKING BACKWARD FORWARD SIMULTANEOUS$EFFECTS
6906    BINAURAL$MASKERS SINE-WAVE$MASKERS
6906    COMMENTS MONAURAL$LOUDNESS$FUNCTIONS MASKING
6906    EFFECT PULSED$MASKING SP$MATERIALS
6906    EFFECTS PT$MASKING LOW-PASS$HIGH-PASS$NOISE
6906    MASKING CONTINUOUS PULSED SINUSOIDS
6906    MASKING SILENT$PERIODS NOISE
6906    NOISE$MASKING CHANGE RESIDUE$PITCH
6906    PERCEP PITCH WHITE-NOISE$MASK
6906    PERCEP$MASKING SOUND$BACKGROUNDS
6906    RELEASE MULTIPLE$MASKERS EFFECTS INTERAURAL$TIME$DISPARITIES

6906    THR DURATION LEVELS CONTINUOUS GATED$MASKER
7006    BINAURAL$MASKING TONE TONE$PLUS$NOISE
7006    MASKING-LEVEL$DIFFERENCES PULSED$TONAL$MASKER
7006    NARROW-BAND$FM$NOISE MASKING$NOISE
7011    MASKING-LEVEL$DIFFERENCES FUNCTION NOISE$SPECTRUM
        $LEVEL FREQ
7106    ADDITIVITY FORWARD$AND$BACKWARD$MASKING FUNCTION SIGNAL
        $FREQ
7106    AUD CRITICAL$BANDWIDTH SHORT-DURATION$SIGNALS
7106    AUD$MASKING PT PORPOISE
7106    AURAL COMBINATION$TONES AUD$MASKING
7106    BINAURAL$UNMASKING VOCALIC$SIGNALS
7106    CORRELATION$MODEL BINAURAL$MASKING LEVEL DIFFERENCES
7106    FORWARD$BACKWARD$MASKING TESTING PERCEP-MOMENT$HYPOTHESIS
        AUDITION
7106    FORWARD$BACKWARD$MASKING INTERACTIONS ADDITIVITY
7106    INFLUENCE PULSED$MASKING SPONDEES
7106    MASKER
7106    MASKING TONES TRANSIENT$SIGNALS IDENTICAL ENERGY$SPECTRA
7106    MASKING$NOISE SP-ENVELOPE$CHARACTERISTICS STUDYING
        INTELLIGIBILITY
7106    ON-FREQ$MASKING CONTINUOUS$SINUSOIDS
7106    SIGNAL$PROCESSING COCKTAIL$PARTY$EFFECT
7106    TWO-VS-FOUR-TONE$MASKING
7111    COMPARISON MASKING$SP-MODULATED$AND$WHITE$NOISE
7111    TRANSDUCER AUD$MASKING
7206    AUD$TEMPORAL$INTEGRATION HIGH$MASKED-THR$LEVELS
7206    AURAL$HARMONICS MONAURAL$PHASE$EFFECTS TONE-ON-TONE
        $MASKING
7206    COMBINATION$BANDS EVEN$ORDER MASKING$EFFECTS ESTIMATIONS
        $LEVEL
7206    CRITICAL$MASKING$INTERVAL
7206    MACH$BANDS AUD$MASKING
7206    MASKING CONTINUOUS$GATED$SINUSOIDS
7206    MASKING COMBINATION$BANDS ESTIMATION LEVELS COMBINATION
        $BANDS
7206    MASKING NARROW$BANDS$NOISE INTENSE$PT$HIGH$FREQ APPLICATION
        MEAS
7206    MLD FORWARD$BACKWARD$MASKING
7206    MONAURAL$BINAURAL$MASKING LOW-FREQ$TONE
7206    PHYSIOLOGICAL$NOISE MASKER LOW$FREQ CARDIAC$CYCLE
7206    POSTMASKING$RECOVERY HUMAN CLICK ACTION$POTENTIALS
        CLICK$LOUDNESS
7206    SUPRATHR$BINAURAL$MASKING
7206    THEORY CENTRAL$AUD$MASKING
7206    TONE-ON-TONE$MASKING BINAURAL$LISTENING$CONDITIONS

7211    EFFECT MASKING VOCAL$INTENSITY VOCAL$WHISPERED$SP
7211    MASKING INTERFERENCE PITCH$PERCEP
7304    RELEASE$FROM$MULTIPLE$MASKERS ELDERLY$PERSONS
7306    CONSEQUENCES PERIPHERAL$FREQ$SELECTIVITY NONSTIMULATING
        $MASKING
7306    CRITICAL$MASKING$INTERVAL TEMPORAL$ANALOG CRITICAL
        $BAND
7306    INFLUENCE INTERAURAL$PHASE FORWARD$MASKING
7306    INTERACTION FORWARD$BACKWARD$MASKING MEAS INTEGRATING
        $PERIOD AUD$S
7306    MASKING PRODUCED SINUSOIDS SLOWLY$CHANGING$FREQ
7306    THR CLICK$PAIRS MASKED BAND-STOP$NOISE
7311    BINAURAL$SUMMATION FUNCTION MASKING$LEVEL
7311    EFFECTS MOTION$MASKER BINAURAL$MASKING$FUNCTION
7404    PT$OCTAVE$MASKING
7406    BINAURAL$MASKING$LEVEL$DIFFERENCES PULSE$TRAINS INTERAURAL
        $CORRELA
7406    DICHOTIC$RELEASE MASKING SP
7406    EFFECT MASKER$DURATION MASKER$LEVEL FORWARD$BACKWARD
        $MASKING
7406    HIGH-FREQ$MASKING$LEVEL$DIFFERENCES NARROW-BAND$NOISE
        $SIGNALS
7406    MASKING NARROW-BAND$FM$NOISE
7406    MASKING$PATTERNS BAND-REJECTED$NOISE
7413    EFFECT NOISE ACOUS$PARAMETER$SP
7504    MARGOLIS MEAS CRITICAL$MASKING$BANDS
7506    BORDELON PRESERVATION INFO MATRIX$FILTERING SIGNAL
7506    CLACK SUBJECTIVE$TONES TONE-ON-TONE$MASKING
7506    JEFFRESS MASKING TONE$BY$TONE DURATION
7506    KAPLAN DISTRACTORS$EXPERIMENT CRITICAL$BAND CONTAMINATED
        $WHITE$NOISE
7506    LESHOWITZ MASKING$PATTERNS SINUSOIDS
7506    MASSARO BACKWARD$RECOGNITION$MASKING
7506    MOORE MECHANISMS MASKING
7506    REPP DICHOTIC$MASKING CONSONANTS VOWELS
7506    REPP DICHOTIC$FORWARD BACKWARD$MASKING CV$SYLLABLES
7506    SEATON COMPARISON CRITICAL$RATIOS CRITICAL$BANDS MONAURAL
        CHINCHILLA
7506    SMALL MACH$BANDS AUDITORY$MASKING
7506    SMIAROWSKI TEMPORAL$RESOLUTION FORWARD$MASKING SIMULTANEOUS
        $MASKING
7506    TAYLOR MONAURAL$DETECTION CONTRALATERAL$CUE
7506    TERHUNE MASKED$HEARING$THRESHOLDS RINGED$SEALS
7511    SMIAROWSKI EFFECT PROBE-TONE$ENVELOPE$SHAPE FORWARD
        $MASKING
7511    SMIAROWSKI PROBE-TONE$ENVELOPE$SHAPE FORWARD$MASKING

7521   HARDCASTLE SP$PROD ORAL$ANAESTHESIA AUD$MASKING
7604   GARBER MASKING LOMBARD SIDETONE$AMP
7604   SORENSON BINAURAL$MASKING BC$NOISE
7606   BERG TEMPORAL.MASKING CLICK DIOTIC+DICHOTIC$LISTENING
       $CONDITIONS
7606   LAKEY TEMPORAL$MASKING-LEVEL$DIFFERENCES EFFECT MASK
       $DURATION
7606   MASSARO RECOGNITION$MASKING AUD$LATERALIZATION PITCH
       $JUDGEMENTS
7606   PARKER INFLUENCE AUDITORY$FATIGUE MASKED$PURE-TONE
       $THRESHOLDS
7606   PHIPPS EFFECT SIGNAL$PHASE DETECTABILITY TONE$MASKED
       $BY$
7606   REPP DICHOTIC$MASKING VOT
7606   SCHACKNOW NOISE-INTENSITY$DISCRIM BANDWIDTH$CONDITIONS
       MASKER$PRESENT
7606   SHANNON TWO-TONE$UNMASKING SUPPRESSION FORWARD-MASKING
7606   SPARKS TEMPORAL$RECOGNITION$MASKING
7606   WIER DETECTION TONE$BURST MASKERS DEFECTS FREQ DURATION
       MASKER$LEVEL
7606   ZWICKER MASKING$PERIOD$PATTERNS HARMONIC$COMPLEX$TONES
7704   MCCLEAN AUD$MASKING LIP$MOVEMENTS
7704   RICHARDS LOUDNESS$PERCEP SHORT-DURATION$TONES
7706   BILLINGS LOW-FREQUENCY$CENTRAL$MASKING
7706   DALLOS ANALOG TWO-TONE$SUPPRESSION WHOLE$NERVE$RESPONSES
7706   ERDREICH INTERMODULATION$PRODUCT MASKING GROWTH
7706   FASTL DURATION TEMPORAL$MASKING$PATTERNS BROAD-BAND
       $IMPULSES
7706   HAFTER LATERALIZATION$MODEL TIME-INTENSITY$TRADINGS
       BINAURAL$MASKING
7706   HOUTGAST AUD-FILTER$CHAR RIPPLED-NOISE$MASKER
7706   KOENIG DETERMINATION MASKING-LEVEL$DIFFERENCES REVERBERANT
       $ENVIRONMENT
7706   LYNN INTERACTIONS BACKWARD FORWARD$MASKING
7706   TERRY SUPPRESSION$EFFECTS FORWARD$MASKING
7706   TYLER TWO-TONE$SUPPRESSION BACKWARD$MASKING
7706   WEBER GROWTH MASKING AUD$FILTER
7706   YOST HIERARCHY MASKING-LEVEL$DIFFERENCES TEMPORAL
       $MASKING
7806   BLAND BACKWARD$MASKING DETECTION RECOGNITION
7806   DON CLICK-EVOKED$BRAINSTEM$POTENTIALS HIGH-PASS MASKING
7806   HALL MODEL ZWICKER'S"MASKING$PERIOD$PATTERNS"
7806   MOORE PSYCHOPHYSICAL$TUNING$CURVES MASKING
7806   NABELEK TEMPORAL$SUMMATION MASKED$AUDITORY$THRESHOLD
7806   NIELSEN MONKEY TTS LOW-FREQUENCY$NOISE
7806   SMALL ADDITIVE$MASKING$EFFECTS NOISE$BANDS DIFFERENT
       $LEVELS

7806    VOGTEN SIMULTANEOUS$PURE-TONE$MASKING
7806    VOGTON PT$MASKING TUNING$CURVES SIMULTANEOUS$FORWARD
        $MASKING
7806    WEBER TEMPORAL$FACTORS SUPPRESSION BACKWARD+FORWARD
        $MASKING
7806    YOST MASKING-LEVEL$DIFFERENCES FILTERED$TRANSIENTS
7821    FARMER EFFECTS AUDITORY$MASKING CEREBRAL$PALSIED$SPEAKERS
7827    HOFFMAN SIMULTANEOUS INTERLEAVED MASKING


## 0113


5703    REL EEG$PATTERNS ELECTRODERMANL$R
5904    ELECTROPHYSIOLOGIC$R SOUND FUNCTION INTENSITY EEG
        $PATTERNS SEX
6003    METHODS EVAL ELECTROENCEPHALIC$R TONES
6004    ELETROPHYSIOLOGIC$R ALPHA$RHYTHM CHIL
6006    FREQ$MEAS EEG
6111    REL EDR$EEG$ALPHA$RHYTHM PATH$ANXIETY
6206    AVERAGE$R CLICKS HUMAN$SCALP
6404    EVOKED$R AUD$STIMULI SUMMING$COMPUTER
6404    TEMPLATE EEG$R SOUND
6404    TEMPLATE EEG$R SOUND
6411    AMPLITUDE$CHANGES EVOKED$POTENTIALS INFERIOR$COLLICULUS
        ACOUSTIC
6411    EVOKED$R$LATENCY STIMULUS$RISE-TIME AUD$CORTEX
6411    STUDIES AUD$ADAPTATION AMPLITUDE$DECLINE EVOKED$AUD
        $POTENTIAL
6504    ANALYSIS EVOKED$ONGOING$ELECTRICAL$ACTIVITY SCALP
        HUMAN
6511    ACOUS$EVOKED$R CESSATION$STIMULUS
6511    UNANESTHETIZED$CATS AUD$EVOKED$POTENTIALS TEST$CAGE
        $ACOUS STUDY
6604    AVERAGED$EVOKED$R
6604    CHARACTERISTICS PEAK$LATENCY PEAK$AMPLITUDE ACOUS
        $EVOKED$R
6604    SUMMED$EVOKED$R PT
6606    ACOUS$REL HUMAN VERTEX$POTENTIAL
6704    AVERAGED$ER SYNTHETIC$SYNTAX$SENTENCES
6704    CHANGES PARAMETERS AVERAGED$AUD$EP REL NUMBER DATA
        $SAMPLES$ANALYZE
6704    INFLUENCE SIGNAL$VARIABLES ER SOUND
6711    FREQ$INTENSITY$EFFECTS BC AVERAGE$EVOKED$AUD$POTENTIALS
6804    AVERAGED$ER LOUDNESS ANALYSIS R$ESTIMATES
6804    EFFECTS SIGNAL$DURATION RISE$TIME AUD$EVOKED$POTENTIAL

6806    EFFECTS CHANGES STIMULUS$FREQ INTENSITY HABITUATION
        HUMAN$VERTEX$P
6806    EFFECTS DURATION RISE$TIME TONE$BURSTS EVOKED$V$POTENTIALS
6806    EFFECTS INTERSIGNAL$INTERVAL HUMAN AUD$ER
6806    MLD PHASE$ANGLE$ALPHA
6811    EFFECTS FREQUENCY AUD$EVOKED$RESPONSE
6904    AUD$EVOKED$R
6904    AUD$EVOKED$R NORMAL$HNG$ADULTS CHIL SEDATION
6904    STABILITY EARLY$COMPONENTS AVERAGED$ELECTROENCEPHALIC
        $R
6906    REL SOUND$INTEN AMPLITUDE AER STIMULUS$FREQS
6911    AUD$EVOKED$R MICE BRAIN$WEIGHTS
6911    EFFECTS HABITUATION AUD$EVOKED$R
6911    EFFECTS STIMULUS$DURATION AVERAGED$ACOUS$EVOKED$CORTICAL
        $R
6911    EVOKED$R AUD$CORTEX MONKEY
6911    RATE$STIMULUS$CHANGE EVOKED$R SIGNAL$RISE-TIME
7004    HABITUATION DISHABITUATION AVERAGED$AUD$EVOKED$R
7006    CRITICAL$BAND$THEORY AUD-EVOKED SLOW-WAVE$POTENTIAL
7006    EFFECTS HIGH$FREQS INTERSUBJECT$VARIABILITY AUD-EVOKED
        $CORTICAL$R
7011    AUD$ACUITY BEAGLE EEG$EVOKED$POTENTIAL
7011    AUD$EVOKED$R RECRUITING$EARS
7011    RATE$FREQ$CHANGE ACOUS$EVOKED$R
7104    COMPARISON AVERAGED$EVOKED$R$AMPLITUDES AFFECTIVE
        $VERBAL$STIMULI
7104    EFFECTS SIGNAL$RISE$TIME DURATION EARLY$COMPONENTS
        AUD$EVOKED$R
7104    PROBLEMS IDENTIFYING ACOUS$EP SINGLE$STIMULUS
7104    WITHIN$AVERAGE$VARIABILITY ACOUS$ER
7111    ELECTROENCEPHALIC$R SWEEP$FREQS
7111    ELIMINATION MOVEMENT$ARTIFACTS EVOKED$RESPONSE$AUD
        INFANTS
7111    LATERAL$SPECIFICITY ACOUSTICALLY-EVOKED$EEG$RESPONSES
7204    BEHAVIORAL$HUMAN$ER$THR FUNCTION FUND$FREQ
7204    EFFECTS STIMULUS$RATE NUMBER EARLY$COMPONENTS AVERAGED
        $ER
7204    RECOVERY$CYCLE ACOUS$EP
7204    REL LOUDNESS AMPLITUDE EARLY$COMPONENTS AVERAGED$ELECTROENCEPHAL
7204    SHORT-TERM$HABITUATION AVERAGED$ELECTROENCEPHALIC
        $R INF
7206    AREA$PROBE
7206    RECORDINGS AVERAGED$ER GUINEA$PIG
7211    AVERAGED$ENCEPHALIC$R LINGUISTIC$AUD$STIMULI
7211    COMPARISON AVERAGED$EVOKED$R FM$AM$TONES
7304    AUD$EVOKED$R VERTEX

7304  AVERAGED$ELECTROENCEPHALIC$R CLICKS
7304  EFFECT ALCOHOL EARLY LATE$COMPONENTS AVERAGE$ELECTROENCEPHALIC
      $R$C
7304  INFLUENCE BACKGROUND$NOISE EARLY$COMPONENTS
7304  SHORT-TERM$HABITUATION INF AUD$EVOKED$R
7404  AVERAGED$ELECTROENCEPHALIC$R CLICKS SLEEP
7404  INFLUENCE STIMULUS$LEVEL SLEEP$STAGE EARLY$COMPONENTS
7511  GUSTAFSON EFFECT DURATION ONSET$RAMP OFFSET$AERS
7511  WANG EEG$DESYNCHRONIZATION PITCH$DISCRIM
7606  MASSARO CONTRIBUTION FF VOT TO /ZI/-/SI/ DISTINCTION
7611  DECKER EFFECTS LISTENER$STATE POTENTIALS MISSING$AUDITORY
      $STIMULI
7611  WEISS EFFECT GENERAL$ANESTHESIA COCHLEAR$POTENTIALS
7629  SEITZ R$REQUIREMENTS LANGUISTIC$CONTEXT ELECTROENCEPHALIC
      $R CLICKS
7704  THORNTON STIMULUS$FREQ$INTENSITY MIDDLE$COMPONENTS
      AER
7706  MILLER PROPERTIES FEATURE$DETECTORS VOT


                              0114


5406  AUD$SENSITIZATION
5406  EFFECTS WHITE$NOISE$BURSTS THR$
5406  LOUDNESS$REL TWO-COMPONENT$TONES
5406  MECHANICAL$IMPED HEAD$MASTOID
5406  METHOD$REPROD IDENTIFICATION AUD$DISPLAYS
5406  NOTE ACOUS$ATTENUATION EARS
5406  OBSERVATION TARTINI$PITCH
5406  PITCH$SHIFTS THR$SHIFTS
5406  REMARKS MULTIPLE$HELMHOLTZ$RESONATORS
5407  EFFECT VISUAL AUD COMBINED$VISUAL-AUD STIMULATION
      SP$R
5506  ABSOLUTE$PITCH
5506  ACOUS$LOCI TRANSITIONAL$CUES CONSONANTS
5506  EFFECT STATIC$AIR$PRESSURE EAM HNG$ACUITY
5506  FUSION INTERMITTENT$WHITE$NOISE
5506  IDENTIFICATION DISCRIM AUD$SIGNALS
5506  LONGTIME$DIFFERENTIAL$INTENSITY$SENSITIVITY
5506  LOUDNESS$REDUCTION EXPERIMENT
5506  MECHANICAL$IMPED FOREHEAD$MASTOID
5506  NOTE OBSERVATION TARTINI$PITCH
5506  NOTE THR$PULSED$SIGNALS FUNCTION DUTY$CYCLE CARRIER
      $FREQ
5506  PARAMETERS PERCEP AM$SIGNALS

5506    PITCH$PERCEP PERIODIC$AUD$STIMULI
5506    STEREOPHONIC$HNG ONE$EARPHONE
5606    AUD$DETECTION SIGNALS$IN$NOISE
5606    HISTORICAL$NOTE HAAS$EFFECT
5606    IDENTIFICATION SOUND$LEVEL MATCHING$FROM$SAMPLE
5606    MEAS INTERAURAL$TIME$DIFFERENCES$THR
5606    MEMORIZING$ABSOLUTE$PITCH
5606    SENSITIVITY CHANGES INTERRUPTION$RATE WHITE$NOISE
5606    THEORY$RECOGNITION
5606    VOBANC TWO-TO-ONE$SP$BANDWIDTH$REDUCTION$SYSTEM
5615    POTENTIALITIES AUD$PERCEP
5703    PITCH SIDE-TONE
5706    AURAL$HARMONICS
5706    BASIS ACOUS$STUDY SINGING
5706    CRITICAL$BANDWIDTH LOUDNESS$SUMMATION
5706    INADEQUACY METHOD$BEATS MEAS AURAL$HARMONICS
5706    INAPPLICABILITY THR$CONCEPT DETECTION$SIGNALS$NOISE
5706    INFLUENCE NOISE EQUIVALENCE INTENSITY$DIFFERENCES
        SMALL$TIME$DELAY
5706    NEURAL$VOLLEYS SIMILARITY SENSATIONS TONES SKIN$VIBRATIONS
5706    OBSERVATION PITCH TIME$DIFFERENCE PULSE$TRAINS
5706    PERFORMANCE VIGILANCE$TASK NOISE$QUIET
5706    SENSATIONS SKIN DIRECTIONAL$HNG BEATS HARMONICS EAR
5706    SENSATION$BEATS TWO$TONES$SIMPLE$RATIO
5706    SIGNAL$DETECTION FUNCTION SIGNAL$INTENSITY DURATION
5804    PROPERTIES GLOTTAL$SOUND$SOURCE
5806    BINAURAL$FUSION LOW-HIGH-FREQ$SOUNDS
5806    DETECTION MULTIPLE$COMPONENT$SIGNALS NOISE
5806    LOUDNESS PERIODICALLY$INTERRUPTED$WHITE$NOISE
5806    MINIMUM$AUDIBLE$ANGLE
5806    PHYSIOLOGICAL$PSYCHOLOGICAL$ACOUS
5806    PITCH BINAURAL$INTERACTIONS
5806    PROPAGATION$VELOCITY SOUND HUMAN$SKULL
5806    SEMANTIC$APPROACH PERCEP$COMPLEX$SOUNDS
5806    SIGNAL$DETECTION FUNCTION FREQ$ENSEMBLE
5806    TONAL$MEM
5814    EFFECT REDUNDANCY SHADOWING DICHOTIC$MESSAGES
5814    EFFECT RELATIVE$INTENSITIES DICHOTIC$MESSAGES SP$SHADOWING
5906    AUD$PERCEP TEMPORAL$ORDER
5906    AUD$PERCEP SUBMERGED$OBJECTS PORPOISES
5906    AUD$PERCEP TEMPORAL$ORDER
5906    BEATS COCH$MODELS
5906    BINAURAL$INTERACTION HIGH-FREQ$COMPLEX$STIMULI
5906    BINAURAL$LISTENING INTERAURAL$NOISE$CROSS$CORRELATION
5906    BINAURAL$COMM$SYSTEMS
5906    CONTINUITY$EFFECTS ALTERNATELY$SOUNDED$TONES

| 5906 | CRITICAL$BANDS LOUDNESS COMPLEX$SOUNDS THR |
| 5906 | DETECTION PULSED$SINUSOIDS NOISE FUNCTION FREQ |
| 5906 | DIFFERENCE$SOUNDS |
| 5906 | DIRECT$MEAS ACOUS$RATIO |
| 5906 | EFFECTIVE$ONSET$DURATION AUD$STIMULI |
| 5906 | GRAPHICAL$DATA$PRESENTATION THEORY$SIGNAL$DETECTABILITY |
| 5906 | IDENTIFICATION AUD$DISPLAYS METHOD RECOGNITION$MEMORY |
| 5906 | INTERAURAL$NOISE$CORRELATION |
| 5906 | MEAS EFFECTS INTERCHANNEL$INTENSITY TIME$DIFFERENCES TWO$CHANNEL |
| 5906 | MONAURAL$TEMPORAL$INTERACTIONS |
| 5906 | REL HNG$THR DURATION TONE$PULSES |
| 5906 | REL LOUDNESS DURATION TONAL$PULSES R PT CLICK-PITCH $THR |
| 5906 | STEREOPHONIC$BINAURAL$COMPROMISE$SYSTEM |
| 5906 | TYPES ROC$CURVES DEFINITIONS PARAMETERS |
| 5914 | HAPAX$LEGOMENON |
| 6004 | ALTERNATE$SIMULTANEOUS$BINAURAL$BALANCING PT |
| 6006 | AIR$DAMPED ARTIFICIAL$MASTOID |
| 6006 | AUD$DETECTION NOISE$SIGNAL |
| 6006 | AUD$FACILITATION STIMULATION LOW$INTENSITIES |
| 6006 | AUDIBILITY SWITCHING$TRANSIENTS |
| 6006 | BINAURAL$LOUDNESS$SUMMATION |
| 6006 | BINAURAL$INTERACTIONS IMPULSIVE$STIMULI PT |
| 6006 | COMPENSATORY$TRACKING PURSUIT$TRACKING LOUDNESS |
| 6006 | DETECTION SIGNAL NOISY$STORED$REFERENCE$SIGNAL |
| 6006 | DETECTION$SIGNALS FREQ |
| 6006 | DETERMINATION ABSOLUTE-INTENSITY$THR FREQ-DIFFERENCE $THR CATS |
| 6006 | DYNAMICS VIBRATION$SENSE LOW$FREQ |
| 6006 | EXPLORING$TONES SIREN$EXPERIMENTS |
| 6006 | HELMHOLTZ MONAURAL$PHASE EFFECTS |
| 6006 | LOW-FREQ$TONES |
| 6006 | PITCH PERIOIDC$PULSES FUND$COMPONENT |
| 6006 | PITCH PERIODIC$PULSES |
| 6006 | REL LOUDNESS DURATION TONAL$PULSES R ABNORMAL$LOUDNESS $FUNCTION |
| 6006 | REL LOUDNESS DURATION TONAL$PULSES R NORMAL$EARS SOUNDS NOISE |
| 6006 | TEMPORAL SAMPLING PARAMETERS INTERAURAL NOISE CORRELATIONS |
| 6006 | THEORY$SIGNAL$DETECTABILITY |
| 6104 | LOW$SENSATION$LEVEL DELAYED$CLICKS KEYTAPPING |
| 6106 | AUD$DETECTION UNSPECIFIED$SIGNAL |
| 6106 | AUDIBILITY PERIODIC$PULSES MODEL THR |
| 6106 | BINAURAL$INTERACTION CLICKS FREQ$CONTENT |
| 6106 | DEPENDENCE SUCCESSIVE$JUDGMENTS DETECTION$TASKS CORRECTNESS $R |

```
6106    DETECTION AUD$SINUSOIDS FREQ
6106    DETECTION COMPLEX$SIGNALS FUNCTION SIGNAL$BANDWIDTH
        DURATION
6106    FUNDAMENTAL$COMPONENT PERIODIC$PULSE$PATTERNS MODULATED
        $VIBRATIONS
6106    INTERVAL TIME$UNCERTAINTY AUD$DETECTION
6106    INVEST EFFECTS INTENSITY PITCH PT
6106    MEM WAVEFORM TIME$UNCERTAINTY AUD$DETECTION
6106    NOTE USE ULTRASONIC$PULSE$COMPRESSION BATS
6106    OPERATING$CHARACTERISTICS SIGNAL$DETECTABILITY METHOD
        $FREE$R
6106    PITCH$SENSATION REL PERIODICITY STIMULUS HNG SKIN
        $VIBRATIONS
6106    PROCEDURE CALCULATING LOUDNESS
6106    REMARKS DETECTION$SIGNAL NOISY$STORED$REFERENCE$SIGNAL
6106    SEQUENTIAL$EFFECTS SIGNAL-DETECTION$SITUATION
6106    SUBDIVISION AUDIBLE$FREQ$RANGE CRITICAL$BANDS
6106    USES SINGLE$SIDEBAND$SIGNALS FORMANT$TRACKING$SYSTEMS
6111    EFFECT BINAURAL$BEATS PERFORMANCE
6111    METHOD$MODALITY$JUDGEMENTS BRIEF$STIMULUS$DURATION
6111    VIGILANCE CUTANEOUS$AUD$SIGNALS
6114    DISCRIM VOWEL$SOUNDS HARMONIC$ADDITION$SYNTHESIS
6114    PERCEP VOWEL$COLOR FORMANTLESS$COMPLEX$SOUNDS
6204    FACTORS AUD$PERCEP PT SP
6204    LOW$SENSATION$LEVEL EFFECTS PT$DAF
6206    ABSOLUTE$PITCH
6206    AMPLITUDE$MODULATION
6206    ASPECTS BINAURAL$SIGNAL$SELECTION
6206    BANDWIDTH$ERROR SYMMETRICAL$BANDWIDTH$FILTERS ANALYSIS
        NOISE VIBRA
6206    BINAURAL$DETECTION SINGLE-FREQ SIGNALS NOISE
6206    CALCULATION DIMENSIONS TRAVELING-WAVE$ENVELOPES SPECIES
6206    COMPARISON SENSATIONS PRODUCED FREQ$MODULATION
6206    CREATION PITCH BINAURAL$INTERACTION
6206    CRITICAL$BANDWIDTH
6206    DEMONSTRATING SUFFICIENCY EXCITATIONS PITCH$PERCEP
6206    EFFECT INTERAURAL CORRELATION PRECISION CENTERING
        NOISE
6206    EFFECT PHASE QUALITY TWO-COMPONENT TONE
6206    EFFECT REVERBERATION ASSESSMENT REPETITIVE IMPULSE
        $NOISE
6206    EFFECT SWITCHING$EARPHONE$CHANNELS PRECISION$CENTERING
6206    ENERGY-DETECTION$MODEL MONAURAL$AUD$DETECTION
6206    EXISTENCE$REGION TONAL$RESIDUE
6206    EXPERIMENTS AIR$PUFFS UNIQUENESS SINUSOIDAL$WAVE
6206    FORMULAS COEFFICIENT INTERAURAL$CORRELATION NOISE
```

6206    FOURIER$COEFFICIENTS SP$POWER$SPECTRA MEAS AUTOCORRELATION
        $ANALYSI
6206    GENERALIZED SHORT-TIME POWER$SPECTRA AUTOCORRELATION
        $FUNCTIONS
6206    LEARNING IDENTIFY NONVERBAL$SOUNDS APPLICATION COMPUTER
6206    LOUDNESS$SUMMATION SPECTRUM$SHAPE
6206    LOUDNESS FUNCTION SIGNAL$DURATION
6206    METHODS CALCULATION USE ARTIC$INDEX
6206    PERCEP STEADY$INTERMITTENT$SOUNDS ALTERNATING NOISE-BURST
        $STIMULI
6206    PERCEP TWO-COMPONENT NOISE$BURSTS
6206    SENSITIVITY UNIDIRECTIONAL FREQ$MODULATION
6206    SMALL$AMPLITUDE
6206    STIMULUS$PARAMETERS
6304    FACTORS PT$DAF
6306    APPLICATION RELATIVE$PROCEDURE PROBLEM BINAURAL-BEAT
        $PERCEP
6306    BINAURAL$INTERACTION CLICK CLICK$PAIR
6306    CHANGE REPETITIVE NOISE$BURSTS
6306    COMPENSATORY$PURSUIT$TRACKING PITCH
6306    DAMPED$SINUSOIDS
6306    DETECTION NOISE$SIGNAL DURATION
6306    DIFFRACTION$EFFECTS RANDOM SOUND$FIELD
6306    EFFECT NOISE DEPENDENCE CORRELATION DETECTION MEAS
6306    EFFECT VARYING INTERAURAL$NOISE$CORRELATION DETECTABILITY
        TONAL$SI
6306    EFFECTS WAVEFORM$CORRELATION SIGNAL$DURATION DETECTION
        NOISE$BURST
6306    EFFECTS SPECTRAL$CONTENT DURATION PERCEIVED NOISE
        $LEVEL
6306    EFFECTS FILTERING VOCAL$DURATION IDENTIFICATION$SPEAKERS
        AURALLY
6306    ENERGY-DETECTION$MODEL MONAURAL$AUD$DETECTION
6306    EXISTENCE$REGION TONAL$RESIDUE
6306    IDENTIFICATION AUD$DISPLAYS EFFECT UNBALANCED PROBABILTIES
        $OCCURRE
6306    INFLUENCE TIME$INTERVAL EXPERIMENTALLY INDUCED PITCH
        $SHIFTS
6306    LOUDNESS$JUDGMENTS BASED DISTANCE$ESTIMATES
6306    LOWER$LIMITS AUD$PERIODICITY$ANALYSIS
6306    MONAURAL$LOUDNESS$FUNCTION
6306    OUTPUT$PROBABILITY$DISTRIBUTION CORRELATION$DETECTOR
6306    OUTPUT$PROBABILITY$DISTRIBUTION MULTIPLIER-AVERAGER
6306    PARTIALLY-CORRELATED$INPUTS
6306    PERCEP TEMPORAL$ORDER LOUDNESS$JUDGMENTS DICHOTIC
        CLICKS

6306    PERIODICITY$PERCEP USING GATED$NOISE
6306    PERIODICITY$PERCEP USING GATED$NOISE
6306    PITCH TIME$DELAY TWO PULSE$TRAINS
6306    TEMPORAL$SUMMATION TONES NARROW-BAND$NOISE
6404    FACTOR$ANALYTIC$STUDY SIGNAL$DETECTION$ABILITIES
6406    BRIEF$IMPULSIVE$STIMULI
6406    BROAD-BAND$NOISE
6406    DETECTION MARKOVIAN$SEQUENCES SIGNALS
6406    DETECTION TONE$PULSE DURATIONS NOISE VARIOUS$BANDWIDTHS
6406    EAR FREQ$ANALYZER
6406    ECHOLOCATION MEAS PITCH DISTANCE SOUNDS$REFLECTED
        $FLAT$SURFACE
6406    EFFECT NOISE$CROSSCORRELATION BINAURAL$SIGNAL$DETECTION
6406    EXPERIMENT SPEECHLIKE$PHASE
6406    EXPERIMENTS RISE$TIME LOUDNESS
6406    INFORMATION$RATE TRANSMIT PITCH-PERIOD$DURATIONS CONNECTED
        $SP
6406    INTEGRATION$ENERGY THR GRADUAL RISE-FALL$TONE PIPS
6406    MEAS AUD$DENSITY
6406    MODIFICATION NOY$TABLES
6406    PITCH FM$SIGNALS
6406    PITCH FM$SIGNALS
6406    PITCH HIGH-PASS-FILTERED PULSE$TRAINS
6406    PROPAGATION ACOUS$TRANSIENTS WATER
6406    ROC DETERMINED MECHANICAL$ANALOG RATING$SCALE
6406    SINGLE-NUMBER$CRITERIA ROOM$NOISE
6406    STIMULUS-ORIENTED$APPROACH DETECTION
6406    SYSTEMATIC$SHIFTS JUDGMENT OCTAVES HIGH$FREQ
6406    TEMPORAL$INTEGRATION FUNCTION FREQ
6406    TIME$REQUIREMENTS TONAL$FUNCTION
6406    VECTOR$PITCH$DETECTION
6504    THR SIGNAL$DETECTION$THEORY
6504    THR SIGNAL$DETECTION$THEORY
6506    BANDPASS$SAMPLING BASEBAND$SIGNAL
6506    BANDPASS$SAMPLING BASEBAND$SIGNAL
6506    BINAURAL$INTERACTIONS CLICKS
6506    BINAURAL$BEATS BINAURAL$AM$TONES COMPARISON LOUDNESS
        $FLUCTUATIONS
6506    CENTRAL$PERIODICITY$PITCH
6506    CONTINUITY$EFFECTS ALTERNATELY$SOUNDED$NOISE TONE
        $SIGNALS FUNCTION
6506    DETECTABILITY$THR COMBINATION$TONES
6506    EFFECT FILTER$TYPE ENERGY-DETECTION$MODELS AUD$SIGNAL
        $DETECTION
6506    EFFECT REPETITION$RATE LOUDNESS TRIANGULAR$TRANSIENTS
6506    FEEDBACK NOISE-SIGNAL$DETECTION PERFORMANCE$LEVELS

6506    JUDGED NOISINESS RANDOM$NOISE$BAND AUDIBLE PT
6506    LEARNING IDENTIFY COMPLEX$SOUNDS PROMPTING CONFIRMATION
6506    LOUDNESS$CHANGE PT CONTRALATERAL$NOISE$STIMULATION
6506    NARROW-BAND$NOISE TONES SIGNALS BINAURAL$DETECTION
6506    SIGNAL NOISE
6506    STIMULUS-IDENTIFICATION OVERLAP LEARNING IDENTIFY
        COMPLEX$SOUNDS
6506    TIME-SEPARATION$PITCH CORRELATED$NOISE$BURSTS
6506    TONAL$CONSEQUENCE CRITICAL$BANDWIDTH
6506    UNCERTAIN$SIGNAL$DETECTION SIMULTANEOUS$CONTRALATERAL
        $CUES
6511    ECHOLOCATION$SIGNALS BAT
6511    EFFECT PEAK$LEVEL$TRIANGULAR$TRANSIENTS
6514    EFFECTS SHARED$REFERENTIAL$EXPERIENCE ENCODER-DECODER
        $AGREEMENT
6514    PREFERENCES PHONETIC$STIMULI
6604    DIFFERENTIAL$SENSITIVITY DURATION ACOUS$SIGNALS
6606    CRITICAL$BANDS RESIDUE
6606    DETECTION AUD$SIGNALS NOISE
6606    DICHOTICALLY$PRODUCED$TONAL$IMAGE
6606    DICHOTICALLY$PRODUCED TONAL$IMAGE
6606    EFFECT NOISE SYSTEM$GAIN ASSIGNED$TASK TALKING$LEVELS
6606    EFFECT PROLONGED$EXPOSURE BINAURAL$INTENSITY$MISMATCH
6606    EFFECT PROLONGED$EXPOSURE BINAURAL$INTENSITY$MISMATCH
        LOCUS
6606    EFFECT PROLONGED$EXPOSURE BINAURAL$INTENSITY$MISMATCH
        LOCUS
6606    EFFECTS WAVEFORM$CORRELATION SIGNAL$DURATION DETECTION
        NOISE$BURST
6606    EVEN$ORDER$SUBHARMONICS PERIPHERAL$SYS
6606    EXAM BINAURAL$INTERACTION
6606    EXTENSION EXAMINATION BINAURAL$INTERACTION
6606    FACTORS PERCEP$CONTINUITY ALTERNATELY$SOUNDED TONE
        NOISE$SIGNALS
6606    FEEDBACK PSYCHOPHYSICAL$VARIABLES SIGNAL$DETECTION
6606    GENERATION ODD-FRACTIONAL$SUBHARMONICS
6606    HUMAN$SIDETONE MEAS FREQ$R FREQ$EQUALIZING DEVICES
6606    IMPLEMENTATION PITCH$EXTRACTOR DOUBLE-SPECTRUM-ANALYSIS
        $TYPE
6606    INFLUENCE RISE-FALL$TIME SHORT-TONES$THR
6606    LOCUS DICHOTICALLY-PRODUCED TONAL$IMAGE
6606    LOW-INTENSITY$LEVELS
6606    MEAS PERCEIVED$ACOUS$QUALITY SOUND-REPRODUCING$SYSTEMS
        FACTOR$ANAL
6606    MEAS PERCEIVED$ACOUS$QUALITY SOUND-REPRODUCING$SYSTEMS
        FACTOR$ANAL

6606    MEAS STRUCTURE$HARMONICS SELF-GENERATED ACOUS$BEAM
6606    PITCH PERIODICALLY$INTERRUPTED$TONE
6606    POWER-GRP$TRANSFORMATIONS GLARE MASKING RECRUITMENT
6606    RESIDUE$PITCH EXPLANATION
6606    RESIDUE$PITCH EXPLANATION
6606    SIGNAL-DETECTION$ANALYSIS EQUALIZATION$CANCELLATION
        $MODEL
6606    TIME$SEPARATION$PITCH NOISE$PULSES
6606    TIME-FREQ$ANALYSIS HNG$PROCESS
6606    TWO-STATE$THRS$MODEL RATING-SCALE EXPERIMENTS
6617    OUTLINE SIGNAL$DETECTION$THEORY
6704    BINAURAL$MONAURAL$INTELLIGIBILITY REVERBERATION
6704    COMFORT$LEVEL LOUDNESS$MATCHING CONTINUOUS$INTERRUPTED
        $SIGNALS
6704    METHODOLOGY DIGIT$MEM$TESTING COLLEGE$STUDENTS
6704    REL HNG REACTION$TIME AGE
6706    APPLICATION MOSSBAUER$METHOD EAR$VIBRATIONS
6706    ASYMMETRIES CUMULATIVE$PROBAILITY$DISTRIBUTIONS SP
        $WAVEFORM AMP
6706    ASYNCHRONY PERCEP TEMPORAL$GAPS PERIODIC$AUD$PULSE
        $PATTERNS
6706    ASYNCHRONY PERCEP TEMPORAL$GAPS PERIODIC$JITTERED
        $PULSE$PATTERNS
6706    AUD$CONTINUITY$EFFECTS FUNCTION DURATION TEMPORAL
        $LOCATION
6706    AUD$NONLINEARITY
6706    AUD$SENSITIZATION
6706    AUD$SPECTRAL$FILTERING MONAURAL$PHASE$PERCEP
6706    BEATS MISTUNED$CONSONANCES
6706    CRITICAL$BAND BINAURAL$DETECTION
6706    DETECTION M$ORTHOGONAL$SIGNALS
6706    DETECTION IN-PHASE$SIGNAL UNCERTAINTY INTERAURAL$PHASE
        MASKING$NOI
6706    DEV AUD NARROW-BAND$FREQ$CONTOURS
6706    DOMINANT$FREQ PERCEP PITCH COMPLEX$SOUNDS
6706    EFFECTS INTENSITY CRITICAL$BANDS TONAL$STIMULI DETERMINED
        BAND$LIM
6706    EFFECTS STIMULUS$DURATION DETECTION SINUSOIDS CONTINUOUS
        $PEDESTALS
6706    ESTIMATION OBSERVED$CRITERION BETA
6706    HUMAN$PERFORMANCE LOW-SIGNAL-PROBABILITY$TASKS
6706    INTEGRATION ENERGY REPEATED$TONE$PULSES MAN GOLDFISH
6706    INTENSITIES AURAL$DIFFERENCE$TONES
6706    INTERPOLATED$SIGNAL
6706    LOUDNESS$DETERMINATION LOW$SOUNDS$FREQ
6706    MODEL$SECONDARY$RESIDUE$EFFECT PERCEP COMPLEX$TONES

6706 PERCEIVED$RATE MONOTIC$DICHOTICALLY$ALTENATING$CLICKS
6706 PERCEP$INDEPENDENCE RECOGNITION TWO-DIMENSIONAL$AUD
      $STIMULI
6706 PITCH COMPLEX$TONES
6706 PITCH NOISE$BANDS
6706 PITCH$PERCEP PULSE$PAIRS RANDOM$REPETITION$RATE
6706 SIGNAL-DETECTION$THEORY SELECTIVE$LISTENING
6706 STIMULUS-ORIENTED$APPROACH DETECTION
6706 TEMPORAL$SUMMATION CRITICAL$BANDWIDTH$SIGNALS
6706 THEORY SIGNAL$DETECTABILITY ADAPTIVE$OPTIMUM$RECEIVER
      $DESIGN
6706 TIME-DOMAIN BANDWIDTH-COMPRESSION$SYSTEM
6713 EFFECTS AUD$FEEDBACK
6804 AUD$GELLE$TEST NEW$TRANSDUCER
6804 INTENSITY$FREQ$INTERACTIONS
6806 ADAPTIVE$OPTIMUM$DETECTION SYNCHRONOUS-RECURRENT$TRANSIENTS
6806 AUD$FLUTTER$FUSION SIGNAL$ENVELOPE
6806 BINAURAL$SYSTEM TEMPORAL$INFO JITTER
6806 CLIPSTRUM$PITCH$DETERMINATION
6806 COMPARISONS TRNG$TECHNIQUES COMPLEX$SOUND$IDENTIFICATION
6806 DETECTION NOISELIKE$SOUNDS TELEPHONE$SP
6806 DETECTION AUD$SIGNAL RESTRICTED$SETS REPRODUCIBLE
      $NOISE
6806 DETECTION MONAURAL$SIGNALS FUNCTION INTERAURAL$NOISE
      $CORRELATION
6806 EAR FREQ$ANALYZER
6806 EFFECT SIGNAL$DURATION DETECTION GATED$NOISE CONTINUOUS
      $NOISE
6806 EFFECT SIGNAL$DURATION DETECTION GATED$NOISE CONTINUOUS
      $NOISE
6806 EFFECT SOUND SUBSEQUENT$DETECTION
6806 EQUIVALENT$PEAK$LEVEL THR$INDEPENDENT$SP$LEVEL$MEAS
6806 FREQ$DEPENDENCY AURAL$DIFFERENCE$TONES
6806 FREQ-K$CHARACTERISTICS AUD$OBSERVERS SIGNALS SINGLE
      $FREQ NOISE
6806 HISTORICAL$BACKGROUND HAAS$PRECEDENCE$EFFECT
6806 INTERAURAL$AMPLITUDE EFFECTS BINAURAL$HNG
6806 MONAURAL$PHASE$EFFECTS AUD$SIGNAL$DETECTION
6806 PRACTICE$EFFECTS ABSOLUTE$JUDGMENT$PITCH
6806 PREDICTION MONAURAL$DETECTION
6806 PROBE-SIGNAL$METHOD
6806 ROC INTERAURAL$CONDITIONS LISTENING
6806 SENSORY$INTERACTION PERCEP LOUDNESS VISUAL$STIMULATION
6806 SIGNAL$FREQ
6806 TASK-INDUCED$STRESS ACOUS$SP$SIGNAL
6806 TWO-STATE$THR$THEORY MULTIPLE-LOOK$K-ALTERNATIVE$FORCED-CHOICE

6806   USE AVERAGE$R$COMPUTER REPRODUCIBLE$BURSTS$NOISE
6806   USE NOISE$BANDS ESTABLISH NOISE$PITCH
6807   TASKS SCIENTIFIC$CONFERENCE PROBLEM UTILIZATION DEV
       ACOUS$PERCEP
6811   INDENTIFYING$MEANING LESS$TONAL$COMPLEXES
6904   EFFECT SPATIALLY$SEPARATED$SOUND$SOURCES SP$INTELLIGIBILITY
6904   EFFECTS VARIABLE-INTERVAL FIXED-INTERVAL SIGNAL$PRESENTATION
       $SCHED
6904   QUANTITATIVE$ANALYSIS FIELD$STUDY$DATA
6906   ACOUS$STIMULATION CONTRALATERAL$EAR
6906   AUD$DETECTION RECOGNITION CONDITIONS LATERAL TEMPORAL
       COMPOSITE
6906   AUD$SENSITIZATION
6906   BINAURAL$INTERACTION TRANSIENTS INTERAURAL$INTEN$ASYMMETRY
6906   COMMENTS HISTORICAL$BACKGROUND HAAS$AND/OR$PRECEDENCE
       $EFFECT
6906   CONSONANCE COMPLEX$TONES CALCULATION$METHOD
6906   CONTINUITY ALTERNATELY$SOUNDED$TONE NOISE$SIGNALS
       FREE$FIELD
6906   DICHOTIC$SUMMATION LOUDNESS
6906   DIFFERENTIAL$ASYNCHRONY THR PULSE$TRAINS
6906   DISTANCE$ESTIMATION SP$SIGNALS ANECHOIC$SPACE
6906   EFFECT PHASE TIMBRE COMPLEX$TONES
6906   EFFECTS SIGNAL$QUANTIZATION PERFORMANCE MULTICHANNEL
       $PROCESSING$SY
6906   ENVELOPE MICROSTRUCTURE FUSION DICHOTIC$SIGNALS
6906   ESTIMATION PERIODIC$SIGNALS NOISE
6906   ESTIMATING AURAL$HARMONICS
6906   FROC$CURVE OBSERVERS$PERFORMANCE METHOD FREE$R
6906   INTERAURAL$TIME INTERAURAL$INTENSITY
6906   LIMITS DETECTION BINAURAL$BEATS
6906   LOUDNESS$JUDGMENTS SP NONSP
6906   MACH$BANDS HNG
6906   MONAURAL$LOUDNESS-INTEN$REL
6906   MONAURAL$DETECTION CONTRALATERAL$CUE ENERGY$DETECTOR
       $PERFORMANCE
6906   NOTE COMMENTS USE NOISE$BANDS NOISE$PITCH
6906   PERIODICITY$PITCH INTERRUPTED$WHITE$NOISE ARTIFACT
6906   PERSTIMULATORY$TRACKING PITCH$PERCEP SENSATION$LEVEL
6906   PITCH FM$SINUSOIDS
6906   PITFALLS ADAPTIVE$TESTING TEMPORAL$INTEGRATION PERIODICITY
       $PITCH
6906   RECOGNITION REPEATED$PATTERNS STUDY SHORT-TERM$AUD
       $STORAGE
6906   REL CRITICAL$BANDS HNG PHASE$CHARACTERISTICS CUBIC
       $DIFFERENCE$TONE

6906    ROC PSYCHOMETRIC$FUNCTIONS SIMPLE-AND-PEDESTAL$DETECTION
        $CONDITION
6906    SIGNAL$DURATION SIGNAL$FREQ REL AUD$SENSITIVITY
6906    STIMULUS$LEVEL DICHOTICALLY$PRESENTED$TONES
6906    SUBJECT$ORIENTATION JUDGMENT$DISTANCE SOUND$SOURCE
6906    TECHNIQUE ENHANCING SIGNALS AUD$DETECTION
6906    TEMPORAL$INTEGRATION PERIODICITY$PITCH
6906    TEMPORAL$SUMMATION LOUDNESS ANALYSIS
6906    TEMPORAL$SUMMATION ACOUS$SIGNALS CHINCHILLA
6907    SUBJECTIVE$RATINGS$NOISE
6911    SIGNAL$PROCESSING BAT
7006    AMPLITUDE PHASE
7006    AUD ELECTRONIC$ENVELOPE PERIODICITY$DETECTION
7006    AUD$THR VISUAL$STIMULATION FUNCTION SIGNAL$BANDWIDTH
7006    AUDIBILITY HIGH$HARMONICS PERIODIC$PULSE
7006    BINAURAL$FUSION LIMITS SIGNAL$DURATION SIGNAL$OUTSET
7006    CHOICE SOUND$DURATION SILENT$INTERVALS TEST COMPARISON
        SIGNALS MEA
7006    COMMENT PITCH NOISE$BANDS
7006    DC$POLARIZATION
7006    EFFECT NOISE$BANDWIDTH LOUDNESS
7006    FORWARD$BACKWARD$ENHANCEMENT SENSITIVITY AUD$SYSTEM
7006    INHARMONIC AM$SIGNALS
7006    INTENSITY$CHANGES EAR FUNCTION AZIMUTH TONE$SOURCE
7006    INTERACTION ELECTRICAL$POLARIZATION ACOUS$STIMULATION
7006    INTRODUCTORY$EXPERIMENTS AUD$TIME$SHARING DETECTION
        INTENSITY
7006    LATERAL$PREFERENCES IDENTIFICATION PATTERNED$STIMULI
7006    LIMITS DETECTION BINAURAL$BEATS
7006    LOUDNESS$LEVEL
7006    MONAURAL$PROCEDURE PSYCHOACOUS$CALIBRATION EARPHONES
7006    MONAURAL$DETECTION PHASE$DIFFERENCE CLICKS
7006    MONAURAL$DETECTION FILTERING
7006    PARAMETERS PERCEPTIBILITY PITCH
7006    PITCH NOISE$BANDS
7006    PITCH TONE$BURSTS CHANGING$FREQ
7006    PITCH$PERCEP TWO-FREQ$STIMULI
7006    ROLE PHASE AUDIBILITY OCTAVE$COMPLEXES
7006    ROLE WEAK$SIGNALS ACOUS$STARTLE
7006    SENSORY$FUNCTION MULTIMODAL$SIGNAL$DETECTION
7006    SUBJECTIVE$OBJECTIVE$MEAS LOUDNESS$LEVEL REPEATED
        $IMPULSES
7006    TECHNIQUE INVEST MONAURAL$PHASE$EFFECTS
7006    TIME$SHARING AUD$PERCEP EFFECT STIMULUS$DURATION
7006    VALIDATION SINGLE-IMPULSE$CORRECTION$FACTOR CHABA
        IMPULSE$NOISE

7011   FACTORS BINAURAL$LOUDNESS$BALANCE
7011   PERCEP ACOUS$STIMULI$NEAR$THR
7011   PERCEP$ASYMMETRY DICHOTICALLY$PRESENTED$CLICK-SENTENCE
       $STIMULI
7011   SIGNAL$DURATION
7011   SIGNAL$INTERAURAL$LEVEL$DIFFERENCES EFFECTS BINAURAL
       $CRITICAL$BAND
7103   OBSERVATIONS REL THR$PT THR$SP
7104   DURATION$PT
7104   ECHO-REACTION APPROACH SEMANTIC$RESOLUTION
7104   FUNCTION FREQ$DISTORTION
7104   TEMPORAL$SEGMENTATION INFLUENCE ENVELOPE$FUNCTION
       PERCEP
7106   ACOUS$LEVEL VOCAL$EFFORT CUES LOUDNESS SP
7106   AMPLITUDE TIME$JITTER$THR RECTANGULAR-WAVE$TRAINS
7106   AUD$THR FUNCTION SIGNAL$DURATION SIGNAL$FILTERING
7106   AUD$THR SHORT$DURATION PULSES
7106   AUDIBILITY HIGH$HARMONICS PERIODIC$PULSE TIME$EFFECT
7106   COMPARISON PREFERENCE$MEAS$METHODS
7106   CONTINUITY ALTERNATELY$SOUNDED$TONAL$SIGNALS FREE
       $FIELD
7106   DETECTION BINAURAL$TONES FUNCTION MASKER$BANDWIDTH
7106   DETECTION NARROW-BAND$NOISE FUNCTION INTERAURAL$CORRELATION
       SIGNAL
7106   EFFECT INTERAURAL SIGNAL-FREQ$DISPARITY SIGNAL$DETECTABILITY
7106   ESTIMATE INHERENT CHANNEL$CAPACITY EAR
7106   FREQ INTENSITY EFFECTS
7106   INTERAURAL$CORRELATION$DETECTION AUD$PULSE$TRAINS
7106   LATERAL$SHIFT
7106   LOUDNESS-INTENSITY$REL LEVELS CONTRALATERAL$NOISE
7106   MCL PT NOISE SP
7106   MEAS TWO-CLICK$THR
7106   MODULATION$DATA
7106   MONAURAL$DETECTION CONTRALATERAL$CUE SINUSOIDAL$SIGNALS
       CONSTANT
7106   MONAURAL$DETECTION CONTRALATERAL$CUE
7106   MONAURAL$DETECTION CONTRALATERAL$CUE INTERAURAL$DELAY
       CUE SIGNAL
7106   PATTERN$REVERSAL AUD$PERCEP
7106   RECOGNITION PHASE$CHANGES OCTAVE$COMPLEXES
7106   RELIABILITY RATINGS AUD SIGNAL-DETECTION EXPERIMENT
7106   SIMULTANEOUS$BINAURAL$SIGNAL$DETECTION COMMENTS TIME
       $SHARING
7106   SPATIAL$PATTERNS COCH$DIFFERENCE$TONES
7106   SPECTRAL$BASIS AUD$JITTER$DETECTION
7106   STIMULUS$FEATURES SIGNAL$DETECTION

7106  TRANSFORMED UP-DOWN$METHODS PSYCHOACOUS
7111  BEHAVIORAL$THR INTERAURAL$PHASE$DIFFERENCES
7111  ECHO$RANGING$SIGNALS SONAR SEA$LION
7111  EXPERIMENTAL$DETERMINATION GROWTH AUD$SENSATION
7111  PRECEPTION CLICKS$EMBEDDED$IN$SENTENCES HANDEDNESS
      MODE$PRESENTATI
7111  SIGNAL$GENERATOR PSYCHOACOUSTIC$EXPERIMENTS
7111  VIGILANCE$EFFECTS DURATION$JUDGMENT
7117  AUD$PERCEP WALKING PILOT$STUDY
7204  MISLEADING$TEXTBOOK$ILLUSTRATIONS SIMPLE$HARMONIC
      $MOTION
7206  ALGORITHM ANALYSIS PHASE$EFFECTS APPLICATION MONAURAL
      $DISTORTION
7206  AUD$DISTORTION$PRODUCTS
7206  AUDIBILITY$REGION COMBINATION$TONES
7206  BINAURAL$INTERACTION LOW-FREQ$STIMULI INABILITY TRADE
      $TIME INTENSI
7206  COMBINATION$BAND$LEVELS COMPARISONS MASKING COMBINATION
      $NOISE
7206  COMBINATION$TONES ORIGIN
7206  CONSTRUCTION DUMMY$HEAD MEAS HNG$THR
7206  DETECTABILITY INTERAURAL$TIME$DIFFERENCES INTERAURAL
      $LEVEL$DIFFERE
7206  DETECTION BINAURAL$TONE$STIMULI TIME$SHARING CRITERION
      $CHANGE
7206  DETECTION TONES ABSENCE EXTERNAL$MASKING$NOISE EFFECT
      SIGNAL$INTEN
7206  DEV CRITICAL$BAND
7206  DIFFERENCE$BANDS
7206  DIRECT$ESTIMATION MULTIDIMENSIONAL$TONAL$DISSIMILARITY
7206  EFFECT SIGNAL$FREQ MLD UNCORRELATED$NOISE
7206  EXPLORATORY$STUDIES ZWICKERS$NEGATIVE$AFTERIMAGE HNG
7206  FUNCTION SIGNAL$DURATION
7206  HYPERBARIC$CHAMBER$NOISE DIVE
7206  INFLUENCE RISE$TIME LOUDNESS
7206  INFORMATION$ANALYSIS CHOICE$BEHAVIOR PROD ACOUS$SIGNALS
7206  INTENSITY FREQ DURATION EFFECTS MEAS
7206  LOUDNESS$ENHANCEMENT CONTRALATERAL$STIMULATION
7206  LOUDNESS$BALANCE SIGNALS UNEQUAL$DUTY$CYCLES
7206  MEMORY WAVEFORM$AUD
7206  MISSING$FUND PERIODICITY$DETECTION HNG
7206  MONAURAL$PHASE$EFFECTS LOW-TONE$SIGNALS
7206  MONAURAL$PHASE$EFFECT CANCELLATION RF DISTORTION$PRODUCTS
7206  NOTE PSYCHOMETRIC$INVARIANCE DETECTION$FUNCTIONS
7206  PITCH COMPLEX$TONES MUSICAL$INTERVAL$RECOGNITION
7206  PRESERVATION CONSTANT$LOUDNESS INTERAURAL$AMP$ASYMMETRY

7206   SIGNAL$DETECTION FUNCTION CONTRALATERAL$SINUSOID-NOISE
       $RATIO
7206   SIGNAL$FREQ
7206   SIMULTANEOUS TWO-CHANNEL SIGNAL$DETECTION SIMPLE$BINAURAL
       $STIMULI
7206   SIMULTANEOUS$TWO-CHANNEL$SIGNAL$DETECTION CORRELATED
       $SIGNALS
7206   UNCORRELATED$CORRELATED$NOISE
7211   EFFECTS INTENSITY DICHOTICALLY$PRESENTED$DIGITS
7211   PROCESSING NON-SYMBOLIC$AUD$INFO
7304   CALIBRATION$DATA
7306   AUD$DETECTION FREQ$TRANSITION
7306   BINAURAL$INTERACTION TRANSIENTS INTERAURAL$TIME$INTEN
       $ASSYMMETRY
7306   EFFECTS RELATIVE$PHASE NUMBER COMPONENTS RESIDUE$PITCH
7306   INTERAURAL$AMP
7306   INTERFERENCE TWO-TONE$INHIBITION
7306   MINMUM$AUDIBLE$ANGLE UNDERWATER REPLICATION DIFFERENT
       $ACOUS$ENVIRO
7306   MULTIDIMENSIONAL$ENCODING TEMPORAL$MICROSTRUCTURE
       AUD$DISPLAYS
7306   MULTIDIMENSIONAL$CODING TEMPORAL$MICROSTRUCTURE AUD
       $DISPLAYS
7306   NUMBER NONREVERBERANT$IMPULSES
7306   OPTIMUM$PROCESSOR$THEORY CENTRAL$FORMATION PITCH COMPLEX
       $TONES
7306   PATTERN-TRANSFORMATION$MODEL PITCH
7306   PERCEP$CONFUSIONS FOUR-DIMENSIONAL$SOUNDS
7306   PHASE$VARIATION SIGNAL
7306   PITCH SOUND$BURSTS CONTINUOUS$DISCONTINUOUS$CHANGE
       $FREQ
7306   PITCH STIMULUS$FINE$STRUCTURE
7306   QUANTITATIVE$MODEL EFFECTS STIMULUS$FREQ SYNCHRONIZATION
7306   SHIFT EAR$SUPERIORITY DICHOTIC$LISTENING
7306   SIMULTANEOUS$TWO-CHANNEL$SIGNAL$DETECTION
7306   TEMPORALLY$PATTERNED$NONVERBAL$STIMULI
7306   TEMPORAL$OFFSET$EFFECTS
7311   AUD$AUTOKINESIS
7311   BINAURAL$SUMMATION FUNCTION MASKING$LEVEL
7311   COMPLEX$NOISE$STIMULI VIBRATION
7311   INSTABILITY AUD$PERCEP$EXPERIENCE
7311   TEST-RETEST$STABILITY AUD$FLUTTER$PERCEP SYNTHETIC
       $STIMULI
7404   EFFECT LOUDSPEAKER$POSITION EARPHONE$AND$FREE-FIELD
       $THRESHOLDS MAP
7406   ACOUS$TRACING SUBSONIC$OBJECTS

7406   AUD$FILTER$SHAPE
7406   BILATERAL$HNG$ASYMMETRY
7406   BINAURAL$INTERACTION CAT MAN SIGNAL$DETECTION NOISE
       $CROSS$CORRELAT
7406   CALIBRATION$METHODS
7406   DETECTION INTERAURAL$ONSET OFFSET$DISPARITIES
7406   DETECTION BINAURALLY$MASKED$TONES CAT
7406   EFFECT LISTENING$INTERVAL AUD$DETECTION
7406   EFFECTIVENESS LINEAR$PREDICTION$CHARACTERISTICS SP
       $WAVE
7406   EQUAL$AVERSION$LEVELS PT OCTAVE$BANDS$NOISE
7406   EQUAL$LOUDNESS$PRESSURES DECAYING$OSCILLATORY$WAVEFORM
7406   ESTIMATION TWO-DIMENSIONAL$SPECTRUM SPACE-TIME NOISE-FIELD
       LINE$AR
7406   FEASIBILITY CRITICAL$BANDWIDTH ESTIMATES
7406   IDENTIFICATION TEMPORAL$ORDER THREE-TONE$SEQUENCES
7406   LOUDNESS$SUMMATION TONES LOUDSPEAKERS
7406   MODIFICATION DIF$SUMMATING$POTENTIAL STIMULUS$BIASING
7406   PERCEP$INTEGRATION DICHOTICALLY$ALTERNATED$PULSE$TRAINS
7406   PHASE$EFFECTS THREE-COMPONENT$SIGNAL
7406   PITCH CONSONANCE HARMONY
7406   PITCH DICHOTICALLY$DELAY$NOISE SPECTRAL$BASIS
7406   PITCH DICHOTICALLY$DELAY$NOISE SPECTRAL$BASIS
7406   SENSORIMOTOR$DOMINANCE RIGHT-EAR$ADVANTAGE MANDIBULAR-AUD
       $TRACKING
7406   TEMPORAL$SUMMATION LOUDNESS DELAYED$PERCEP OFFSET
       BRIEF$STIMULI
7406   TIME-INTENSITY$TRADING$FUNCTIONS PT HIGH-FREQ$AM$SIGNAL
7406   VARIATIONS SOUND$INTENSITY MISTUNED$CONSONANCES
7406   WITHIN-AND-BETWEEN-MODALITY CORRELATION DETECTION
7412   AUD$PROCESSES
7414   EFFECT SP-SOUND$CUE EAR$ASYMMETRY DICHOTIC$LISTENING
7504   RICHARDS MCL PT SP MASKING
7504   SUSSMAN PURSUIT$AUD$TRACKING DICHOTIC$TONAL$AMPLITUDES
7504   THURLOW LOCALIZATION NOISE OVERLAPPING$TIME
7506   ALTES MECHANISM AURAL$PULSE$COMPRESSION MAMMALS
7506   BERGLUND SCALING$LOUDNESS NOISINESS ANNOYANCE AIRCRAFT
       $NOISE
7506   ELMASIAN LOUDNESS$ENHANCEMENT
7506   MILLER PERCEPTUAL$SPACE MUSICAL$STRUCTURES
7506   OSMAN SIGNAL-NOISE$DURATION INTERAURAL$CONFIGURATION
       PSYCHOMETRIC$FUNC
7506   RAAB AUD$INTENSITY$DISCRIM BURSTS REPRODUCIBLE$NOISE
7506   SCHROEDER AMPLITUDE$BEHAVIOR CUBIC$DIFFERENCES$TONE
7506   TAYLOR MONAURAL$DETECTION CONTRALATERAL$CUE
7511   CAZALS LOUDNESS$FUNCTION CLICK$STIMULI

7511   CAZALS LOUDNESS$FUNCTION CLICK$STIMULI
7511   MCPHERSON LOUDNESS BRIGHTNESS CROSS$MODALITY$MATCHING
7511   MCPHERSON LOUDNESS BRIGHTNESS CROSS$MODALITY$MATCHING
7511   RUSSELL LOUDNESS$BALANCING COMPLEX$SOUND$LOCALIZATION
7511   SMIAROWSKI EFFECT PROBE-TONE$ENVELOPE$SHAPE FORWARD
       $MASKING
7511   WANG EEG$DESYNCHRONIZATION PITCH$DISCRIM
7511   YOUNG FUSED$IMAGE LOW-FREQ$SINUSOID HIGH-FREQ$AM$SIGNAL
7511   YOUNG FUSED$IMAGE LOW-FREQUENCY$SINUSOID HIGH-FREQUENCY
       $AM$SIGNAL
7526   BRENNAN SCALING APPARENT$ACCENTEDNESS
7526   GUIRAO IDENTIFICATION ARGENTINE$SPANISH$VOWELS
7526   KRULEE SCANNING$PROCESSES SENTENCE$RECOGNITION
7527   GOLDMAN AUD$PERCEP COGNITIVE$SKILLS
7527   PANTALOS SENTENCE$LENGTH-DURATION$RELATIONSHIPS AUD
       $ASSEMBLY$TASK
7532   BLUMSTEIN EAR$ADVANTAGE DICHOTIC$LISTENING
7532   BRYDEN SP$LATERALIZATION DICHOTIC$LISTENING
7532   PORTER DEV$CHANGES DICHOTIC$RIGHT-EAR$ADVANTAGE
7532   SATZ DEV$PARAMETERS EAR$ASYMMETRY
7532   SHANKWEILER LATERALIZATION SP$PERCEP
7604   DIRKS PSYCHOMETRIC$FUNCTIONS LOUDNESS$DISCOMFORT MCL
7604   YOUNG TIME-INTENSITY$TRADING$FUNCTIONS PT
7606    YOST LATERALIZATION REPEATED$FILTERED$TRANSIENTS
7606   &
7606   ABBAS
7606   AYLOR PERCEP NOISE TRANSMITTED THROUGH BARRIERS
7606   BERGLUND SCALING$LOUDNESS NOISINESS ANNOYANCE COMMUNITY
       $NOISES
7606   BILSEN BINAURAL$PITCH$PHENOMENON
7606   BRAUN TIME-DOMAIN$FORMULATION DOPPLER$EFFECT
7606   DANNENBRING EFFECT SILENCE TONES AUD$STREAM$SEGREGATION
7606   EFRON EAR$DOMINANCE INTENSITY$INDEPENDENCE PERCEP
       DICHOTIC$CHORDS
7606   FADDEN LATERALIZATION HIGH$FREQ BASED ON INTERAURAL
       $TIME$DIFFERENCES
7606   GEESA BINAURAL$INTERACTION CAT MAN
7606   GILLIOM GAP$DETECTION TWO-CHANNEL$DETECTION MISSING
       $EVENT
7606   GILLOM CONTRALATERAL$CUES DETECTION SIGNALS UNCERTAIN
       $FREQ
7606   GREENWOOD TWO-TONE$SUPPRESS COMB-TONE$DRIVE COCH$NUCLEUS
       CAT
7606   GRIFFIN SUBJECTIVE$EQUIVALENCE SINUSOIDAL RANDOM WHOLE-BODY
       $VIBRATION
7606   GUIRAO PERCEIVED$ROUGHNESS AMPLITUDE-MODULATED.TONES
       NOISE

7606   HECOX BRAINSTEM$EVOKED$R RISE-FALL$TIME DURATION
7606   HELLMAN GROWTH LOUDNESS
7606   LIPPMANN INTENSITY$PERCEP EFFECT PAYOFF$MATRIX ABSOLUTE
       $ID
7606   MASSARO RECOGNITION$MASKING AUD$LATERALIZATION PITCH
       $JUDGEMENTS
7606   MILLER DISCRIM LABELING NOISE-BUZZ$SEQUENCES
7606   NUETZEL LATERALIZATION COMPLEX$WAVEFORMS FINE$STRUCTURE
       AMP DURATION
7606   PHIPPS EFFECT SIGNAL$PHASE DETECTABILITY TONE$MASKED
       $BY$
7606   PICKLES AUDITORY-NERVE-FIBER$BANDWIDTHS CRITICAL$BANDWIDTHS
       CAT
7606   POLLACK ID RANDOM$AUD$WAVEFORMS INTERAURAL$RELATIONSHIPS
7606   POLLACK ID RANDOM$AUD$WAVEFORMS EFFECT INTERFERENCE
7606   POPELKA ACTIVATING$SIGNAL$BANDWIDTH ACOUSTIC-REFLEX
       $THRESHOLDS
7606   RABINOWITZ INTENSITY$PERCEP DEVIATIONS WEBER,S$LAW
7606   RAJCAN AUD$DISCRIM ONSET-OFFSET$PHASA TONE$BURSTS
7606   REPP ID DICHOTIC$FUSIONS
7606   ROMER DIMENSIONLESS$PARAMETERS ACOUSTICAL$DATA
7606   SACHS PHENOMENOLOGICAL$MODEL TWO-TONE$SUPPRESSION
7606   SCHACKNOW NOISE-INTENSITY$DISCRIM BANDWIDTH$CONDITIONS
       MASKER$PRESENT
7606   SCHARF AR LOUDNESS$SUMMATION CRITICAL$BAND
7606   SPARKS TEMPORAL$RECOGNITION$MASKING
7606   STEVENS EQUAL-SENSATION$FUNCTIONS MAGNITUDE$ESTIMATION
7606   VAN DEN BRINK DICHOTIC$PITCH$FUSION
7606   WILLIAMS GAP$DETECTION SINGLE-CHANNEL$PROCESS
7606   WOOD DISCRIMINABILITY R$BIAS PHONEME$CATAGORIES DISCRIM
       VOT
7606   ZUREK MEAS COMBINATION$TONES
7606   ZWICKER PSYCHOACOUSTIC$EQUIVALENT PERIOD$HISTOGRAMS
7611   HALL MEASUREMENT COMBINATION$TONES
7611   MORDAUNT EFFECTS DUTY$CYCLE LOUDNESS PULSED AND CONTINUOUS
       $TONES
7621   LEHISTE INFLUENCE FUNDAMENTAL$FREQ$PATTERN PERCEP
       DURATION
7627   CARPENTER DEV ACOUS$CUE$DISCRIM CHILDREN
7632   CATLIN MONAURAL$RIGHT-EAR$ADVANTAGE TARGET-IDENTFICATION
7632   DONNENFELD EFFECTS EXPECTANCY ORDERS$OF$REPORT AUD
       $ASYMMETRIES
7704   MILLAY RELIABILITY DICHOTIC$LISTENING RESPONSE$MODES
7704   RICHARDS LOUDNESS$PERCEP SHORT-DURATION$TONES
7704   SUSSMAN RESPIRATORY$TRACKING TONAL$AMPLITUDES
7706   AHROON SELECTIVE$ATTENTION TWO-CHANNEL$SIMULTANEOUS
       $FREQ$DL

7706   BILSEN PITCH NOISE$SIGNELS EVIDENCE CENTRAL$SPECTRUM
7706   BLOCK STATISTICALLY$BASED$MEASURE ACOUSTIC$REFLEX
       STIMULUS$LOUDNESS
7706   COOK HISTORY AMERICAN$ACOUSTICS
7706   DIVENYI EAR$DOMINANCE DICHOTIC$CHORD EAR$SUPERIORITY
       FREQUENCY$DISCRIM
7706   GANS OLIVOCOCHLEAR STIMULATION COCHLEAR$SUMMATING
       $POTENTIAL
7706   GREY MULTIDIMENSIONAL$PERCEPTUAL$SCALING MUSICAL$TIMBRES
7706   HAFTER LATERALIZATION$MODEL TIME-INTENSITY$TRADINGS
       BINAURAL$MASKING
7706   HALL DETECTION$THRESHOLD TWO-TONE$COMPLEX
7706   JENNINGS REPRODUCTION FAMILIAR$MELODIES PERCEPTION
       TONAL$SEQUENCES
7706   LIM INTENSITY$PERCEPTION LOUDNESS$COMPARISONS DIFFERENT
       TYPES STIMULI
7706   MCFADDEN ACOUS$INTEGRATION LATERALIZATION HIGH$FREQ
7706   MEHRGARDT TRANSFORMATION$CHAR  EXTERNAL$HUMAN EAR
7706   NAKATANI COMPUTER-AIDED$SIGNAL$HANDLING SP$RESEARCH
7706   NOORDEN MINIMUM$DIFFERENCES LEVEL FREQ PERCEP$FISSION
       TONE$SEQUENCES
7706   PENNER DETECTION TEMPORAL$GAPS MEASURE DECAY AUDITORY
       $SENSATION
7706   PERROTT ROTATING$TONES BINAURAL$BEATS
7706   POLLACK MONAURAL BETWEEN-EAR$TEMPORAL$GAP$DETECTION
7706   POLLACK PITCH$RATINGS HARMONIC$SERIES
7706   REPP MEASURING LATERALITY$EFFECTS DICHOTIC$LISTENING
7706   SMALL LOUDNESS$PERCEPTION SIGNELS CHANGING$SOUND$PRESSURE
7706   WIER DETECTION TONE$BURST MASKERS DEFECTS FREQ DURATION
       MASKER$LEVEL
7706   YOST LATERALIZATION PULSED$SINUSOIDS TEMPORAL$DIFFERENCES
7706   YUND MODEL RELATIVE$SALIENCE PITCH PURE$TONES PRESENTED
       DICHOTICALLY
7711   BOTHE FREQ-LOUDNESS$EFFECTS NEAR$FIELD
7711   ELFNER EFFECT FREQ AURAL$ACUITY LATERALIZATION
7711   HAWKES R$DELAY$EFFECTS CROSS-MODALITY$DURATION$JUDGEMENTS
7721   PARKER PERCEPTUAL$CUES PHONOLOGICAL$CHANGE
7725   JOHNSON MUSIC$EAR$SUPERIORITY TONE$SEQUENCES
7732   GATES CEREBRAL$HEMISPHERES MUSIC
7732   HEILMAN EAR$ASYMMETRIES SELECTIVE$ATTENTIONAL
7732   MORAIS LISTENING SP RETAINING$MUSIC RIGHT-EAR$ADVANTAGE
7732   WOLF PROCESSING FUNDAMENTAL$FREQ DICHOTIC$MATCHING
       $TASK
7806   ABBAS EFFECTS FREQ TWO-TONE$SUPPRESSION
7806   BURNS CATEGORICAL$PERCEP MELODIC$MUSICAL$INTERVALS
7806   COLBURN THEORY BINAURAL$INTERACTION AUD-NERVE$DATA

7806  COLLINS TEMPORAL$INTEGRATION TONE$GLIDES
7806  CROW PHASE$LOCKING MEDULLARY$NEURONS BINAURAL$PHENOMENAA
7806  CULLEN TEMPORAL$INTEGRATION TONE$GLIDES
7806  DEUTSCH LATERALIZATION FREQ REPEATING$SEQUENCES DICHOTIC
      $TONES
7806  DIVENYI FIGURAL$PROPERTIES AUDITORY$PATTERNS
7806  FLORENTINE LOUDNESS COMPLEX$SOUNDS STIMULUS NUMBER
      $COMPONENTS
7806  FOSTER AUD$R CATS PULSED$ULTRASOUND
7806  GERSON CENTRAL$OPTIMAL$PROCESSING PITCH COMPLEX$TONES
7806  GOLDSTEIN COMPATIBILITY MEAS AURAL$COMBINATION$TONES
7806  GOLDSTEIN AURAL$PROCESSING PITCH COMPLEX$TONES
7806  GRANTHAM DETECTABILITY INTERAURAL$TEMPORAL$DIFFERENCES
7806  GREY PERCEP$EFFECTS SPECTRAL$MODIFICATIONS MUSICAL
      $TIMBRES
7806  GREY TIMBRE$DISCRIM MUSICAL$PATTERNS
7806  HALL ADAPTATION RESIDUE$PITCH
7806  HARTMANN AMPLITUDE$ENVELOPE PITCH SINE$WAVE$TONES
7806  HELLMAN DEPENDENCE LOUDNESS$GROWTH EXCITATION$PATTERNS
7806  JOHNSON INTENSITY GUITAR$PLAYING AUD$FEEDBACK
7806  KILLION REVISED$ESTIMATE MINIMUM$AUDIBLE$PRESSURE
7806  KLEIN LATENCY$SHIFTS BSER
7806  MARKS BINAURAL$SUMMATION LOUDNESS PT
7806  MCFADDEN BINAURAL$DETECTION HIGH$FREQ TIME-DELAYED
      $WAVEFORMS
7806  NABELEK TEMPORAL$SUMMATION MASKED$AUDITORY$THRESHOLD
7806  OHGUSHI TEMPORAL$SPACIAL$CUES PERCEPTION PITCH COMPLEX
      $TONES
7806  PARKER VISUAL-FIELD$DISPLACEMENTS HUMANS ACOUSTICAL
      $TRANSIENTS
7806  PATTERSON AM$NOISE DETECTION MODULATION MODULATION
      $RATE
7806  PENNER POWER$LAW$TRANSFORMATION TIME-INTENSITY$TRADES
      NOISE$BURSTS
7806  POLLACK PERIODICITY$MEAS RANDOM$AUD$PATTERNS
7806  POLLACK TEMPORAL$SWITCHING BINAURAL$INFO$SOURCES
7806  REPP SINGLE+DOUBLE-CORRECT$R DICHOTIC$TWO-R$PARADIGM
7806  SR
7806  STERN THEORY BINAURAL$INTERACTION BASED AUD-NERVE
      DATA
7806  THIESSEN INTERMITTENT$TRUCK$NOISE DEEP$SLEEP
7806  TRAHIOTIS REGRESSION$INTERP TIME-INTENSITY$TRADING
      LATERALITY
7806  WATKINS PSYCHOACOUSTICAL$ASPECTS VERTICAL$LOCALE$CUES
7806  YOST PITCH$DISCRIM BROADBAND$SIGNALS RIPPLED$SPECTRA
7806  YOST STRENGTH PITCHES RIPPLE$NOISE

7825    SPELLACY DIRECTED$ATTENTION PERCEP$ASYMMETRY MONAURAL
        $TONES
7829    MUELLER LISTENER$ID SPEAKER$SEX CHILD


                              0115


5603    EFFECT ACOUS$ENVIRONMENT SPEAKER$INTELLIGIBILITY
5606    SP$COMM NOISE EQUIPMENT
5606    UNDERWATER$COMM
5706    EFFECT LOUDSPEAKERS FREE$SPACE$CONDITIONS
5706    PERFORMANCE VIGILANCE$TASK NOISE$QUIET
5706    UNDERWATER$HNG$THR
5806    COMPARISON HNG$THR AIR$WATER
5906    AUD$PERCEP SUBMERGED$OBJECTS PORPOISES
5906    DISTRIBUTION SOUND$SOURCES JET$STREAM
5906    EFFECT BRIEF$LOUD$NOISE DECISION$MAKING
6106    SENSITIVITY WATER-IMMERSED$EAR HIGH-LOW$LEVEL$TONES
6206    EFFECTS AMBIENT$NOISE TALKERS FACE-TO-FACE$COMMU$TASK
6206    EFFECTS BACKGROUND$NOISE AUD$DETECTION NOISE$BURSTS
6206    UNDERWATER HNG$THR
6406    COVARIANCE NOISE ATTENUATING$MEDIA
6406    PERCEP RETENTION VERBAL$INFORMATION AUD$SHADOWING
6406    SINGLE-NUMBER$CRITERIA ROOM$NOISE
6506    SP$COMM LIMITED AMBIENT$NOISE
6606    ACOUS$HAZARDS CHILDREN$TOYS
6606    ANALYSIS$SP HELIUM-OXYGEN$MIXTURE PRESSURE
6706    PHONEMIC$ANALYSIS CONSONANTS HELIUM$SP
6706    UNDERWATER HNG$THR MAN
6804    INF$R RECORDED$SOUNDS
6811    UNDERWATER SRT DISCRIM
6904    EFFECTS HYPNOSIS SUGGESTION AUD$THR
6906    EFFECT AIR$BUBBLES EAM UNDERWATER HNG$THR
6906    UNDERWATER HNG$THR MAN FUNCTION WATER$DEPTH
6907    EFFECTS NOISE SP$INTELLIGIBILITY
6907    SP$INTERFERENCE COMMUNITY$NOISE
6911    EFFECT AUDIO-FREQ$STIMULATION CRYING$BABY
6911    GENERATING$CALIBRATING UNIFORM$AQUATIC$SONIC$FIELD
7006    EFFECT AMBIENT-NOISE$LEVEL THR$SHIFT MEAS EAR-PROTECTOR
        $ATTENUATIO
7011    AUD$SENSITIVITY NOISE$DENTAL$DRILLS
7106    OBSERVATIONS UNDERWATER$HNG
7116    EFFECT CLASSROOM$LISTENING$CONDITIONS SP$INTELLIGIBILITY
7206    PERCEIVED$LEVEL$NOISE
7214    R$LATENCY$DIFFERENCES SP$SHADOWING INDICATOR DISTINCTIVE
        $FEATURES

7306   MINMUM$AUDIBLE$ANGLE UNDERWATER REPLICATION DIFFERENT
       $ACOUS$ENVIRO
7406   AMBIENT$NOISE$FIELD EDGE$EFFECTS PRODUCT$ARRAY$PROCESSING
7406   INTERACTION CONTINUOUS$AND$IMPULSE$NOISE
7506   ARCTANDER NOISE-REDUCTION$CONCEPTS AIRPLANES
7506   BERANEK ACOUSTICS CONCERT$HALL
7506   BERMAN BOUNDED$SPACE
7506   BISHOP VARIABILITY AIRCRAFT$FLYOVER$NOISE$MEAS
7506   BLUMENTHAL AIRCRAFT$COMMUNITY$NOISE$RESEARCH
7506   FRASCA NOISE-REDUCTION$PROGRAMS AIRPLANES
7506   HILLQUIST MOTOR$VEHICLE$NOISE$SPECTRA CHARACTERISTICS
7506   HOLLIEN EXTERNAL$AUDITORY$MEATUS AUDITORY$SENSITIVITY
       $UNDERWATER
7506   HRUSKA FREE-FIELD$METHOD SOUND-ATTENUATION$MEASUREMENT
7506   JENKINS MEAS FREEWAY$NOISE COMMUNITY$R
7506   LAUCHLE RADIATION SOUND LOUDSPEAKER CIRCULAR$BAFFLE
7506   LEASURE TIRE-ROAD$NOISE
7506   LEE NOMOGRAM ESTIMATING NOISE$PROPAGATION URBAN$AREAS
7506   LUKAS NOISE SLEEP LIT$REVIEW
7506   MAESTRELLO MECHANISMS NOISE$GENERATION RADIATION SUBSONIC
       $JET
7506   MALCHAIRE COMMUNITY$NOISE$SURVEY CINCINNATI
7506   MILLS NOISE CHILD REVIEW LITERATURE
7506   MOORE UNDERWATER$LOCALIZATION CLICK PULSED$PT$SIGNALS
       CALIF$SEA$LION
7506   NELSEN NOISE-REDUCTION$CONCEPTS
7506   SCHULTZ MEASUREMENT ACOUSTIC$INTENSITY SOUND$FIELD
7506   SEKYRA VALIDITY AIRCRAFT$NOISE$DATA
7506   VER LOW-NOISE$CHAMBERS AUDITORY$RESEARCH
7511   ALLUISI REACTIONS AIRCRAFT$NOISES
7606   BERGLUND SCALING$LOUDNESS NOISINESS ANNOYANCE COMMUNITY
       $NOISES
7606   BIES IMPEDANCE-TUBE$CALIBRATION REVERBERANT$ROOM SOUND
       $POWER TONES
7606   CERMAK MULTIDIMENSIONAL$ANALYSES JUDGEMENTS TRAFFIC
       $NOISE
7606   CORLISS METHOD ESTIMATING AUDIBILITY EFFECTIVE$LOUDNESS
       SIRENS SP AUTO
7606   GALAITSIS PREDICTION NOISE$DISTRIBUTION FREE-FIELD
       $MEASUREMENTS
7606   MCPHERSON MIDDLE$EAR$PRESSURE EFFECTS AUD$PERIPHERY
7606   SANTON NUMERICAL$PREDICTION ECHOGRAMS INTELLIGIBILITY
       SP$IN$ROOMS
7706   ANGEVINE IMPROVING ACOUSTIC$ENVIRONMENT NOISE$MEASUREMENTS
7706   CORNILLON SIMPLE$MODEL SIMULATING TRAFFIC$NOISE$SPECTRA
7706   HODGSON SURFACE$ACOUSTICAL$INTENSITY$METHOD NOISE
       $POWER

7706   HRUSKA ENVIRONMENTAL$EFFECTS MICROPHONES VARIOUS$CONSTRUCTIONS
7706   KOENIG DETERMINATION MASKING-LEVEL$DIFFERENCES REVERBERANT
       $ENVIRONMENT
7806   SCHOMER HUMAN$R HOUSE$VIBRATIONS SONIC$BOOMS AIR$BLASTS
7806   SCHOMER AMPLITUDE SPECTRUM BLASTS ATMOSPHERE
7806   SCHULTZ SYNTHESIS SOCIAL$SURVEYS NOISE$ANNOYANCE
7806   THIESSEN DISTURBANCE SLEEP NOISE

## 0116

5603   CARDIAC$REFLEX TONES THR$INTENSITY
5703   TERMS ELECTROPHYSIOLOGIC$TESTS$HNG
5804   GSR AUD$THR$MECHANISMS EFFECT TONAL$INTENSITY AMPLITUDE
       LATENCY
5804   GSR$AUD$THR$MECHANISMS INSTRUMENTATION SPONTANEOUS
       $R THR$DEFINITIO
5904   UNCONDITIONED$STIMULUS$STRENGTH GSR
6006   TEMPORAL$IRREGULARITY EXCITATIONS BRAIN REPORTING
       $PITCH
6111   EFFECT STIMULUS$RISE$TIME EVOKED$R CEREBRAL$CORTEX
       $CAT
6204   NEONATAL$EKG$R SOUND METHODOLOGY
6304   EEG$R AUD$STIMULI WAKING$CHIL
6304   HNG MICE GSR$AUDIOMETRY
6411   CHANGES$RESPIRATION AUDITORY$STIMULI
6411   EMG HNG$R
6504   FACTORS ELECTROPHYSIOLOGICAL$R NORMAL$ADULTS
6511   COMPARISON SINGLE$UNIT$RESPONSES AUD$NERVE GSR$THR
       MICE
6604   USE COMPOUND$UNCOND$STIMULUS EDA
6606   ELECTROPHYSIOLOGICAL$ANALOG INTERAURAL$TIME-INTENSITY
       $TRADE
6704   EARLY$COMPONENTS AVERAGED$ER RAPIDLY$REPEATED$AUD
       $STIMULI
6804   HNG MICE GSR$AUDIOMETRY MAGNITUDE UNCONDITIONED$GSR
       FUNCTION
6804   HNG$MICE GSR$AUDIOMETRY MAGNITUDE UNCONDITIONED$GSR
6807   USE CUTANEOUS-GALVANIC$REACTIONS OBJECTIVITY$STUDY
       LOUDNESS$PERCEP
6904   EFFECT TEST$CONDITIONS EARLY$COMPONENTS AVERAGED$ELECTROENCEPHA
6911   GSR CONDITIONABILITY BRAIN$WEIGHTS
6911   INVEST OCULAR$MOVEMENTS FORMS SOUND$FIELD$AUD$STIMULATION
7003   TECHNIQUES REDUCE NEGATIVE$EFFECTS HIGH$VOLTAGE$ELECTRICAL
       $ARTIFAC

7004  EVOKED$CORTICAL$R STIMULUS$CHANGE
7004  SENSITIVITY TONGUE ELECTRICAL$STIMULATION
7104  EARLY$COMPONENTS AVERAGED$ELECTROENCEPHALIC$R REL
      RISE-DECAY$TIME
7104  EARLY$COMPONENTS AVERAGED$ELECTROENCEPHALIC$R CLICKS
      SLEEP
7206  PSYCHOPHYSICAL$EVIDENCE LATERAL$INHIBITION HNG
7211  AVERAGED$ELECTRO-OCULAR$R ACOUS$STIMULI
7504  GOLDENBERG AVERAGE$EP CATS LESIONS$AUDITORY$PATHWAY
7506  BAUER LOUDNESS$ENHANCEMENT MAN BRAINSTEM-EVOKED$RESPONSE
      $CORRELATES
7506  BOTTE ELECTROENCEPHALIC$RESPONSE LOUDNESS$ESTIMATIONS
7511  GUSTAFSON DURATION ONSET$RAMP OFFSET$AER
7606  BOSTON AC$DC$COMPONENTS LATERAL$LINE MICRIPHONIC$POTENTIALS
7606  EGGERMONT AP TONE$BURSTS HUMAN + GUINEA$PIG$COCHLEA
7606  HECOX BRAINSTEM$EVOKED$R RISE-FALL$TIME DURATION
7606  MOORE R COCHLEAR-NUCLEUS$NEURONS SYNTHETIC$SP
7606  MOORE RECORDING ELECTROCOCHLEOGRAPHIC$R HUMANS
7606  OZDAMAR INPUT-OUTPUT$FUNCTIONS COCHLEAR$ACTION$POTENTIALS
7606  PRICE AP LOW$INTENSITIES
7606  PRICE INTERRUPTING$RECOVERY LOSS COCHLEAR$MICROPHONIC
      $SENSITIVITY
7606  YATES LOCALIZED$COCHLEAR$MICROPHONICS SPIRAL$LAMINA
7703  SKINNER ELECTROPHYSIOLOGIC$RESPONSE$AUDIOMETRY
7706  ALLEN COCHLEAR$MICROMECHANICS MECHANISM TRANSFORMING
      $TUNING COCHLEA
7706  BUUNEN PSYCHOPHYS$ELECTROPHYSIO COMBINATION$TONES
      PERCEP PHASE$CHANGES
7706  DALLOS ANALOG TWO-TONE$SUPPRESSION WHOLE$NERVE$RESPONSES
7706  EGGERMONT TUNING$CURVES NORMAL PATHOLOGICAL$HUMAN
      $EARS
7706  SCHMIEDT SOUND-TRANSMISSION CM$CHAR MONGOLIAN$GERBIL
      GUINEA$PIG
7722  ROBINSON ABNORMALITIES AUD$EP PATIENTS MULTIPLE$SCLEROSIS
7729  TYLER ACTION$POTENTIALS R LOW$FREQ$STIMULI
7804  COBB EFFECTS SIGNAL$RISE-TIME FREQUENCY BRAINSTEM
      $EVOKED$RESPONSE
7804  GUTNICK CONTRALATERAL$NOISE MIDDLE$COMPS ELECTROENCEPH
      $R
7804  WOLFE SOUND$INTENSITY LATENCY AMPLITUDE BRAINSTEM
      $EVOKED$RESPONSE
7806  DALLOS AP SINGLE$UNIT$THR ABNORMAL$EARS
7806  DON CLICK-EVOKED$BRAINSTEM$POTENTIALS HIGH-PASS MASKING

0117

5406  R SIMULTANEOUS$MESSAGES

5509    LISTENING SPEAKING
5703    LISTENER$PREFERENCE
5706    MONITORING$TASK SP$COMM
5806    MAINTENANCE$ALERTNESS LOUD$AUD$SIGNAL
6109    LISTENER$JUDGMENTS STATUS$CUES SP
6209    PROPOSAL LISTENING$TRNG
6306    EFFECTS LISTENER ACCURACY COMPETING$MESSAGES VARIED
        NUMBER RATE LE
6504    AUDIO-VISUAL$TEST EVAL ABILITY$RECOGNIZE$PHONETIC
        $ERRORS
6714    ATTENTION SIMULTANEOUS$TRANSLATION
6804    EFFECTS EAR$PREFERENCE ORDER$BIAS RECEPTION VERBAL
        $MATERIALS
7006    LISTENER$RELIABILITY
7011    EFFECTS LOW$PASS$FILTERING EAR$ASYMMETRY DICHOTIC
        $LISTENING
7106    EFFECTS INTERSTIMULUS$INTERVAL LISTENERS$ABILITY PERCEIVE
7214    LEVEL$LISTENING$COMPREHENSION FUNCTION PROCESS$VARIABLES
        SYNTAX
7306    SHIFT EAR$SUPERIORITY DICHOTIC$LISTENING
7506    NACHSHON STIMULUS$FAMILIARITY EAR$SUPERIORITY DICHOTIC
        $LISTENING
7508    COLEMAN LISTENING
7520    ROSENFELD LISTENER$PERSONALITY WINTER
7526    BARON SEMANTIC$FEATURES RETREVIAL$SPEED
7526    WERTSCH INFLUENCE PERCEP SPEAKER RECOGNITION$MEMORY
7532    BLUMSTEIN EAR$ADVANTAGE DICHOTIC$LISTENING
7532    BRYDEN SP$LATERALIZATION DICHOTIC$LISTENING
7532    PORTER DEV$CHANGES DICHOTIC$RIGHT-EAR$ADVANTAGE
7532    SATZ DEV$PARAMETERS EAR$ASYMMETRY
7532    SHANKWEILER LATERALIZATION SP$PERCEP
7632    CATLIN MONAURAL$RIGHT-EAR$ADVANTAGE TARGET-IDENTFICATION
7632    DONNENFELD EFFECTS EXPECTANCY ORDER$OF$REPORT AUD
        $ASYMMETRIES
7710    DELIA LISTENER-ADAPTED$COMM SIX TWELVE-YEAR-OLD BOYS
7713    BROWN SEX$IDENTIFICATION CONSTANT$LARYNGEAL$SOURCE
7723    FRENCH COMPREHENSION BEFORE AFTER LOGICAL ARBITRARY
        $SEQUENCES
7723    KUCZAJ INFLUENCES CHILDREN'S$COMPREHENSION 'YOUNGER'
        'OLDER'
7727    FENSTER ACCURACY$EMOTIONAL COMM
7732    HEILMAN EAR$ASYMMETRIES SELECTIVE$ATTENTIONAL
7732    MORAIS LISTENING SP RETAINING$MUSIC RIGHT-EAR$ADVANTAGE
7810    BEATTY SITUATIONAL$DETERMINANTS COMMUNICATION$APPREHENSION
7813    ROTHENBERGER DICHOTIC$LISTENING
7818    BEHNKE SP$ANXIETY PREDICTOR TREMBLING

7820   INFANTE PREDICTORS SP$ANXIETY
7829   MANZER INTENSITY$PRESENTATION$LEVELS DICHOTIC$LISTENING


## 0118

5804   AUD$SKILLS BLIND TRNG$PILOT$DOGS
5804   AUD$SKILLS BLIND TRNG$PILOT$DOGS
6204   VOCAL$R DAF CONGENITALLY$BLIND$ADULTS
6604   AUD$DISCRIM MR$CHIL
6813   AUD$PROBLEMS MR$CHIL
6911   AUD$ABILITIES BLIND
7314   SP$DISCRIM BLACK$CHIL
7627   HESSE PSYCHOTIC$CHILDREN$ SELECTION NATURAL$DISTORTED
       $SP
7722   ROBINSON ABNORMALITIES AUD$EP PATIENTS MULTIPLE$SCLEROSIS
7825   MAZZUCCHI DICHOTIC$LISTENING TEMPORAL$EPILEPTICS


## 0201

5403   CONDITIONED$GSR RF
5403   CONSIDERATIONS GSR MEAS AUD$SENSITIVITY
5403   MEAS$HNG$LOSS ADULTS GSR
5403   SRT TEST CHIL
5403   USE ELECTRO-MECHANICALLY$DST$ AUD$TESTING
5406   NOTE DEFINITION HNG$BC
5503   DIFFERENTIAL$INTENSITY$SENSITIVITY LOUDNESS$RECRUITMENT
5503   DIFFICULTY CONDITIONING$ELECTRODERMAL$R TONE CHIL
5506   BASIC$PROBLEMS A
5506   USE PGSR PT$AUDIOMETRY
5515   DETECTION ASSESSMENT AUD$DIS CHIL$LESS$THREE$YRS
5603   A$EXAM INNER$EAR AURAL$OVERLAOD$TEST
5603   CONDITIONED$EYELID$R TONE OBJECTIVE$TEST$HNG
5603   EVAL PT$AUDIOGRAM
5603   EVAL PT$AUDIOMETRY PRESCH$CHIL
5603   TESTING HNG MR
5615   GSR$AUDIOMETRY CHIL
5703   MILITARY$AUDIOMETRY VETERANS$COMPENSATION HNG$LOSS
5703   MILITARY$AUDIOMETRY
5703   MILITARY$AUDIOMETRY CLASSIFICATION$HNG$TESTS
5703   MILITARY$AUDIOMETRY DIAGNOSTIC$AUDIOMETRY
5703   MILITARY$AUDIOMETRY PRACTICAL$LIMITATIONS
5703   MILITARY$AUDIOMETRY

5703    NOISE$BANDS PT STIMULI AUDIOMETRY
5703    PROBLEMS MILITARY$AUDIOMETRY AUTOMATIC$AUDIOMETRY
5703    PROBLEMS MILITARY$AUDIOMETRY
5703    SKIN-RESISTANCE$AUDIOMETRY PRESCH$CHIL
5706    BC$THR FREE$FIELD
5706    COMPARISON AUD$THR MEAS INDIV$PT BA
5706    IMPED$MEAS PATHOLOGICAL$EARS
5706    MEAS IMPED$EARDRUM
5706    METHOD$SINGLE$DESCENT GRP$AUDIOMETRY
5706    METHODS$MEAS$HNG MAN
5803    PUP-SHOW MODIFICATION PEEP-SHOW
5804    GSR
5804    INTENSITIES SHOCK CONDITIONED$TONE EXTINCTION$TONE
5804    METHOD ELECTRODERMAL$R
5804    SKIN$RESISTANCE SIDETONE$TEST$AUD$MALINGERING
5815    SELF-RECORDING$AUDIOMETRY
5903    ABBREVIATED$SWEEP-CHECK$PROCEDURES SCH$HNG$TESTING
5903    AUDIOMETRIC$CONSIDERATIONS STAPES-MOBILIZATION$SURGERY
5903    CONDITIONING GSR$AUDIOMETRY CHIL
5903    METHOD DETERMINATION PT$THR
5903    PROBLEMS CONDITIONING GSR$AUDIOMETRY
5903    SCREENING$HNG$TESTS
5903    SINGLE$DOUBLE$FREQ$AUDIOMETRY SCH
5904    CONDITIONED$GSR SP$THR
5904    VALIDITY ONE-FREQ$SCREENING SCH$CHIL
5906    MASKING THR$LEVEL
6003    APPROACH DIAGNOSTIC$A
6003    CLINICAL$EFFICIENCY COMPENSATION$AUDIOMETRY
6003    DOUBLE$FREQ$AUD$SCREENING SCH
6003    INSTRUMENTAL$AVOIDANCE GSR$AUDIOMETRY
6004    BA ANALYSIS AUD$DIS
6004    ELECTRODERMAL$R DEAF$CHIL
6005    IDENTIFICATION$AUDIOMETRY$CONFERENCE
6006    DETERMINATION HNG$THR NAVAL$RECRUITS BRITISH$USA$STANDARDS
6006    TECHNIQUE MEAS IMPED
6011    A$FINDINGS EIGHTH$NERVE$LESION
6011    AUDIOMETRIC$TESTING CHIL$SCH
6015    HNG$EVAL BRAIN-DAMAGED$CHIL
6103    AUDIOMETRIC$PROCEDURES CHIL
6103    BA
6103    ELECTRODERMAL$AUDIOMETRIC$PROCEDURE ADULTS
6103    EVAL SCH$HNG$TESTING$PROCEDURES
6103    LIMITED$FREQ$SCREENING EAR$PATH
6103    MEAS BC
6104    ELECTRODERMAL$R$AUDIOMETRY MR$CHIL
6104    HNG CHIL ACOUS$ENVIRONMENT AUDIOMETER$PERFORMANCE

6104    MEAS AUD$THR ANALOG$COMPUTER
6104    RELIABILITY CONDITIONED$GSR$PT$AUDIOMETRY ADULT$MALES
6106    LOW-FREQ$PT$MASKING
6106    SRT METHODS$ADMINISTRATION
6107    HNG$LEVELS CHIL IDENTIFICATION$AUDIOMETRY
6107    IDENTIFICATION$AUDIOMETRY
6107    LAWS$REGULATIONS IDENTIFICATION$AUDIOMETRY
6111    ALTERATIONS$PT$THR CHANGES$PRESSURES$EAR
6111    COMPARISON METHODS$ADMINISTRATION$BA
6111    EVAL REGER-NEWBY$GRP$HNG$TEST
6111    REACTION$TIME DL AMPLITUDE$EXCURSION BA
6111    RECRUITMENT ALLIED$PHENOMENA DIFFERENTIAL$DIAGNOSIS
6114    PREDICTION WORD-RECOGNITION$THR STIMULUS$PARAMETERS
6115    PUBLIC$SCH$AUDIOMETRY
6115    TESTING$HNG PRESCH$CHIL
6203    ACCURACY$INDICATOR TESTING$HNG
6203    CONDITIONING CHIL PT$TESTING
6203    USE CARDIAC$RATE AUDIOMETRIC$APPRAISAL MR$CHIL
6203    USE SINGLE-FREQ$AUDIOMETRY SCH$SCREENING
6204    COMPARISON BC$THR CONVENTIONAL$RAINVILLE$METHODS
6204    EVAL AUD$MEAS
6204    MASKING$BC$TESTING
6204    PLACEMENT$VIBRATOR BC$TESTING
6205    EFFECTS LISTENING$TRNG AUD$THR MR$CHIL
6205    HNG$TESTS OTOLOGIC$DIAGNOSIS
6206    AUD$THR FUNCTION FORCED-CHOICE$TECHNIQUE FEEDBACK
        MOTIVATION
6206    BA
6206    EVAL VARIABILITY AUDIOMETRIC$PROCEDURES
6211    AUDIOMETRIC$SCREENING PSYCHIATRIC$HOSPITAL
6211    EFFECTS REVERSED$FREQ$SWEEP BA
6211    MEAS SAL CONDUCTIVE$HNG$LOSS
6211    PT$MASKING NARROW-BAND$NOISE HI
6211    RELIABILITY INDUSTRIAL$AUDIOMETRY
6211    SSW CENTRAL$AUD$NERVOUS$SYSTEM
6213    DIAGNOSTIC$PROCEDURES AUD$DIS CHIL
6215    A$ASPECTS DEAF$MR
6303    A$EVAL STAPES$SURGERY PERICHONDRIUM-POLYETHYLENE$PROSTHESIS
6303    DETECTION ASSESSMENT PSEUDOHYPOACUSIS SCH$CHIL
6303    ELECTROENCEPHALIC$AUDIOMETRY CHIL
6303    MODIFIED$SISI$TECHNIQUE ACOUS$NEURINOMA
6303    MODIFIED$TONE$DECAY$TEST SCREENING$PROCEDURE EIGHTH
        $NERVE$LESION
6303    NONORGANIC$HNG$LOSS CHIL BA
6303    PROBLEMS AUD$TESTING NEUROSURGICAL$DIAGNOSIS
6303    USE SLIDE$PROJECTORS PT$AUDIOMETRIC$TESTING

6304    ACOUS$METHOD CLINICAL$EXAM$EAR
6304    BA CHIL
6304    IMPED$MEAS EAR-DRUM DIAGNOSIS
6304    OBSERVATIONS TYPE$V$BEKESY$TRACINGS
6304    SRT SCHIZOPHRENIC$CHIL
6304    THR$TESTING BA
6306    BC$THR SONIC$ULTRASONIC$FREQ
6315    A$ASSESSMENT CHIL
6319    SINGLE-FREQ$HNG$SCREENING COLLEGE
6403    BEKESY$TRACINGS SITE$LESION
6403    CLINICAL$MASKING AC$BC$STIMULI
6403    CLINICAL$COMMENT SAL
6403    DAF$AUDIOMETRY
6403    EVAL PROGRAM IDENTIFICATION$AUDIOMETRY SCH$CHIL
6403    PSEUDOAUD$BC$THR
6403    REPORT USE BA STENGER$TEST
6403    SIS$TEST
6403    SPONDEE$THR$MEAS COMPARISON METHODS
6403    TONE$DECAY EIGHTH$NERVE COCH$LESIONS
6403    USE MASKED$BC$SP DETECTION FEIGNED$UNILATERAL$HNG
        $LOSS
6403    VARIABLE$INTENSITY$PULSE$COUNT$METHOD DETECTION MEAS
        PT$THR CHIL
6404    CHANGES BC$THR MASKING NON-TEST$EAR
6404    EVAL BEKESY$ASCENDING$DESCENDING$GAP
6404    INTENSITY$GENERALIZATION EDR$AUDIOMETRY
6404    INTERNATIONAL$STANDARD$REFERENCE$ZERO PT$AUDIOMETERS
        REL EVAL$HI
6404    LOUDNESS$TRACKING BA
6406    AUDIOGRAM$AVERAGE$METHODS SRT$SCORES
6406    AUDIOGRAM-AVERAGED$METHODS SRT
6406    BA FREQ
6406    RELIABILITY MEAS ZWISLOCKI$ACOUS$BRIDGE
6406    RELIABILITY MEAS ZWISLOCKI$BRIDGE
6411    BA ANIMAL$RESEARCH
6411    BA SRT
6411    CLINICAL$COMPARISON METHODS MEASURING$ABNORMAL$AUD
        $ADAPTATION BA
6411    INSTRUMENTAL$AVOIDANCE CLASSICAL$CONDITIONING GSR
        $SP$AUDIOMETRY
6411    RELATIONSHIPS BEKESY$FIXED$FREQUENCY CONVENTIONAL
        $AUDIOMETRY CHIL
6411    RELIABILITY IMPEDANCE EARDRUM
6411    SAL$TECHNIQUE NARROW$BAND$NOISE
6411    TYPE$II BA MODIFIED$TONE$DECAY$TEST
6415    AUDIOLOGICAL$EXAMINATION CHIL

```
6415   METHOD TEST$HNG MR$CHIL
6503   A$MANIFESTATIONS NEURAL$LESION CASES MENIERES$DISEASE
6503   ABNORMAL$BEKESY$TRACINGS
6503   ASA-ISO$TRANSITION NOTE USE SAL$TECHNIQUE
6503   ASA-ISO$TRANSITION NOTE USE SAL$TECHNIQUE
6503   AUD$TEST$RESULTS RETROCOCH$LESIONS
6503   BEKESY$TRACINGS TONE$DECAY LOUDNESS$RECRUITMENT
6503   CLINICAL$FINDINGS SAL$AUDIOMETRY OBSERVATIONS
6503   DILEMMAS IDENTIFICATION$AUDIOMETRY
6503   EXAM NORMAL$HEARERS$R SISI
6503   SISI$TEST EIGHTH$NERVE$COCH$INVOLVEMENT
6503   SISI$TEST LOUDNESS$RECRUITMENT ABLB
6503   TYPE$V BA
6503   USE BA AUD$DIAGNOSIS
6504   CRITICAL$EVAL SAL$AUDIOMETRY
6504   EFFECTS BC$MASKING
6504   OCCLUSION$EFFECT BC$HNG
6504   PARAMETERS FIXED-FREQ$BA
6506   MEAS AUD$THR
6506   RATING$SCALES TWO-STATE$THR$MODELS
6511   BA HI$CHIL
6511   EFFICIENCY AUDIOMETRIC$MEAS FUNCTIONAL$HNG$LOSS
6511   EVAL PT$AUDIOGRAM$CONFIGURATION IDENTIFYING$ADULTS
       FUNCTIONAL$HNG$
6511   PATIENT$ERRORS SPONDEE$PURE-TONE$THR$MEAS
6511   RELIABILITY HIGH-FREQ$THR
6511   RELIABILITY FREQUENCY$THR
6511   VALIDITY RELIABILITY SAL$TECHNIQUE
6515   BIBLIOGRAPHY PUBLICATIONS TESTING$HNG$INF
6515   HNG$TESTS SUPERMARKET
6515   LIGHT UNCONDITIONED$STIMULUS EDR$AUDIOMETRY
6515   METHOD LIMINAL$AUDIOMETRY
6603   AVERAGE$ER MEAS AUD$SENSITIVITY CHIL
6603   BEHAVIORAL$AUDIOMETRY OPERANT$PROCEDURE
6603   CLINICAL$USE EEA AVERAGE$R$COMPUTER CASE$REPORT
6603   COLLAPSE EAR$CANAL AUDIOMETRY
6603   COLLAPSE EAR$CANAL AUDIOMETRY
6603   COMMENTS DILEMMAS IDENTIFICATION$AUDIOMETRY
6603   MISDIAGNOSIS CHIL AUD$PROBLEMS
6603   MODIFICATIONS TYPES BA
6603   SAL$TECHNIQUE GRASON-STADLER$SP$AUDIOMETER
6604   BC$THR AUDIOMETRY
6604   COLLAPSING$EAR$CANALS
6604   CRITICAL$OFF-TIME EIGHTH$NERVE$DIS
6604   EFFECTS PARAMETER$VARIATIONS BA ACOUS$NEURINOMA
6604   RELIABILITY SP$AUDIOMETRY INSTITUTIONALIZED$MR$CHIL
```

6606    AMPLITUDE BEKESY$TRACING ATTENUATION$RATES
6606    DECISION$RULES THR$DETERMINATION
6606    INTERIM$BC$THR AUDIOMETRY
6606    NOTE DATA$LOGGING AUDIOMETRIC$MEAS
6606    OBJECTIVE$AUDIOMETRY
6615    DIAGNOSIS MEANING DEAFNESS
6703    A$EVAL ACOUS$NEURINOMAS
6703    CLINICAL$MASKING NONTEST$EAR
6703    ENG CLINICAL$A
6703    EVAL CHIL HNG$LOSS
6703    INTEREST$VARIABILITY AC$BC$GAP
6703    MIDDLE$EAR$REFLEX$MEAS PSEUDOHYPACUSIS
6703    MODIFICATION BING$TEST BA
6703    RISING$AUDIOMETRIC$CONFIGURATION
6703    TEST COLLAPSE EXTERNAL$EAR$CANAL AUDIOMETRY
6704    CLINICAL$APPLICATION EVOKED$R$AUDIOMETRY
6704    CROSS—MODAL$GENERALIZATION CONDITIONED$GSR$AUDIOMETRY
6704    CROSS—MODAL$GENERALIZATION CONDITIONED$GSR$AUDIOMETRY
6704    ELECTROENCEPHALIC$AUDIOMETRY CORTICAL$CONDITIONING
6704    RELIABILITY ELECTRODERMAL$AUDIOMETRY APHASIC$ADULTS
6704    SPONDEE$THR MEAS ASCENDING$
6704    SPONDEE$THR MEAS ASCENDING$
6704    TYPE$V$BEKESY$PATTERN INTERPRETATION CLINICAL$UTILITY
6704    VALIDATION ER$AUDIOMETRY
6706    CORRECTIONS ATTENUATOR$TRANSIENT$EFFECTS DATA SELF—RECORDED
        $AUDIO$
6711    AUDIOMETRIC$SCREENING PSYCHIATRIC$STATE$HOSPITAL
6711    BEKESY$LOUDNESS$TRACING$WIDTH DIFFERENTIAL$INTENSIVE
        $LIMEN
6711    EFFECT R$MODE SRT MR$CHIL
6711    HAND$PREFERENCE BA
6711    INTERAURAL$ATTENUATION CROSS$HNG AIR$CONDUCTION$AUDIOMETRY
6711    SIGNIFICANCE SISI$TEST
6715    AUDIOMETRIC$SCREENING
6715    CHIL$AUDIOGRAM
6715    CLINICAL$AUDIOMETRY
6803    A$VESTIBULAR$MANIFESTATIONS MENINGIOMAS CEREBELLOPONTINE
        $ANGLE
6803    OPERANT$AUDIOMETRIC$PROCEDURE DIFFICULT—TO—TEST$PATIENTS
6803    SSW$TEST INTERMIM$REPORT
6803    SYSTEM CLINICAL$ER$AUDIOMETRY
6804    CLINICAL$MEAS TEMPORAL$AUD$SUMMATION
6804    EFFECTS METHOD$MEAS MCL$SP
6804    JUDGE$RELIABILITY INF$TESTING
6804    REPROACHING$STYLI SP$AUDIOMETRY
6804    SIGNAL$DETECTION$AUDIOMETRY EXPLORATORY$STUDY

```
6804   SIGNAL$DETECTION$AUDIOMETRY EXPLORATORY$STUDY
6804   TYPE$V$BEKESY EFFECTS LOUDNESS$MEM
6806   EFFECTS ATTENUATION$RATE STARTING$INTEN BA$THR
6811   BEHAVIORAL$MEASUREMENTS PURE$TONE$THRESHOLD
6811   BEKESY$SWEEP$FREQUENCY CONVENTIONAL$AUDIOMETRY HNG
       $IMP$CHIL
6811   COMPARISON SP$BEKESY$TRACINGS CLINICAL$AUD$MEASURINGS
6811   EEG$AUDIOMETRY COCHLEAR$PATHOLOGY
6811   EFFECT OFF-TIME AMPLITUDE$THRESHOLD BEKESY$TRACINGS
6811   EFFECTS MASKING$NOISE SISI
6811   EFFECTS IPSILATERAL$MASKING BEKESY$AMPLITUDE
6811   EXPERIMENTAL$STUDIES SISI TEST
6811   HOLLEIN$THOMPSON GROUP$SCREENING$TEST$HEARING
6813   METHOD SORTING$OUT MR$CHIL DEAF$CHIL
6816   HNG$CAPACITY MEAS CALCULATION
6903   CLINICAL$IMPRESSIONS PORTABLE$MASKING$UNIT
6903   COMPARISON STUDIES BC$THR HAIC$INTERIM$STANDARD BC
       $AUDIOMETRY
6903   ER$AUDIOMETRY CONSIDERATIONS
6903   EVIDENCE USE OCCLUDED$FOREHEAD$BC
6903   PROGRAMMED$APPROACH OPERANT$AUDIOMETRY LOW-FUNCTIONING
       $CHIL
6903   VALIDATION OBSERVER$JUDGMENT BEHAVIORAL$OBSERVATION
       $AUDIOMETRY
6904   BA TEMPORAL$SUMMATION
6904   COMPARATIVE$BEKESY$TYPING BROAD$NARROW-BAND$NOISE
6904   COMPARISON FRONTAL$MASTOID$BC$THR CONDUCTIVE$LESIONS
6904   DIFFERENTIAL$EFFECT CONDUCTIVE$HNG$LOSS THR-DURATION
       $FUNCTION
6904   LOUDNESS$DISCOMFORT$LEVEL$MODIFICATION
6904   STIMULI$INTENSITY$FACTORS TESTING$INF
6904   TEST-RETEST$RELIABILITY SERIAL$PT$AUDIOGRAMS CHIL
       DEAF$SCH
6906   COMPARISON CONTINUOUS$PULSED-TONES BA$THR MEAS
6906   FREQ$PATTERN RESIDUAL$MASKING PT MEAS BA
6906   INFLUENCE PULSED$MASKING THR SPONDEES
6911   BC$THR LOCATIONS$SKULL
6911   CONTINUOUS$TONE$MASKING$TEST IDENTIFYING$SITE$LESION
6911   EFFECTS EXPERIMENTER$BIAS PT$SP$AUDIOMETRY
6911   EST SRT PT$HNG$LOSS
6911   FACTORS SCREENING$HNG NEWBORN
6911   OCCLUSION$EFFECT BC$VIBRATOR MASTOID$VS$FOREHEAD
6911   PERSONALITY AUDIOMETRIC$CONSISTENCY
6911   R$VARIABILITY PERSONALITY AUTOMATED$AUDIOMETRY
6911   THR$TONE$DECAY$TEST CENTRAL$AUD$PATHOLOGY
6915   BIBLIOGRAPHY TESTING$HNG$INF
```

7003    AUD$SCREENING SCH$CHIL VA$C
7003    AVERAGED$ELECTROENCEPHALIC$AUDIOMETRY
7003    IMPED PATHOLOGICAL$EARS
7003    LENGTHENED$OFF-TIME SELF-RECORDING$SCREENING$DEVICE
7003    USE BOTTLE-FEEDING INF$HNG$TESTING
7004    COMPARISON SYSTEMS HIGH-FREQ$AC$AUDIOMETRY
7004    COMPARISON APPROACHES BOA
7004    IMPED MEAS
7004    IMPED MEAS
7004    NARROW-BAND$NOISE$AUDIOMETRY HARD-TO-TEST$PATIENTS
7004    OCCLUSION$EFFECT UNILATERAL$FUNCTIONAL$HNG$LOSS
7004    REACTION$TIME PEDIATRIC$AUDIOMETRY
7004    STIMULUS$R$OBSERVER$VARIABLES AUD$SCREENING NEWBORN
        $INF
7004    VARIABLE$BANDWIDTH$MASKING AUTOMATIC$AUDIOMETRY
7004    WARBLED$TONE$MASKING BC$AUDIOMETRY
7005    SYMBOLS PT$AUDIOMETRY
7006    MEAS$SYSTEM FETAL$AUDIOMETRY
7011    AUD$EVOKED$R RECRUITING$EARS
7011    AUD$TESTING NEWBORNS EYEBLINK$CONDITIONING
7011    AVERAGED$ELECTROENCEPHALIC$AUDIOMETRY MEDICATED$MR
        $ADULTS SLEEP
7011    CLINICAL$APPLICATION TEMPORAL$SUMMATION
7011    COMPARISON ASCENDING$DESCENDING$MODES PT$STENGER$TEST
7011    DESCENDING$ASCENDING$BEKESY$THR ATTENUATION$RATED
        $OFFTIMES
7011    EFFECTS DIRECTION FREQ$SWEEP BA
7011    IDENTIFICATION FUNCTIONAL$HNG$LOSS EFFICIENCY STENGER
        $TESTS
7011    INF$HNG$SCREENING RUBELLA$EPIDEMIC
7011    REL AUD$REACTION$TIME TRACING$AMPLITUDE BA
7011    REL VIBRATOR$PLACEMENT BC$MEAS MONAURALLY$DEAF
7011    SISI$TEST SUBJECTIVE$LOUDNESS
7011    SP$IN$NOISE DIAGNOSTIC$AUDIOMETRY
7011    TONE-IN-NOISE$TEST
7011    VALUE DOERFLER-STEWART$TEST
7015    COMPUTER TEST$HNG$INF
7103    AVERAGED$ELECTROENCEPHALIC$AUDIOMETRY INF
7103    BA FUNCTIONAL$HNG$LOSS
7103    BA SIMULATED$HNG$LOSS
7103    CRITIQUE NEONATAL$HNG$EVAL
7103    RELEVANCE VASCULAR$DIS A$FINDINGS
7104    AUDIOMETRIC$EVAL ADULT$APHASICS
7104    DEV LOT$BEKESY$TEST NONORGANIC$HNG$LOSS
7104    DICHOTIC$THR$TEST BRAIN$DAMAGE
7104    EFFECT INCREMENT$SIZE SISI

7104   INDUCED$BIOPHYSICAL$ARTIFACTS AER$AUDIOMETRY
7104   TIME-OUT$PUNISHMENT BUTTON$PUSHING
7104   TONE$DECAY HNG$THR SENSORINEURAL$LOSS
7104   USE ALTERNATED$STIMULI REDUCE$R$DECREMENT AUD$TESTING
        NEWBORNS$INF
7104   VALIDITY RELIABILITY BA PRESCH$CHIL
7106   ANSI-STANDARD$REFERENCE$THR SPL AUDIOMETERS COMMENTS
7106   AUDIOMETRIC$THR$LEVEL$STANDARDS
7106   EFFECTS UNILATERAL$MENIERES$DISEASE MASKING-LEVEL
        $DIFFERENCES
7106   EFFECTS ATTENUATION DESCENDING$BEKESY$THR
7106   REVERSALS PERCEP NOISE TONE$PATTERNS
7111   ATTENTION$DIVERSION AUD$THR
7111   EVOKED$R$AUDIOMETRY TEMPORAL$LOBE$PATH
7111   INVESTIGATION SPONDEE$THR CHIL
7111   OCCLUSION$EFFECT
7111   PEDIATRIC$AUDIOLOGY
7111   PROPOSED$SYSTEM TESTING$EXTRA-HIGH$FREQUENCIES
7111   SCHEMATIC$REPRESENTATION NONTEST$EAR$MASKING$PROBLEM
7203   AVERAGED$ELECTROENCEPHALIC$AUDIOMETRIC$SENSITIVITY
        PROCEDURE
7203   CLINICAL$EQUIPMENT MEAS MIDDLE-EAR$MUSCLE$REFLEXES
        TYMPANOMETRY
7203   OPERANT$AUDIOMETRY CONSIDERATION SHORTCOMINGS A$TESTING
        CHIL
7203   SP$AUDIOMETRY EARPHONE SOUND$FIELD
7203   UNUSUAL$FINDINGS BA
7204   ANSI-
7204   EFFECTS PRACTICE SISI$SCORES NORMAL$HNG$SUBJECTS
7204   EVAL EFFICIENCY VASC
7204   NOISE$AUDIOMETER
7204   R$INF$CHIL FUNCTION AUD$STIMULI TEST$METHODS
7205   AUDIOMETRIC$PRACTICES TESTS$SITE$LESION
7206   HIGH-FREQ$AUDIOMETRIC$THR$LEVELS
7211   AUDIOMETRIC$PROCEDURES THR$ABOVE$
7211   BA MEAS THR$INTELLIGIBILITY CONNECTED$DISCOURSE
7211   BA$THR TDH-
7211   CONTINUOUS$TONE$MASKING$TEST
7211   CONTRALATERAL$MASKING$EFFECTS AUD$THR
7211   DESCENDING$BEKESY$THR FREQ$MODULATED$TONES
7211   FEASIBILITY COMPUTERIZED$AUDIOMETRY
7211   LINEAR$EXTRAPOLATION ELECTROENCEPHALIC$R$AUDIOMETRY
7211   NORMAL$OTOADMITTANCE$VALUES
7211   PTA SRT REL SIMULATED$HNG$LOSS
7211   TEMPORAL$INTEGRATION MEAS BRIEF-TONE$AUDIOMETRY

7212    COMPUTERIZED$SCREENING$BATTERY
7303    ACOUSTIC$NEUROMAS IMPED
7303    GROUP$AUDIOMETRY PATIENT-CONTROLLED$AUDIOMETERS
7303    INFLATABLE$PROBE$ASSEMBLY ELECTROACOUSTIC$IMPED$BRIDGES
7303    SRT$PROCEDURE
7304    BC$THR$SENSITIVITY MASTOID$SCLEROSIS
7304    COMPUTERIZED$PT$AUDIOMETRIC$PROCEDURES
7306    ANOMALOUS$LOUDNESS$FUNCTION SP
7306    BC$THR HUMAN$TEETH
7306    EFFECT ASCENDING$DESCENDING$MEAS$METHODS COMFORTABLE
        $LOUDNESS$LEVE
7311    INF$R PT$STIMULATION
7311    INFLUENCE LOMBARD$TEST DAF$TEST FUNCTIONAL$HNG$LOSS
7311    INVEST RELIABILITY WEBER$TEST
7311    PREDICTING SRT PRESCH$CHIL
7311    SIGNIFICANCE BRIEF$TONE$AUDIOMETRY
7311    VALIDITY RELIABILITY FUSION$INFERRED$THR
7311    VISUAL$IDENTIFICATION$R RESPIRATION$AUDIOMETRY
7315    EVOKED$R$AUDIOMETRY
7315    FREQ$COMPONENTS NOISEMAKERS PEDIATRIC$A$EVAL
7403    AUDIOMETRIC$BING$TEST DETERMINATION$MINIMUM$MASKING
        BC
7403    BRIEF-TONE$AUDIOMETRY NORMAL DEAF SCH$CHIL
7403    CLINICAL$PROCEDURE$EVAL AL
7403    MINIMUM$EFFECTIVE$MASKING THR$AUDIOMETRY
7403    NEWBORN$HNG$SCREENING COUNTY$HOSPITAL
7403    R$INF$CHIL BA
7404    COMPUTER$AUDIOMETRY
7404    EFFECTS FREQ$DETECTION BRIEF-TONE$AUDIOMETRY
7404    PT$OCTAVE$MASKING SENSORINEURAL$HNG$LOSS
7404    THR$MEAS BRIEF-TONE$AUD
7405    A$EVAL GUIDELINES AUD$SYMBOLS
7405    IMPEDANCE$MEASUREMENT HOUSTON
7406    LOUDNESS$DISCOMFORT$LEVEL METHODS STIMULI
7406    PASS-FAIL$RATIOS IDENTIFICATION$AUDIOMETRY FUNCTION
7406    SIMULATION EFFECT RECRUITMENT LOUDNESS$REL SP
7408    DUAL$HNG$SCREENING IDENTIFYING$CHIL PHONIC$READING
        $PROBLEMS
7408    IDENTIFICATION$AUDIOMETRY$ACCURACY SCH-AGE$CHIL
7415    VIDEO$TAPE EARLY$DETECTION$INTERVENTION HEARING$ALERT
7503    COOPER IMPEDANCE$BRIDGE$TECHNIQUE SCHOOL$SCREENING
7503    DOCKUM WARBLE$TONE AUDIOMETRIC$STIMULUS
7503    FULTON HEARING$ASSESSMENT CHIL
7503    MARTIN EFFECTS TYPE$V$BEKESY$PATTERNS SIMULATED$HNG
        $LOSS
7503    MEYER HIGH-RISK$REGISTER NEWBORN$HNG$SCREENING

7503    MOORE AUDITORY$LOCALIZATION INFANTS REINFORCEMENT
        $CONDITIONS
7504    BILLINGS PT$THR DAF ELECTRODERMAL$AUDIOMETRY VOLUNTARY
        $R$AUDIOMETRY
7504    CHIAL COST-BENEFIT$ANALYSIS DECISION$CRITERIA SPONDEE
        $THR$MEAS
7504    DIRKS BONE$VIBRATOR$MEAS PHYSICAL$CHAR BEHAVIOR$THR
7504    GALAMBOS BS$AUD$ER PREMATURE$INFANTS
7504    IVEY TYMPANOMETRIC$CURVES OTOSCLEROSIS
7504    MARGOLIS STATIC+DYNAMIC$IMPEDANCE INFANT
7504    WILEY AR+R SUSTAINED$SIGNALS
7505    GREENBERG ACOUSTIC$IMPEDANCE ADMITTANCE$MEAS OCTOBER
7505    HANNAH AUDIOLOGIST$MODEL TEST$SELECTION FEBRUARY
7505    JACOBSON CLINICAL$APPLICATION GRASON-STADLER$OTOADMITTANCE
7505    YANTIS AUDIO ASSOCIATION OCCUPATIONAL$HRING$CONSERVATION
7511    LIEBMAN SISI$SCORES NORMAL-HEARING
7511    LIEBMAN SISI$SCORES NORMAL$POPULATION
7511    SIEGENTHALER RELIABILITY BEKESY$EXCURSION$SIZE
7511    SIEGENTHALER RELIABILITY BEKESY$EXCURSION$SIZE NORMAL
        $ADULTS
7511    WOOTEN IMPEDANCE$AUDIOMETRY RETARDATES
7511    WOOTEN IMPEDANCE$AUD RETARDATES
7512    WOOD ASSESSMENT AUD$PROCESSING
7515    LING THR$VARIATIONS REPEATED$AUDIOGRAMS
7515    TWEEDIE VIDEOAUDIOMETRY
7516     CHILD HL REPORTING DIAGNOSIS
7516     SP$DETECTION$THRESHOLDS
7527    SIEGENTHALER RELIABILITY TIP DIP SP-HNG$TESTS CHILDREN
7529    MENCHER EARLY$IDENTIFICATION HL A REVIEW
7603    BEATTIE RELIABILITY DISCRIM$TESTS WHITE$NOISE HEARING
        $AIDS
7603    BEATTIE RELIABILITY DISCRIM$TESTS WHITE$NOISE HEARING
        $AIDS
7603    DANCER STIMULUS$PRESENTATION INSTRUCTIONS PT$THRESHOLDS
        FALSE-ALARM
7603    ERBER AUDIOLOGIC$EVALUATION DEAF$CHILDREN
7603    MARTIN TANGIBLY$REINFORCED$SRT CHIL
7603    SANDERSON-LEEPA ARTICULATION$FUNCTIONS TEST-RETEST
        CHIL SP$DISCRIM
7603    SEIDEMANN SYSTEM REPORTING TYMPANOMETRIC$RESULTS
7603    VENTRY PT$SRT FUNCTIONAL$HNG$LOSS
7604    FREEMAN LEAD+LAG$EFFECTS SSW
7605    FELLENDORF BELL'S$AUDIOMETER
7611    CHERRY ASCENDING-DESCENDING$GAP IDENTIFYING SUPRATHRESHOLD
        $RESPONSE
7611    GELFAND TRACKING$ABLB RECRUITMENT$TESTING

7611   KEYDAR HEBREW$VERSION SSW$TEST
7615   LLOYD DETECTION DIAGNOSIS HI CHILD
7616    ELECTROPHYSIOLOGICAL$TEST INFANT$HRING
7629   GILBERT HEMISPHERECTOMIZED$SUBJECTS DICHOTIC$BINAURAL
       $FREQ$FUSION
7629   TYLER TEMPORAL$INTEGRATION COCHLEAR$HL
7629   ZINK NOISE$ALLOWABLE AUDIOMETRIC$TEST$AREAS
7703   ABAHAZI ACOUSTIC$REFLEX INFANTS
7703   ANDREWS ASSESSMENT PITCH$DISCRIM CHIL
7703   COLEMAN HIGH-FREQUENCY$HEARING$LOSS CHIL IDENTIFICATION
7703   MONRO EFFECTS SOPHISTICATION TESTS NON-ORGANIC$HEARING
       $LOSS
7703   MOORE VISUAL$REINFORCEMENT HEAD-TURN$RESPONSES INFANTS
7703   ORCHIK BEKESY$COMFORTABLE$LOUDNESS
7703   SEIDEMANN TYMPANOMETRIC$ASSESSMENT EUSTACHIAN$TUBE
       $PATENCY CHIL
7703   SKINNER ELECTROPHYSIOLOGIC$RESPONSE$AUDIOMETRY
7704   MARGOLIS PREDICTING$HL ACOUSTIC$REFLEX
7704   MARGOLIS MEAS TEMPORAL$CHAR FILTER$R IMPEDANCE$INSTRUMENTS
7704   MARGOLIS INTERACTIONS TYMPANOMETRIC$VARIABLES
7704   MARGOLIS TYMPANOMETRIC$ASYMMETRY
7704   MCFARLAND MIDDLE$COMPONENTS AER TONE-PIPS
7704   MENCHER OBSERVER$BIAS NEONATAL$SCREENING
7704   MUSKET CIRCUMAURAL$ENCLOSURES CHILD
7704   WOOD AUD$REACTION$TIMES HL
7705   EGAN HIGH-RISK$REGISTERS
7706   EGGERMONT TUNING$CURVES NORMAL PATHOLOGICAL$EARS
7716    TYMPANOMETRIC OTOSCOPIC$EVALUATIONS
7729   MENCHER CRIB-O-GRAM CLINICAL$DIAGNOSIS
7803    VENTRY EVAL CLINICAL$METHOD MEAS COMFORTABLE$LOUDNESS
7803   GREENBERG VISUAL$REINFORCEN
7803   GREENBERG VISUAL$REINFORCEMENT$AUD DOWNS$SYNDROME
       $CHILD
7803   HUMES AURAL-OVERLOAD$TEST
7803   LUCKER EFFECTS INSTRUCTIONAL$SET COMFORTABLE$LOUDNESS
       $RANGE
7803   OLSEN SIGNAL$MONITOR AUDIOMETRY
7804   KAMM EFFECT SENSORINEURAL$HEARING$LOSS LOUDNESS$DISCOMFORT
       $LEVEL MCL
7804   MARGOLIS SIGNIFICANCE ASYMMETRICAL$TYMPANOGRAM
7804   PEARLMAN SIGNIFICANT$ASYMMETRICAL$TYMPANOGRAM
7805   MARTIN STATUS AUDIOMETRIC$PRACTICE
7805   ROBINSON CALIBRATION$CHARACTERISTICS IMPEDANCE$BRIDGES
7806   SILMAN SN$HEARING$LOSS ACOUSTIC$REFLEX GROWTH$FUNCTIONS
7815   RUBEN DELAY DIAGNOSIS
7827   GEFFNER SP LANG$ASSESSMENT DEAF$CHIL

7827  LEVITT ASSESSMENT TRAINING TECHNOLOGY DEAF

## 0202

5406  ARTIFICIAL$VOICE MINIATURE$ANECHOIC$CHAMBER HA$MEAS
5406  WINDSCREEN EARS
5415  HA ACCEPTANCE USE
5415  HA DEAF$CHIL
5515  CHIL HA
5515  HA CHIL
5515  HA SELECTION USE
5515  LISTENING HA
5515  USE AMPLIFICATION SCH$DEAF
5615  GROUP$HA SCH
5615  GUIDE GROUP$HA
5615  HA PRESCH$CHIL
5615  HA$GARMENTS
5706  SP$COMM HIGH$NOISE$LEVELS ROLES NOISE-OPERATED$AUTOMATIC
      $GAIN$CONT
5715
5716  GRP$WEARABLE$HA RESIDENTIAL$SCH$DEAF
5803  BINAURAL$HA
5815  REL AUDIO$FINDINGS USE HA
5818  HAS
5903  INDIV$HA EARLY$THERAPY PRESCH$CHIL
5906  INFLUENCE DIFFRACTION SOUND$WAVES HUMAN$HEAD CHARACTERISTICS
      HA
6003  HA$SELECTION
6003  HAE RELIABILITY REPEATED$MEAS
6003  TEST-RETEST$CONSISTENCY CLINICAL$HA$TESTS
6004  HA CHIL
6005  HAIC UNIVERSITY$CONFERENCE
6005  PRELIMINARY$REPORT IMPLEMENTATION OREGON$HA$LAW
6015  BINAURAL$HA CHIL
6104  BINAURAL$HA SP$INTELLIGIBILITY
6105  STANDARD MEAS HA$PERFORMANCE
6106  BINAURAL$HA
6111  REL SP$INTELLIGIBILITY ELECTRO-ACOUS$CHARACTERISTICS
      LOW$FIDELITY
6117  GAIN$PRESCRIPTION HAS
6203  MEAS PERFORMANCE GRP$HA
6203  SURVEY REACTIONS USERS BINAURAL$MONAURAL$HA
6204  APPROACH HAS
6205  IMPLEMENTATION OREGON$HA$LAW

```
6215   VALUE BINAURAL$HA HI$CHIL SCH
6216   WEARABLE$HA
6303   COMPARISON PROCEDURES HAE
6303   COMPARISON PROCEDURES HAE
6303   INFLUENCE ATTACT$RELEASE COMPRESSION$AMPLIFICATION
       UNDERSTANDING$S
6305   HAE
6315   COMPARISON HAE$TEST$INSTRUMENTS AIDS$DEALERS
6316   COMPARISON GRP$HA$SYSTEMS
6403   BINAURAL$HNG ONE$HA
6404   IMPLICATIONS BINAURAL$SIGNAL$SELECTION HAE
6405   CLINICAL$HAS
6415   IMPLICATIONS HA$AMPLIFICATION BELOW$
6415   USE HA HI$CHIL NORMAL$SCH
6503   CASE UNILATERAL$HNG$LOSS HA
6503   REHAB$APPROACH UNILATERAL$HI CROS
6515   ROLE HA$DEALER
6603   HA CHIL SCH
6603   USE MASTER$HA AUD$TRAINER
6604   COMPARISON SP$INTELLIGIBILITY$TESTS EVAL HA$PERFORMANCE
6604   HA$PERFORMANCE HAS
6615   INDUCT$LOOP$AMPLIFICATION TV$DEAF
6703   BATTERY$LIFE NONLINEAR$DISTORTION HA
6703   BODY$TYPE$HA UNILATERAL$HNG$LOSSES
6704   ACOUS$GAIN THR$IMPROVEMENT HAS
6704   HA$DESIGN EVAL DISCRIM$LOSS
6704   INFLUENCE GAIN$CONTROL$ROTATION NONLINEAR$DISTORTION
       HA
6704   LONGITUDINAL$EXAM HARMONIC$DISTORTION HA
6704   NONLINEAR$DISTORTION HA
6704   VARIABILITY GAIN FREQ$CHARACTERISTICS HA
6707   HAE$PROCEDURES
6711   AIDED$SPEECH$DISCRIM NOISE VENTED$UNVENTED$EARMOLDS
6803   APPLICATION LR$TEST HAE
6803   DISTORTED$PERCEP$SP HA$CONSULTATION
6804   EFFECT CONVENTIONAL$VS$NONOCCLUDING$EARMOLD CROS FREQ
       $R HA
6804   EFFECTS HIGH$GAIN$AMPLIFICATION CHIL RESIDENTIAL$SCH
       $DEAF
6804   MODIFIED$EARPIECES CROS HIGH$FREQ$HNG$LOSS
6804   REL VIBRATOR$SURFACE$AREA STATIC$APPLICATION$FORCE
6805   PATIENT$ATTITUDES REACTIONS HAS
6815   AUDIBILITY HA LOW$FREQ
6816   FREQ$SHIFT$TYPE$HA UTTERANCE$TRAINER
6816   USE AMPLIFICATION EDUC$DEAF$CHIL
6903   HA$ORIENTATION STATE$SCH MR
```

6904   BACTERIOLOGY EARPHONE$CONTAMINATION
6904   BINAURAL$HNG$SP AIDED$CONDITIONS
6904   REL AUD$DISTORTION$TEST$RESULTS SP$DISCRIM SELECTIVE
       $AMPLIFYING$SY
6911   EFFECT AGE INTERTEST$TIME$INTERVAL INITIAL$RECHECK
       $SP$DISCRIM HA$U
6911   INFLUENCE HA$GAIN$CONTROL$ROTATION ACOUS$GAIN
7004   ACOUS$COUPLER$EFFECTS SP$AUDIOMETRIC$SCORES CROS$HA
7004   EARMOLD$INFLUENCE AIDED$SP$IDENTIFICATION
7004   EFFECT EARMOLD SP$INTELLIGIBILITY HA
7004   FOLLOW-UP$REPORT MODIFIED$EARPIECES CROS HIGH$FREQ
       $HNG$LOSSES
7004   HA$EFFICIENCY COMPETING$SP$SITUATION
7004   INTELLIGIBILITY SP HA INDUCTANCE$LOOP MICROPHONE$MODES
       SIGNAL$RECE
7004   LISTENER$PREFERENCE SELECTIVE$VS$FLAT$AMPLIFICATION
       HIGH-FREQ$HNG$
7005   INDUCTION$LOOP$AMPLIFICATION$SYSTEMS CLASSROOM$PERFORMANCE
7006   EARMOLD$ALTERATION$EFFECTS MEAS HUMAN$EAM
7006   INVEST ACOUS EARMOLD$VENTS
7011   EFFECT HARMONIC$DISTORTION HA SP$INTELLIGIBILITY
7016   HA$R INDUCTION$LOOP$AMPLIFICATION
7103   EVAL HA DEAF$CHIL
7103   FREQ$R$PROCEDURE EVAL SELECTING$HA DEAF$CHIL
7103   HIGH-FREQ$CONSONANT$DISCRIM$WORD$LIST HAE
7104   EXAM CROS$HA
7104   HA$DISTORTION CONSONANT$IDENTIFICATION
7104   PERFORMANCE INDIV$HA MICROPHONE INDUCTION$COIL$INPUT
7104   QUALITY$JUDGMENTS HA$TRANSDUCED$SP
7111   ACCEPTABLE$S/N$RATIOS AIDED$SP$DISCRIM HI
7111   EFFECT FREQUENCY$RESPONSE$CHARACTERISTICS HNG$AIDS
       SP$INTELLIGIBIL
7111   EFFECTS MODIFIED$EARMOLDS HNG$SENSITIVITY
7111   SP$DISCRIM CROS-AIDED$NORMAL-HNG
7115   CONVENTIONAL$HA
7115   COUPLING$HA$TELEPHONE
7115   SP$ANALYZING$HA
7203   FOLLOW-UP$STUDY CROS$HA
7203   HA$REFERRALS REPORT
7205   SURVEY HAE$PROCEDURES
7211   COMPARATIVE$PERFORMANCE HA$MICROPHONE INDUCTION$COIL
7211   HAE$PROCEDURE
7211   UTOPIAN$HA
7215   EVAL IMPLANTABLE$HA COCHLEAR$POTENTIALS
7215   HA$CHIL LONGITUDINAL$STUDY PERFORMANCE
7215   STUDY AMPLIFICATION$SYSTEMS SCH$DEAF

```
7216   REL EXTENT$HA$USE LANG$ACADEMIC$ACHIEVEMENT
7303   BODY-BAFFLE REAL-EAR$EFFECTS SELECTION$HA$AIDS DEAF
       $CHIL
7303   EARMOLD$NOMENCLATURE SURVEY
7303   HNG$LOSSES HA CHIL LANG$DIS
7304   BACTERIOLOGY CLEANING$METHODS STOCK$EARMOLDS
7311   IMPROVEMENT$SP$DISCRIM COMPRESSION$VS$LINEAR$AMPLIFICATION
7311   MODIFIED$RHYME$TEST HAE
7311   OBJECTIVE$EVAL MONAURAL$BINAURAL$AMPLIFICATION HH
       $CHIL
7315   HA OLDER$AMERICAN
7315   TELECOIL MICROPHONE HA
7316   HA RESIDENTIAL$DEAF$SCH
7317   COMBINATION$AUDITION$VISION HAE CASE$REPORT
7403   HAE$METHODS
7404   MONAURAL$BINAURAL$SP$PERCEP HA NOISE REVERBERATION
       HI
7405   COMMENTS HNG$AID$INDUSTRY SURVEY HARD$HNG
7405   HNG$AID$PROGRAM BRITISH$NATIONAL$HEALTH$SEVERICE
7406   REVERBERATION HA
7415   HA$MONITOR$PROGRAM
7415   TELEPHONE$ADAPTER TELEPHONE$AIDS HH
7415   USE RATING$SCALE COMPARE BINAURAL$MONAURAL$AMPLIFICATION
       HI$CHIL
7503   GENGEL EVALUATE TRANSPOSER$HNG$AID
7503   SHAPIRO MCL HNG$AIDS$EVAL
7504   TONISSON IN-THE-EAR$GAIN HA AR$METHOD
7505   GLADSTONE HISTORY STATUS INCOMPATIBILITY HA+TELEPHONES
       FEBRUARY
7506   SCHELLENG ANOMALY PITCH$PERCEPTION
7511   GREENBERG HEARING$AID$DISTORTION SYNTHETIC$SENTENCE
       $IDENTIFICATION
7511   GREENBERG HA$DISTORTION SSI
7511   MAREING BENEFIT CHIL CROS$HEARING$AIDS
7511   MARELING BENEFIT CHILD CROS$HA
7515   FELLENDORF HA HI CHILD SWEDEN US
7531   GALLOWAY HNG$AID$FITTINGS YOUNG$ADULTS HI
7531   MOOREHNG$CHARACTERSTICS IMPLICATIONS AUD$TRNG
7603   BEATTIE RELIABILITY DISCRIM$TESTS WHITE$NOISE HEARING
       $AIDS
7605   BLOOD NEEDS HEARING$AID$USERS
7615   LYBARGER PERSONAL$HA
7615   PICKETT SP-PROCESSING$AIDS
7631   HARDICK INCLUSION AUD$TRAINING$UNITS RULES HNG AIDS
7631   WARREN HNG$AIDS$REPAIRS MANUFACTURERS ALTERNATIVE$FACILITIES
7703   NAVARRO EARMOLD GERIATRIC$PATIENT
```

7703    ROESER HNG$AID$MALFUNCTION$DETECTION$UNIT
7703    WALDEN COMFORT$LEVEL$METHOD SETTING$HEARING$AID$GAIN
7704    TOWNSEND COMPARISON HEARING$AID$MEAS$SYSTEMS
7706    BURNETT ATTACK RELEASE$TIME AUTOMATIC-GAIN-CONTROL
        HNG$AIDS
7706    FELDMAN SIGNAL-PROCESSING$TECHNIQUES COMPUTERIZED
        $HNG$AID TEST$SYSTEM
7706    MAZOR MODERATE FREQUENCY$COMPRESSION MODERATELY$HNG
        $IMPAIRED
7711    EDGERTON R$BIAS HA$EVALUATIONS
7803    JIRSA RELATIONSHIP ACOUS$GAIN AIDED$THR$IMPROVEMENT
        CHILD
7804    PUNCH MEASUREMENT ATTACK-RELEASE$TIMES COMPRESSION
        $HEARING$AIDS
7806    PLOMP AUD$HANDICAP LIMITED$BENEFIT HA
7815    WILBER AMPLIFICATION ADOLESCENT
7816    EFFECT PROLONGED$HA$USE
7816    WITHROW AMPLFICATION EDUC DEAF
7827    MADELL AMPLIFICATION HNG-IMPAIRED$CHIL
7829    MENEGAUX SCREENING DEAFNESS YOUNG$CHILD


                            0203


5403    SUMMER$RESIDENTIAL$PROGRAM HNG$EDUC
5415    ADJUSTING NORMALLY$HNG
5415    BIBLIOGRAPHY TEACHING$DEAF
5415    DEAF$CHIL$EDUC
5415    DEAF$CHIL$EDUC DAY$SCH STATE$PROGRAM
5415    DEAF$CHIL$EDUC DAY$SCH
5415    DEAF$CHIL$EDUC PARENT
5415    DEAF$CHIL$EDUC PRIVATE$RESIDENTIAL$SCH
5415    DEAF$CHIL$EDUC SCH$PROGRAM
5415    DEAF$CHIL$EDUC
5415    DEAF$CHIL$EDUC RESIDENTIAL$SCH
5415    EMPLOYMENT$COUNSELING HARD$OF$HNG
5415    HOME-SCHOOL$REL
5415    NURSERY$DAY$SCH
5415    PREPARATION TEACHING$VOCAB
5415    READING$PROGRAM DEAF$SCH$CHIL
5415    RHYTHMS MUSIC HI
5415    SCHOOL
5415    SHAKESPEARE HARD$OF$HNG
5415    SOCIAL$STUDIES DEAF
5415    SPECIAL$EDUC DEAF

```
5415   TEACHING$READING HI$CHIL
5415   TEACHING$VOCAB SCH$SHOP
5415   WORKING DEAF$CHIL
5416   A SERVICE SCH$DEAF
5416   ASPECTS SCH$PLACEMENT DEAF$CHIL
5416   MEAS INTELLIGENCE DEAF$CHIL GRP$TEST
5416   STUDY PROCEEDINGS CONVENTION$AMERICAN$INSTRUCTORS
       $DEAF
5416   VOCATIONAL$APTITUDE$TEST$BATTERY DEAF
5503   SCH$ADJUSTMENT CHIL MINIMAL$HNG$LOSS
5515   ACADEMIC$PROGRAM SCH$DEAF
5515   ADVANTAGES ORAL$METHOD
5515   AUSTRALIAN$SCH DEAF$BOYS
5515   DAY$SCH DEAF
5515   DEAF$NURSERY$SCH
5515   EDUC HNG$HIGH$SCH
5515   EDUC PROFOUNDLY$DEAF$CHIL
5515   EDUC$NEEDS HI
5515   EDUCATIONAL$VOCATIONAL$COUNSELING DEAF$STUDENTS
5515   HARD$OF$HNG$CHIL SCH$DEAF
5515   LIFE HNG$WORLD
5515   LOS$ANGELES SCH$CLINICS HI
5515   NURSERY$SCH DEAF$CHIL
5515   PLANNING DEAF$CHIL SCH$AWAY$HOME
5515   READING
5515   READING DEAF$CHIL
5515   REL PERIPHERAL$FIELDS EDUC$DEAF
5515   TEACHER DEAF$CHIL
5515   TEACHING$FIRST$AID DEAF$CHIL
5515   VOCATIONAL$GUIDANCE
5516   AMERICAN$INSTRUCTORS$DEAF
5516   DOCTORS$DISSERTATIONS MA$THESES DEAF$EDUC
5516   EDWARD$MINER$GALLAUDET
5516   STUDY CONVENTION AMERICAN$INSTRUCTORS$DEAF
5516   STUDY PROCEEDINGS CONVENTION$AMERICAN$INSTRUCTORS
       $DEAF
5516   SURVEY CREDENTIAL$REQUIREMENTS TEACHERS$DEAF USA
5516   TEXTILES DEAF
5603   TEACHER$JUDGMENT HNG$LOSS CHIL
5615   EDUC$DEAF SCH$CALIFORNIA
5615   EDUC$DEAF INDONESIA
5615   GUIDING DEAF$CHIL FOLLOWING$INTERESTS READING
5615   HOME$PARENT$GUIDANCE ENGLAND
5615   HUMAN$RELATIONS PARENT$EDUC
5615   OLDER$DEAF$CHIL
5615   ORAL$EDUC DEAF
```

```
5615   PRESCH LANG$EDUC BRAIN-DAMAGED$CHIL
5615   PRESENTATION VISUAL$AIDS UPPER$GRADES
5615   PROGRAM ADULT$DEAF
5615   PSYCHOLOGICAL$DEV DEAF$CHIL PRESCH
5615   READING DEAF$CHIL
5615   READING DEAF$CHIL AUDIO-VISUAL$AIDS
5615   READING DEAF$CHIL TEXTBOOKS
5615   READING DEAF$CHIL TECHNIQUES READING$SKILLS
5615   READINGS$DEAF$CHI
5615   SLOW$LEARNING DEAF$CHIL
5615   TEACHER$TRNG PAKISTAN
5615   TEACHER$COMMENTS EDUC$DEAF ENGLAND
5615   TEACHING$CONCEPTS PRESCH$DEAF
5615   TEACHING$CONCEPTS HI$CHIL
5615   TEACHING$SAFETY HARD$OF$HNG$CHIL
5616   ACTIVITY$METHOD EDUC$DEAF
5616   COMM$THEORY EDUC$DEAF
5616   EDUC LIFE MISSISSIPPI$SCH NEGRO$DEAF PROGRAM
5616   NEW$APPROACHES TEACHING DEAF$CHIL
5616   PREDICTING SCH$ACHIEVEMENT DEAF$CHIL
5703   HOME$TEACHING DEAF$CHIL
5703   SURVEY FAMILIES JOHN$TRACY$COURSE
5715   BENEFITS ORAL$CLIMATE
5715   CHIL SEVERE$HI SCH HNG$CHIL
5715   CURRICULUM SCH DEAF
5715   DAY$SCH
5715   DEAF CLASSROOM$METHODS
5715   LANG$ARTS SCH$DEAF
5715   LIBRARY$WORK DEAF
5715   PARENTS DEAF$CHIL
5715   PROGRAM COMPTON AURAL$EDUCATION
5715   QUALIFICATIONS TEACHER$DEAF
5715   READINGS$LESSON FITZGERALD$KEY$HEADINGS
5715   RESEARCH INTEGRATION DEAF$CHIL
5715   SCH DEAF$CHIL
5715   SEX$EDUC DEAF$CHIL
5715   TEACHING$ENGLISH ADOL
5715   TEACHING USE TELEPHONE
5715   TEMPORARY$ENROLLMENT HARD$HNG$CHIL EDUC$PROGRAM DEAF
5715   TRANSATLANTIC$DIFFERENCES TEACHING DEAF$CHIL
5716   MATHEMATICS DEAF
5716   PERFORMANCE DEAF$COLLEGE$STUDENTS NON-VERBAL$INTELLIGENCE
       $TESTS
5716   PERSONALITY$CHARACTERISTICS RUBELLA$DEAF$CHIL IMPLICATIONS
       TEACHIN
5716   READING KEY PROGRESS DEAF$CHIL
```

5716  VOCATIONAL$EDUC GALLAUDETS
5803  HI$CHIL COMMUNITY$RECREATION$CAMPING$PROGRAMS
5809  EDUC$GUIDANCE DEAF$CHIL
5815  EDUC$DEAF IRON$CURTAIN
5815  EDUC$DEAF IRON$CURTAIN
5815  EDUCATION$DEAF IRON$CURTAIN
5815  IMPROVING$READING DEAF$CHIL
5815  PARENTS DEAF$CHIL
5815  PROBLEMS INSTRUCTION DEAF
5815  PROFILE HNG$SP GALLAUDET$COLLEGE$STUDENTS
5815  REL LANG READING
5815  STUDY PROGRESS ACADEMIC$ACHIEVEMENT CHIL$SCH
5815  TEACHING DEAF$CHIL THINK
5816  FEELINGS ATTITUDES DEAF VOCATIONAL$REHAB
5816  HEALTH$EDUC DEAF SCH
5816  HISTORICAL$BACKGROUND TYPES SCH METHODS COMM
5816  INSTITUTE PERSONAL SOCIAL VOCATIONAL ADJUSTMENT DEAFNESS
5816  MAXIMUM$USE COMMUNITY$RESOURCES DEAF$REHAB
5816  PSYCHIATRIC$ASPECTS
5816  PSYCHOLOGICAL$IMPLICATIONS INTEGRATION DEAF$CHIL HNG
      $CHIL
5816  RESOURCE$NEEDS DEAF
5816  RESOURCE$NEEDS DEAF
5816  VOCATIONAL$REHAB PRIVATE$AGENCY
5816  VOCATIONAL$REHAB OPPORTUNITY DEAF
5817  EDUC HI$CHIL SCH
5915  CAMPING DEAF$CHIL
5915  EDUC$DEAF USSR
5915  LANG SCH$CURRICULUM
5915  LANG$DEV FACTOR SCH$PLACEMENT
5915  ORAL$EDUC COLLEGE
5915  ORAL$EDUC DEAF$CHIL
5915  PREPARING$TEACHERS HARD$HNG SCH
5915  SCH CLASSES DEAF$CHIL
5915  SCREENING GROUP$READINESS
5915  SOCIAL$AWARENESS SOCIAL$STUDIES
5915  SOCIAL$LIFE RESIDENTIAL$SCH
5915  TEACHER DEAF$CHIL PARENTS
5915  TEACHER$PREPARATION COLLEGES
5916  ADMINISTRATIVE$PROCEDURES ADMISSION NEW$STUDENTS RESIDENTIAL
      $SCH$D
5916  EDUC$ACHIEVEMENT DEAF$CHIL
5916  LEGISLATION TEACHERS$DEAF
5916  SUGGESTIONS FAILURE FOLLOW TRADE LEARNED SCH
5916  TEACHING DEAF$CHIL READ
6003  HISTORICAL$ASPECTS MANUAL$COMM

| | |
|---|---|
| 6015 | DEAF$GRADS |
| 6015 | DISCIPLINE DEAF$CHIL |
| 6015 | EDUC$DEAF NEW$YORK |
| 6015 | EDUC$DEAF DENMARK |
| 6015 | EDUC$DEAF ATHENS |
| 6015 | EDUC$DEAF HAWAII |
| 6015 | EDUC$HI |
| 6015 | EXTRACURRICULAR$ACTIVITIES DEAF$CHIL |
| 6015 | OBSERVATIONS EDUC$DEAF NETHERLANDS USA |
| 6015 | ORGANIZATION DAY$CLASS |
| 6015 | PARENTAL$COUNSELING |
| 6015 | RECRUITING$TEACHERS DEAF |
| 6015 | RESIDENTIAL$SCH$CHIL COMMUNITY |
| 6015 | STUDY NEED TEACHERS$DEAF |
| 6015 | TEACHER DEAF$CHIL |
| 6015 | TEACHING$MACHINES DEAF |
| 6015 | TEACHING$DEAF PRESCH SOVIET$UNION |
| 6015 | TV DEAF$CHIL |
| 6016 | ART DEAF$CHIL |
| 6016 | EDUC$DEAF AUSTRALIA |
| 6016 | GRAD$TEACHER$TRNG DEAF$STUDENTS |
| 6016 | HELPING DEAF$CHIL ENG FINGER-SPELLING |
| 6016 | KENTUCKY$SCH$DEAF |
| 6016 | PROJECT FACILITATE TEACHING ARITHMETIC DEAF$CHIL |
| 6016 | PSYCHIATRIC-PREVENTIVE$SOCIOGENETIC$STUDY ADJUSTIVE $CAPACITIES |
| 6016 | USE PICTURES TEACHING DEAF$CHIL HOME |
| 6016 | WORKSHOP IDENTIFICATION VOCATIONAL$REHAB$PROBLEMS DEAF |
| 6103 | PRESCH$EDUC DEAF$CHIL |
| 6103 | URBAN$SCH$SERVICES CHIL$HI |
| 6104 | IDENTIFICATION TRNG INSTITUTIONALIZED$MR$DEAF$PATIENT |
| 6115 | DEAF$CHIL REGULAR$SCH |
| 6115 | FILMSTRIPS DEAF$CHIL |
| 6115 | MUSIC DEAF$CHIL |
| 6115 | NORMALITY DEAF$CHIL |
| 6115 | OFFERINGS TRENDS VOCATIONAL$EDUC |
| 6115 | ORAL$EDUC DEAF$CHIL |
| 6115 | PARENT$GRP SCH$PROGRAM |
| 6115 | SCH$CLASSES DEAF$CHIL |
| 6115 | SLOW-LEARNING DEAF$CHIL |
| 6115 | TEACHER$SHORTAGE NATIONAL$PROBLEM |
| 6115 | TEACHER$ROLE MENTAL$HEALTH |
| 6115 | TEACHING$CHIL DICTIONARY |
| 6115 | TEACHING DEAF$CHIL DANCE |
| 6115 | USE RESIDUAL$HNG EDUC DEAF$CHIL |

6116    GUIDELINES ESTABLISHMENT REHAB$FACILITIES DEAF
6116    INTEGRATION DEAF SCH$HNG
6116    LEADERSHIP$TRNG DEAF
6116    MECHANICAL$DEVICE TEACHING SIGHT$VOCAB DEAF$CHIL
6116    RESEARCH CLASSROOM$TEACHER$DEAF
6116    SIGN$LANG PROGRAMMED$LESSONS
6116    WORKSHOP CATHOLIC$PERSONNEL DEAF
6203    A DEAF$EDUC
6203    INTEGRATION HH$CHIL NORMAL$SCH
6215    ACADEMIC$EXPECTANCIES SLOW-LEARNING$DEAF$CHIL
6215    CHILD$STUDY EDUC$DEAF$CHIL
6215    DEAF$COLLEGE$STUDENT
6215    DEAF$GRADS HNG$GRADS
6215    EDUC$DEAF WESTERN$EUROPE
6215    HARD$HNG$CHIL CLASSROOM GUIDE TEACHER
6215    ORALISM ST.JOSEPH$INSTITUTES$DEAF
6215    READING DEAF
6215    READING$RATE VOCAB COMPREHENSION
6215    READING$RATE VOCAB COMPREHENSION
6215    REASONING$TRNG READING$COMPREHENSION
6215    ROLE AUDIOLOGIST SCH$DEAF
6215    SOCIAL$VOCATIONAL$PLANNING ADOL
6215    SPECIAL$EDUC STATE$RESIDENTIAL$SCH DEAF
6215    STUDY IMPROVING$PROGRAMS PREPARATION$TEACHERS$DEAF
6215    TALKING$DICTIONARY
6215    TEACHER$TRNG
6215    TV DEAF$CHIL CHICAGO
6216    A$SERVICES SCH$DEAF
6216    ADULT$EDUC DEAF
6216    AUDIOMETRIC$TESTING EDUC$SIGNIFICANCE DEAF
6216    CURRICULUM$NEEDS DEAF PRIMARY$LEVEL
6216    CURRICULUM$NEEDS COLLEGE$LEVEL
6216    CURRICULUM$NEEDS SECONDARY$LEVEL
6216    DIFFERENTIAL$EDUC$NEEDS HABILITATION REHAB DEAF
6216    GUIDANCE COUNSELING DEAF
6216    HIGHER$EDUC DEAF USA INVEST
6216    NEBRASKA$TEST$LEARNING$APTITUDE PRESCH$DEAF$CHIL
6216    PHILOSOPHY EDUC$DEAF
6216    PROBLEMS PARENTS DEAF$CHIL
6216    PSYCHIATRIC$CONSIDERATIONS DEAF$CHIL SCH
6216    WORKSHOP EPISCOPAL$WORKERS DEAF
6303    EDUC$STATUS HH$CHIL CLASSROOM
6305    CHANGING$ROLE DEAF$SCH
6315    APPLICATION PROGRAMMED$INSTRUCTION REMEDIAL$READING
        DEAF
6315    ART DEAF$CHIL

```
6315   DEAF$CHIL MR ACADEMIC$EXPECTANCIES
6315   EDUC$DEAF OREGON
6315   HOME$EDUC DEAF$CHIL NETHERLANDS
6315   IMPACT MULTIPLE$HANDICAPPED$DEAF SPECIAL$EDUCATION
6315   INTEGRATION HI
6315   PARENT-TEACHER$COOPERATION COMM DEAF$CHIL
6315   PRESCH$DEAF$CHIL
6315   PSYCHOLOGICAL$VARIABLES TRNG DEAF$CHIL
6315   RESEARCH EDUC$DEAF USA
6315   SOCIAL$VOCATIONAL$ASSESSMENT
6315   TEACHER$TRNG$CENTERS
6315   TELEPHONE DEAF
6316   APPLICATION PROGRAMMED$LEARNING DEAF$CHIL INDUSTRIAL
       $ARTS
6316   CRITIQUE QUESTION COLLEGE$ENROLLMENT DEAF USA
6316   EVOLUTION TEACHER$PREPARATION DEAF
6316   PROBLEMS SELECTION TRNG TEACHERS DEAF$CHIL
6316   ROLE USOE PREPARATION TEACHERS$DEAF
6316   STUDY PREDICTING SCH$ACHIEVEMENT DEAF$CHIL
6403   SEQUENCE$LEARNING APHASIC$CHIL DEAF$CHIL
6415   ACADEMIC$PREPARATION ADJUSTMENT CLASSES$HNG$STUDENTS
6415   ACADEMIC-VOCATIONAL$EDUC HI$CHIL
6415   COMMUNITY$LIVING BASIS CURRICULUM
6415   COMPARISON AUD$AMPLIFIERS CLASSROOM$DEAF
6415   COMPREHENSIVE$PROGRAMMING NEEDS ORAL$DEAF$CHIL
6415   COUNSELING DEAF$STUDENT
6415   CURRICULUM$CONTROL
6415   CURRICULUM SLOW$LEARNING$DEAF$CHIL
6415   ECONOMIC$REHAB EDUC$DEAF
6415   EDUC$PLACEMENT MULTIPLY$HANDICAPPED$HI$CHIL
6415   INFLUENCE PROGRAM$INSTRUCTION CONCEPTUAL$THINKING
       DEAF
6415   INSTITUTE$PARENTS DEAF$CHIL
6415   ISSUES EDUC$DEAF
6415   MR$HI$LEARNER
6415   MULTIPLY$HANDICAPPED WORKING$WORLD
6415   ORIENTATION NEW$TEACHERS
6415   OTOLOGICAL$CONSIDERATIONS PRESCH$HNG$PROGRAM
6415   PAIRED-ASSOCIATES$LEARNING MOVING$SEQUENCES DEAF$CHIL
6415   PAMPHLETS HI PROFESSIONAL
6415   PARENT$GUIDE HA CHIL
6415   PARENT$ROLE EDUC$PLANNING
6415   PARENTS DEAF$CHIL
6415   PARENTS DEAF$CHIL
6415   PERSONAL$HYGIENE ADOL
6415   PROGRAMMING ADOL
```

6415    READING GOALS ACHIEVEMENTS CLARKE$SCH$DEAF
6415    RESIDENTIAL VOCATIONAL$REHAB PROGRAM ADULTS$SEVERELY
        $HI
6415    RESIDENTIAL$SCH$COMMUNITY
6415    ROLE DEAF$TEACHER
6415    ROMAN$ALPHABET TEACHING$DEAF
6415    SCH$SUBJECTS DEAF
6415    SEPARATE$PROGRAMMING DEAF$HH
6415    SERVICES HI SPECIAL$SCH$DISTRICT
6415    SMALL$PERCEP$HNG$LOSS SCH$CHIL
6415    TEACHER$DEAF
6415    TEACHING$ART DEAF NIGERIA
6415    VISUAL$AIDS TEACHERS$DEAF
6415    VOCATIONAL$PREPARATION
6415    VOCATIONAL$COMPETENCE ACADEMIC$PREPARATION
6415    WYOMING$PROGRAM HI
6416    BASES PROGRAM EDUC DEAF$CHIL
6416    EDUC TEACHERS$DEAF
6416    EFFECTS PRESCH$TRNG DEV READING LR DEAF$CHIL
6416    READING$ALOUD SIGN$LANG
6503    CURRENT$STATUS VOCATIONAL$REHAB HNG$SP$DIS
6505    EDUC$HI$CHIL EUROPE
6515    ANALYSIS GROUP DEAF$STUDENTS COLLEGES$HNG
6515    CONTEXT$CLUES READING$PROGRAM DEAF
6515    DEAF$GRADUATES SCH$HNG
6515    EDUC$DEAF TORONTO
6515    EDUC$DEAF USA
6515    EDUC$RECOMMENDATIONS DEAF
6515    FUN DEAF$CHIL
6515    FUTURE VOCATIONAL$TECHNICAL$EDUC
6515    GUIDELINES EDUC$PROGRAMS HI$CHIL
6515    ORAL$EDUC LOUISIANA
6515    PARENT$RESPONSIBILITY DEAF$CHIL SOCIAL$ADJUSTMENT
6515    PROBLEMS INDUCT$LOOP$AMPLIFICATION
6515    READING$CONSULTANT SCH$DEAF
6515    SCH$CLASSES$PRESCH DEAF$CHIL
6515    SCH$CLASSES DEAF$CHIL
6515    SECONDARY$EDUC DEAF$CHIL
6515    TEACHING$MUSIC DEAF$CHIL
6516    DEMONSTRATIONS
6516    EVAL EFFECTIVENESS LEADERSHIP$TRNG$PROGRAM DEAF
6516    FINGERSPELLING ORAL$CLASSROOM
6516    IMPLICATIONS LEARNING$THEORY EDUC HI
6516    PROBLEMS AUDIOVISUAL$EDUC DEAF
6516    PROJECT$LIFE LANG$IMPROVEMENT EDUC HI$CHIL
6516    PURPOSE SCIENCE CURRICULUM DEAF

6516    RESEARCH$BASIS READING$INSTRUCTION DEAF$CHIL
6516    RESPONSIVE$ENVIRONMENTS$PROJECT DEAF
6516    TEACHING CARD$PUNCH$OPERATORS USE FILMED$LESSONS
6516    UNDERACHIEVEMENT DEAF$CHIL
6516    USE EDUC$MEDIA TECHNIQUES DEAF$SCH
6615    CHANGE$TEACHING HI$CHIL
6615    CURRICULUM LOW-ACHIEVING$HI
6615    DEAF$COLLEGE$STUDENT
6615    EDUC$DEAF USA REVIEW$RECOMMENDATIONS
6615    EDUC$HI EUROPE
6615    FEDERAL$PROGRAM TRNG$TEACHERS$DEAF
6615    HH$CHIL EDUC$DEAF
6615    HI$RETARDED$READER
6615    HIGHER$LEARNING DEAF
6615    ORALISM
6615    PROBLEMS DAY$CLASS$PROGRAM
6615    RELIGIOUS$EDUC DEAF STATE$RESIDENTIAL$SCH
6615    STATUS
6615    SUPERVISION EXPERIENCES STUDENT$TEACHING
6615    TADOMA$METHOD
6615    UNITS DEAF$CHIL
6616    ADMINISTRATIVE$PROBLEMS EDUC$DEAF
6616    AUD$CHANNEL EDUC$DEAF$CHIL
6616    EDUC$OPPORTUNITY DEAF$CHIL
6616    MULTI-MEDIA$APPROACH CLASSROOM$DEAF
6616    ROLE RESIDENTIAL$SCH PREPARING$DEAF$ADOL MARRIAGE
6616    VOCATIONAL$NEEDS EDUC$PROGRAMS DEAF$ADOL
6704    EFFECTS DELAY$EARLY$TREAMENT DEAFNESS
6715    CAMPING DEAF$CHIL
6715    DAY$CLASSES DEAF COVINA$PLAN
6715    DEAF$GRAD$SURVEY
6715    DEAF$STUDENTS HNG$COLLEGE
6715    EDUC$DEAF ROLE$LANG
6715    MR HI
6715    NON-LANG$IQ$TESTS DEAF$PUPILS
6715    NYC$ADOL$PROGRAM$DEAF
6715    ORTHOGRAPHIC$SYSTEMS EDUC$DEAF
6715    PARENT$COUNSELING
6715    PARENT-ORIENTED$NURSERY$PROGRAM PRESCH$DEAF$CHIL
6715    PUBLIC$LAW TRNG$TEACHERS$DEAF
6715    TEXAS$FACILITIES DEAF$CHIL
6716    ORAL$MULTISENSORY$APPROACH PRELINGUAL$DEAF$CHIL ROCHESTER
        $METHOD
6804    EFFECTS DELAY$EARLY$TREATMENT DEAFNESS
6807    EXPERIENCE WORK HNG$FIELD SCH$DEAF-MUTE$CHIL
6807    OTIATRIC$OBSERVATION SCH$PRESCH DEAF-MUTE$HH

6815    CALIFORNIA$PROGRAM HI$CHIL
6815    COMPUTER-ASSISTED$INSTRUCTION TEACHING$DEAF
6815    CURRICULUM DEAF
6815    EDUC$TREATMENT DEAFNESS KENT
6815    EDUCATIONAL$MEDIA DEAF$EDUC LITERATURE
6815    HEAD$START$PROGRAM DEAF$CHIL
6815    HI$STUDENTS SUPPORTIVE$PROGRAMS
6815    HOME$DEMONSTRATION PARENTS DEAF$CHIL
6815    IDENTIFICATION TRNG DEAF$CHIL$INF
6815    MCGINNIS HI$CHIL
6815    ORAL$EDUC
6815    ORAL$EDUC
6815    PARENTS$DEAF$CHIL SUGGESTIONS CHILD$MANAGEMENT
6815    PROBLEM$ADOL
6815    PROJECT EMOTIONALLY$DISTURBED$DEAF$BOYS
6815    SOCIAL$STUDIES DEAF$CHIL
6815    SPECIAL$EDUC IMC
6815    STRUCTURED$PROGRAM LEARNING MR$DEAF$ADULTS
6815    VISUAL$IMPAIRMENT DEAF$CHIL EDUC$CONSEQUENCES
6816    DESIGN USE TECHNICAL$AIDS TRNG$DEAF$HH$CHIL
6816    PROGRAMMED$INSTRUCTION SWEDISH$DEAF$CHIL
6904    LEARNING$LIMITS DEAF$CHIL CODED$SP
6915    ADOL$HI$STUDENTS
6915    APPLICATION RESEARCH$ATTITUDE CLASSROOM$TEACHING HI
        $CHIL
6915    CIRCUIT$TV TRAIN$TEACHERS$DEAF
6915    DEAF-BLIND$CENTERS
6915    DENMARK COTTAGE$SYSTEM HOME$ENVIRONMENT DEAF$CHIL
6915    EDUC$DEAF INDIA
6915    FACTORS HI$COLLEGE$STUDENT
6915    FINGER$PAINT HA
6915    GUIDELINES MODEL$PRESCH
6915    PARENTS CINCINNATI RELIGIOUS$EDUC HI$CHIL
6915    PARENTS DEAF$CHIL
6915    PLAY DEAF$CHIL
6915    SUMMER$PROGRAM PARENTS DEAF$CHIL
6915    TEACHING$DEAF OVERHEAD$PROJECTORS
6915    USE MULTIMEDIA WYOMING$SCH$DEAF
6915    VIDEO-TAPE TEACHING$TOOL DEAF$EDUC
6915    VISUAL$SYSTEM TEACHER-GROUP$INTERACTION EDUC$DEAF
        $CHIL
6915    WORK-STUDY$PROGRAM HI$STUDENTS
6916    EDUC$DEAF DEAF$CHIL ENGLAND
6916    GRAMMAR NOUN$PHRASES ARITHMETIC$INSTRUCTION DEAF$CHIL
6916    HISTORY EDUC$DEAF PHILIPPINES
6916    MOTIVATING TRNG INSTITUTIONALIZED$DEAF

```
6916   OPERANT$CONDITIONING$TECHNIQUES DEAF$SCH
6916   PRELINGUAL$DEAF$CHIL ORAL$EDUC
7015   DEAF$CHIL SEVENTIES
7015   DRIVING$STIMULATOR WAY TEACH DEAF$DRIVERS
7015   EDUC$DEAF PENNSYLVANIA
7015   EDUC$PROVISIONS MR$DEAF$STUDENTS RESIDENTIAL$INSTITUTIONS
7015   FREE$PLAY LEARNING$EXPERIENCE
7015   ORAL$METHOD
7015   ORALISM
7015   PARENT$COUNSELING DEAF
7015   PARENTS$CHALLENGE EDUC PARENTS DEAF
7015   POST-SECONDARY$OPPORTUNITIES DEAF$STUDENTS
7015   PUBLIC$SCH MULTIPLY$HANDICAPPED$DEAF$CHIL
7015   RATIONALE ORAL$METHOD
7015   SCH$INTEGRATION DEAF
7015   TEACHING$DEAF INDIA
7015   TECHNICAL$TRNG DEAF$STUDENTS COMMUNITY$COLLEGE
7015   TRADE$TECHNICAL$PROGRAM DEAF$HH$STUDENTS
7015   TREATMENT DEAFNESS ENGLAND USA
7015   USE VIDEO$TAPE PROGRAMS$DEAF
7015   VOCATIONAL$EDUC DEAF$ADOL
7016   TOTAL$COMM
7104   IMITATIVE$ALTRUISM DEAF$CHIL
7104   PAIRED$ASSOC$ROTE$LEARNING DEAF
7104   SOCIAL$CLASS CODE$ELABORATION ORAL$COMM
7115   ACADEMIC-VOCATIONAL$PROGRAM MULTIPLY$HANDICAPPED$DEAF
7115   CHARACTERISTICS SUCCESSFUL$STUDENT$TEACHERS$DEAF
7115   MENTAL$ASSESSMENT DEAF$CHIL
7115   MUSIC TEACHING DEAF
7115   PARENT-ORIENTED$NURSERY$PROGRAM PRESCH$DEAF$CHIL
7115   POLAROID$CAMERA TEACHING LANG
7115   READING$COMPREHENSION HI$ADOL
7115   SEX$EDUC DEAF$CHIL
7115   STUDIES MANUAL$COMM HI$CHIL
7115   SYSTEM$COLOR$CODING$EARMOLDS DEAF$SCH
7115   VOLUNTEER$ASSISTANCE DEAF$PRESCH
7116   EFFECTS ORAL$PRESCH EARLY$MANUAL$COMM EDUC COMM DEAF
       $CHIL
7116   PREVALENCE BEHAVIORAL$PROBLEMS DEAF$SCH$CHIL
7204   COMPARISON RUBELLA NONRUBELLA DEAF$ADULTS IMPLICATIONS
       LEARNING
7205   MANAGEMENT HI SOUTH$VIETNAM
7208   INCIDENCE HI LEARNING$DISABLED$STUDENTS
7214   SOCIAL$CLASS CODE$ELABORATION WRITTEN$COMM
7215   EDUC$HI ILLINOIS
7215   HI$CHIL CLASSROOM
```

7215    MODEL FACILITATIVE$PROGRAM HI$COLLEGE$STUDENTS
7215    NORMALIZATION REALITY
7215    ORALISM$AURALISM TOTAL$COMM
7215    PARENT$APPROACH LANG DAILY$JOURNAL
7215    PARENT$VIEW INTEGRATION
7215    RATIONALE TOTAL$COMM
7215    STATE$CERTIFICATION SERVICES HI
7215    TOTAL$COMM
7215    TUTORING HI$STUDENTS SCH
7216    SIGN$LANG$ACQUISITION TEACHING DEAF$CHIL
7303    TOTAL$COMM
7315    ABILITY$SCREENING PROGRAM$PLACEMENT DEAF-BLIND$CHIL
        $ADULTS
7315    ADJUSTING INTEGRATION HI$CHIL PUBLIC$SCH
7315    COMPETENCIES TEACHERS$DEAF HI$INF PARENTS
7315    CRITICISM DIRECT$DISCOURSE PRIMARY$LEVEL$BASAL$READERS
7315    EDUC$DEAF ST.MICHIELSGESTEL$NETHERLANDS
7315    FAMILY$EDUC DEAF ALASKA
7315    INTEGRATION HI$STUDENTS SCH
7315    LISTEN INTEGRATED$PRESCH
7315    PARENT$EDUC
7315    PARENT$POTENTIAL DEAF
7315    PARENTS DEAF
7315    RESOURCE$ROOM
7315    RESOURCE$ROOM HI$STUDENTS
7315    ROLE$TEACHERS$DEAF
7315    SERVICES PRESCH$HI SWEDEN
7315    SERVICES PRESCH$HI$SWEDEN
7315    SEX$EDUC DEAF CLARKE$SCH
7315    STRATEGIES TEACHERS$DEAF$ORAL$SCH
7403    AURALLY$HANDICAPPED$CHIL
7403    TEACHING$ENGLISH$SECOND$LANG DEAF$CHIL
7405    DISTRIBUTION HNG$LOSS STUDENTS$EDUCATIONAL$PROGRAMS
        HNG$IMP
7408    INTEGRATION CHILDREN LIMITED$HEARING
7415    APPROACHES LEARNING$PROCESSES DEAF
7415    CURRICULUM PRESCH$DEAF
7415    DEAF$EDUC
7415    FACILITATING$INTEGRATION ADOL
7415    ORAL$AURAL TEACHER$PREPARATION
7415    PARENT$PERSPECTIVE DEAF HH
7415    PARENTS DEAF$ADULTS EDUC$OPPORTUNITIES DEAF$CHIL
7415    PARENTS$DEAF TEACHING$RESOURCE
7415    POST-RUBELLA$CHIL SPECIAL$EDUC HI
7415    READING$ACHIEVEMENT DEAF
7415    STUDY SEMANTICS DEAFNESS

7417    DEAF$CHIL SURVEY PROCEDURES OHIO
7417    EDUC PRESCH$HI$CHIL FAMILY
7503    JENSEMA CHIL HNG$IMPAIRED MUMPS
7508    NOBER HI/FI$PROGRAM
7511    CARSON LEARNING DEAF$CHIL
7515    BALDWIN QUALITY$PROGRAMS HI CHILD
7515    BALOW READING ACAD$ACHIEVEMENT GRAD$CLEASSES CALIF
7515    FALLIS INTEGRATED$LEARNING CHILD HI
7515    FELLENDORF TRENDS FUTURE$GOALS
7515    HEHIR COMPETENCE BASED TEACHER$EDUC
7515    ISRAEL HA
7515    JENSEMA EDUC$ACHIEVEMENT OF ODAS$MEMBERS
7515    NAKANO ORAL$EDUC HI CHILD JAPAN
7515    NOBER IN-SERVICE$PROGRAM INTEGRATING$HI CHILD
7515    RISTER DEAF$CHILD MAINSTREAMING$EDUC
7515    ROBINSON TESTING TRAINING PRELINGUISTIC HI
7516     ACHIEVEMENT$TEST$SCORES MULTIPLY$HANDICAPPED$CHILD
7516     ASSESSMENT INSTRUCTION
7516     COMM-BASED EARLY$CHILDHOOD$PROGRAMS DEAF
7516     DAAF CHILD VS BOARD EDUC
7516     DEAF$CHILD SOLVE ADDITION SUBTRACTION
7516     EFFECTS COMM$METHODS LEARNING
7516     ESL$APPROACH TEACHING ENGLISH
7516     HI INSTITUTIONS RETARDED
7516     INTEGRATION DEAF HRING$STUDENTS
7516     MAINSTREAMING
7516     ROCHESTER$METHOD FLORIDA$SCHOOL
7516     SOVIET$RESEARCH EDUC
7516     TELEVISION TEACHING$TOOL DEAF$STUDENTS
7516     USE SIGN$LANG TEACHING$ENGLISH
7531    CRANDALL ASSESSMENT READING+WRITING$ADULT$DEAF
7531    FRISINA CAREERS TECHNOLOGY NTID
7531    JOHNSON COMMUNICATION NTID$STUDENTS
7531    SUBTELNY COMMUNICATION NTID$STUDENTS PLANNING REHAB
7615    CALVERT COMM$PRACTICES AURAL/ORAL VISUAL/ORAL
7615    CRAIG CURRICULUM PERSPECTIVES  PROSPECTS
7615    HEALEY INTEGRATED$EDUC
7615    HOAG TEACHERS DEAF
7615    KINDRED INTEGRATION SECONDARY$SCHOOL
7615    LANE ORAL$ADVOCACY
7615    WENTLING CAREER$EDUC EVAL HI ADOLESCENTS
7616     COMM$TRENDS
7616     COMPARATIVE$STUDIES ACADEMIC$ACHIEVEMENT
7616     COMPARISON RUBELLA NON-RUBELLA$STUDENTS
7616     COUNSELING SCHOOLS DEAF
7616     DEAF$STUDENTS GROUP$PROBLEM$SOLVING$SITUATIONS

7616    EFFECTS TOTAL$COMM ORALISM
7616    HIGH$SCHOOL MAINSTREAMING
7616    MAINSTREAMING COST$ISSUE
7616    TEACHING LANG MR DEAF$CHILD
7616    UPDATE POSTSECONDARY$PROBLEMS
7715    ALLEN PARENT$ROLE PL$
7715    BALDWIN POSITION TEACHER HI$CHIL
7715    BLAIR AMPLIFICATION SPEECHREADING CLASSROOM
7715    CASTLE TELEPHONE$TRNG DEAF
7715    FOLTS DEAF$CHIL MUSICAL$INSTRUMENT
7715    GJERDINGEN UNIVERSITIES DEAF$STUDENTS
7715    LING IEP HI$CHIL
7715    MCCLURE ACAD$ACHIEVEMENT MAINSTREAMED$HI$CHIL RUBELLA
7715    MURPHY COUNSELING
7715    NOBER SUPPORT$SERVICES MAINSTREAMED$HI$CHIL
7715    NORTHCOTT ORAL$INTERPRETER HEARING$IMPAIRED
7715    ROSS GUIDELINES AUDIOLOGY$PROGRAMS EDUCATIONAL$SETTINGS
        HI$CHIL
7715    SAKS VANCOUVER$ORAL$CENTRE DEAF$CHIL
7715    SCHEIN CURRENT$PRIORITIES DEAFNESS
7716    CAPTIONED$FILMS
7716    CONTINUING$EDUC DEAF$ADULTS
7716    EDUC DEAF
7716    EDUCATIONAL$NEEDS BLACK$DEAF$CHILD
7716    INTEGRATION HI$CHILD
7716    MAINSTREAMING DEAF$STUDENTS
7716    MEDIA$EXPERIENCE DEAF$EDUC
7716    MINICOURSES DEAF$STUDENTS
7716    MODEL$EVALUATION$SYSTEM TEACHER$EDUC$PROGRAM
7716    PUBLIC$LAWS
7716    REVIEW LITERATURE INSTRUCTIONAL.TELEVISTION
7716    USE ADAPTED CLASSICS READING$PROGRAM
7815    AUSTIN GUIDANCE CURRICULUM DEAF$ADOLESCENT
7815    BECKER PERSONAL$SOCIAL$MATURITY
7815    CASTLE POSTSECONDARY$EDUCATION$OPPORTUNITIES
7815    CRANDALL READING$WRITING$SKILLS DEAF$ADOLESCENT
7815    DIFRANCESCA THINKING$SKILLS CAREER$EDUCATION
7815    DOEHRING READING$SKILLS INTEGRATED$HI$CHIL
7815    HICKS DEMONSTRATION$SCHOOLS GALLAUDET$COLLEGE
7815    LANE CAPACITY INDEPENDENT$LIVING
7815    LING MATHEMATIC HI$CHIL
7815    MELTZER MAINSTREAMING PARENT
7815    NEYHUS ASSESSMENT IEP
7815    ROSS MAINSTREAMING
7815    SCHMITT TRAINING$PERSONNEL HEARING-IMPAIRED$ADOLESCENTS
7815    SHAH DELAY REFERRAL CHIL IMPAIRED$HEARING

```
7815    STINSON DEAFNESS MOTIVATION ACHIEVEMENT
7816     COMPETENCIES TEACHER$TRAINING
7816     DEAF READ
7816     DEAF$ADOLESCENTS COMP INFO
7816     DEAF$EDUC WEST$GERMANY
7816     DEAF$STUDENTS POSTSECONDARY$SCHOLLS
7816     EDUC$PROGRAMS$SERVICES
7816     IMPACT PL$
7816     IMPULSE$CONTROL
7816     MEASUREMENT$ERROR ACHIEVEMENT$TESTS
7816     PARAPROFESSIONAL$TUTORS NOTETAKERS
7816    ASPECTS TOTAL$COMM
7816    BRANSFORD COMM$SATELLITES APPLICATIONS HI
7816    CACCAMISE SIGN$LANG SIMULTANEOUS$COMM
7816    CAREER$DEV$PROGRAMS RESIDENTIAL$SCHOOLS
7816    CARR
7816    CERF ELECTRONIC$MAILBOX COMM$TCOL HI
7816    CERTIFICATION$REQUIREMENTS TEACHERS DEAF
7816    CURRICULUM DEAF$CHILD BORROWING
7816    DUGDALE COMPUTER-BASED$INSTRUCTION HI$CHILD
7816    EARLY$EDUC HI
7816    KELLY HEMISPHERIC$SPECIALIZATION DEAF$CHILD
7816    MCLEAN STATUS MEDIA$MATERIALS$CENTER
7816    NOMELAND TECHNOLOGY KENDALL$DEMONSTRATION SCHOOL
7816    OUTDOOR$LEARNING$EXPERIENCE
7816    PROPP EDUC$TECHNOLOGY HI
7816    PURVIS VIDEODISC
7816    R STATE$DEPT EDUC
7816    RESIDENTIAL$PROGRAM DEAF$MULTI-HANDICAPPED
7816    RICHARDSON COMPUTER$SUPPORT INSTRUCTIONAL$SYSTEM MATH
7816    SEX$EDUCATOR
7816    STATEWIDE$PLANNING EDUC HI
7816    SURVEY MATERIALS PROCEDURES TEACH READING
7816    THAYN MEDIA$TECHNOLOGY DEV COMM,SKILLS DEAF
7816    TORR GALLAUDET$COLLEGE MEDIA$APPLICATIONS
7816    VOCATIONAL$EVAL$SERVICES HI
7816    WATSON INSTRUCTIONAL$TECHNOLOGY MODEL$SECONDARY$SCHOOL
7827    PERMAN READING$ATTAINMENT HNG-IMPAIRED$CHIL
```

0204

```
5406    VISUAL$CONTRIBUTION SP$INTELLIGIBILITY NOISE
5415    LK$LESSON SHORT$A
5415    READING$LIPS
```

```
5415   TEACHER$LR
5415   VOCAB SPEECHREADING
5515   LR$EXERCISE
5515   LR$FUN
5515   TV$MEDIUM TEACHING$SPEECHREADING$SP
5603   LR$ABILITY PSYCHOLOGICAL$FACTORS
5615   LR TV
5615   SP$SEE
5715   BEGINNING$SPEECHREADING
5715   LR HA COMPREHENSION
5815   LANG$DEV SPEECHREADING
5815   VISUALIZED$LANG
5816   EXPLORATORY$INVEST METHOD IMPROVING$SPEECHREADING
5816   EXPLORATORY$INVEST METHOD IMPROVING$SPEECHREADING
5816   FACTORS LR
5904   FACTORS LR
5904   LR RATE$SPEAKER
5904   REL FILMED$LR$TESTS
5914   AGE$DIFFERENCES ABILITY VISUAL$CUES AUD$COMM
5914   AGE$DIFFERENCES ABILITY VISUAL$CUES AUD$COMM
5915   COMBINING AUD$VISUAL$STIMULI
5915   SPEECHREADING CLOSED$CIRCUIT$TV
5918   EFFECTIVENESS INSTRUCTIONAL$FILMS LR
5920   TV$LR
6004   PHONEME$PERCEP LR
6004   VISUAL$WORD$RECOGNITION DEAF$CHIL
6016   COMM GESTURES
6016   PARENTS HELP DEAF$CHIL SPEECHREADING
6103   SP$READING SP$MATERIALS
6104   DISTANCE FINGERSPELLING
6104   LR LETTER$PREDICTION
6115   LR TV
6203   CONCEPT$ATTAINMENT LR$ABILITY DEAF$ADOL
6203   ITEM$SELECTION SPEECHREADING$TEST SCALOGRAM$ANALYSIS
6216   LR
6303   SELF-ADMINISTERED$TRNG LR
6303   TACTUAL$COMM SP DEAF COMPARISON LR
6403   SENTENCE$FAMILIARITY FACTOR LR
6415   COMPARISON SPEECHREADING HINDI$ENGLISH SCH$DEAF
6515   RATIONALE LR$THERAPY
6516   PROGRAMMED$DISCRIM$TRNG LR
6516   USE AUDIOVISUAL$TECHNIQUES EXPAND LR AUD$EXPERIENCES
       DEAF$CHIL
6603   LR$TEST NONORGANIC$DEAFNESS
6615   SPEECHREADING$LABORATORY DEAF$CHIL
6704   DEV MULTIPLE-CHOICE$TEST LR
```

6704   FACTOR$ANALYTIC$STUDY SPEED$VISUAL$PERCEP LANG$ABILITIES
       DEAF$ADOL
6704   FACTORS IDENTIFICATION ENG$SOUNDS LR
6715   METHOD TEACHING$LR PROGRAMMED$LEARNING
6715   TEACHING$LR SCH$DEAF SOUTH$AFRICA
6716   CUED$SP
6804   CONFUSIONS VISUALLY$PERCEIVED$CONSONANTS
6804   EFFECTS SIMULTANEOUS$SUCCESSIVE$STIMULUS$PRESENTATIONS
       VISUAL$DISC
6804   VISUAL$DISCRIM CONSONANTS
6815   SPEECHREADING$TEST$CHIL
6816   WEARABLE$EYEGLASS$SPEECHREADING$AID
6904   SPEED VISUAL$PERCEP DEAF$CHIL
6909   VISUAL$DISCRIM CONSONANTS
6916   CUED$SP CONSIDERATIONS
7004   LR REL MEAS VISION
7004   MEAS VISUAL$SP$COMPREHENSION
7004   SPEECHREADING SYNTHESIS DISTORTED$PRINTED$SENTENCES
7104   EFFECTS DISTANCE VISUAL$RECEPTION SP
7104   RELATIVE$CONTRIBUTION VISUAL$AUD$COMPONENTS SP SP
       $INTELLIGIBILITY
7104   SENTENCE$FAMILIARITY FACTOR LR DEAF$COLLEGE$STUDENTS
7503   ERBER AUDITORY-VISUAL$PERCEPTION SP
7512   FARRAN PERCEPTUAL$FEATURES SPEECHREADING
7531   JACOBS PROGRAMMED$SELF INSTRUCTION SPEECHREADING
7603   BINNIE VISUAL$INTELLIGIBILITY CONSONANTS LR$SCREENING
       $TEST
7603   JOHNSON ACQUISITON LR DEAF$MULTIHANDICAPPED$CHILD
7604   DANHAUER INDSCAL CONSONANTS VISUAL-TACTILE INPUTS
7604   ERBER EFFECTS SENTENCE$CONTEXT LIPREADING DEAF$CHILDREN
7604   JACKSON PERCEP$DIMENSIONS VOWEL$LIPREADING
7616    EMPIRICAL$INVESTIGATION VISIBLE$ENGLISH
7629   WINKELAAR SPEECHREADING$ABILITIES LIVE RECORDED PRESENTATIONS
7704   SHEPHERD VISUAL-NEURAL$CORRELATE SPEECHREADING
7704   WALDEN EFFECTS TRAINING VISUAL$RECOGNITION CONSONANTS
7711   COZAD SPEECHREADING COMM$DIFFICULTY CHILD ADULTS UNILATERAL
       $HL
7716    INFO$RECEPTION LIVE+VISUAL$MOTION$MEDIA
7806   ERBER VOICE/MOUTH$SYNTHESIS TACTUAL/VISUAL$PERCEPTION
7812   FARRAN PERCEPUAL$FEATURES SPEECHREADING
7815   PERRY LIPREADING$CURRICULUM ADULTS

                        0205

5415   AUD$TRNG POSSIBILITIES$LIMITATIONS

```
5415   AUD$TRNG
5415   AUD$TRNG PRESCH$CHIL
5415   AUD$TRNG HARD$OF$HNG$CHIL
5415   AUD$TRNG DIVERGENT$VIEW
5515   AUD$TRNG$PROGRAM HOUSTON$SCH$DISTRICT
5515   AUD$TRNG
5515   AUD$TRNG ST.$JOSEPHS$INSTITUTE
5515   AUD$TRNG SCH$DEAF
5515   HINTS AUD$TRNG CHIL
5615   AUD$TRNG PRIMARY$GRADES
5615   PROBLEMS AUD PERCEP UNDERSTANDING
5715   APPROACH AUD$TRNG
5715   EXPERIENCE AUD$TRNG
5815   DEAF$CHIL EXPERIENCES AUD$TRNG
5815   EFFECT HNG$OWN$VOICE CHIL$HI
5815   FREQUENCY$DISCRIM DEAF$CHIL REL ACHIEVEMENT AUD$TRNG
5815   GOALS AUD$TRNG SCH$DEAF
5816   CONSIDERATIONS AUD$TRNG
5915   AUD$TRNG TECHNIQUES
5915   AUD$TRNG PRINCIPLES
5915   AUD$TRNG SOURCES$AUD$EXPERIENCES
5915   AUD$TRNG
6204   SOUND$DISCRIM FUNCTION PRETRNG$CONDITIONS
6405   UNISENSORY$PROGRAM HI$CHIL
6415   ACOUPEDICS UNI-SENSORY$AUDITORY$TRNG
6415   AUD$APPROACH PRESCH$DEAF$CHIL
6516   AUD$TRNG$PROGRAM DEAF$CHIL
6615   FORMANTS AUD$TRNG DEAF$CHIL
6710   SELF-ADMINISTERED$TECHNIQUE AUD$TRNG
6711   ELECTRONICS$SP$PROCESSING$METHODS HNG$IMP
6711   INCREASED$INTELLIGIBILITY HYPACUSIC SLOW-PLAY$FREQ
       $TRANSPOSITION
6715   EXPERIENCE AUD$TRNG
6807   AUD$WORK SCH$HH$CHIL
6807   FUNDAMENTALS METHODOLOGY DEV AUD$PERCEP DEAF-MUTE
       $CHIL
6807   PERCEP$SP BLIND$DEAF-MUTES CUTANEOUS$ANALYSOR
6807   STUDY RETRNG HNG CHIL SEVERE$HNG$LOSS
6807   UTILIZATION DEV AUD$PERCEP SCH$HH$CHIL
6816   INSTRUMENT ARTIFICIAL$SP$SPECTRA HH
6915   LOOP$AUD$TRNG PRESCH$HI$CHIL
6915   TAPE$RECORDINGS GERMANY AUD$TRNG AUD$EDUC
6916   CRITIQUE CURRENT$AUD$TRNG$EQUIPMENT
6916   LOOP$INDUCTION$SYSTEM
6920   RESEARCH SLOW-PLAYED$SP LISTENER$TRNG CONSONANT$ERRORS
7004   AUD$TRNG SP$DISCRIM
```

7004   MEAS LISTENING HI$CHIL
7004   ROLE$PRACTICE OBSERVATION$PRACTICE SP$DISCRIM$LEARNING
7011   EFFECTS SYSTEMATIC$RF SP$DISCRIM HI$CHIL
7011   LEARNING$SP$DISCRIM HI$CHIL
7015   PIONEERS AUD$TRNG
7017   AUD$STIMULATION TRNG DEAF
7103   MODIFICATION SP$DISCRIM BINAURAL$ASYMMETRICAL$HNG
       $LOSS
7104   FREQ$TRANSPOSITION TEACHING$SP DEAF$CHIL
7104   PROGRAMMED$INSTRUCTION HI$CHIL AUD$DISCRIM VOWELS
7115   AUD$TRNG
7211   HI$CHIL FILTERED$SP
7215   AUD$TRNG HOME
7215   LISTEN ACOUPEDIC$PROGRAM
7315   PARENT$REPORT AUD$APPROACH
7316   INVEST RADIO$FREQ$AUD$TRNG$UNITS
7415   AUD$TRNG
7503   ERBER AUDITORY-VISUAL$PERCEPTION SP
7504   DANAHER MASKING LOW-FREQ$VOWEL$FORMANTS SENSORINEURAL
       $HL
7504   FRANKLIN COMBINING$LOW + HIGH-FREQ$PASSBANDS CONSONANT
       $RECOG HI
7515   GRAMMATICO DEV LISTENING$SKILLS
7531   MOORE PROGRAMMED$SELF-INSTRUCTION AUD$TRNG
7531   MOOREHNG$CHARACTERSTICS IMPLICATIONS AUD$TRNG
7604   BILGER CONSONANT$CONFUSIONS SENSORI-NEURAL$HL
7611   BALDWIN GENERALIZATION VOWEL$DISCRIM$LEARNING HI$CHIL
7615   CLARKE CUED$SP
7615   ERBER AUDIO$TAPE-CARDS AUD-TRAINING
7803   OWENS CONSONANT$ERRORS REMEDIATION SN$HL
7827   SIGER FORENSIC$APPROACH HNG SP


                        0206


5406   DESIGN VISIBLE$SP$DEVICES
5515   AUDIOLOGY DEAF$CHIL
5515   VISIBLE$SP
5515   VISUAL$AID$TRAINER
5609   HNG$THERAPY CHIL
5615   CALIFORNIA REHAB$DEAF
5615   RESULTS JOHN$TRACY$CORRESPONDENCE$COURSE
5616   FOLLOW-UP ADJUSTMENT$PROBLEMS ACOUS$HANDICAPPED TECHNIQUES
5816   A$ASPECTS REHAB$DEAF
5816   REHAB$DEAF

| | |
|---|---|
| 5903 | SEMIDIAGNOSTIC$TEST$MATERIALS AURAL$REHAB |
| 6003 | DIAGNOSTIC$APPROACH AURAL$REHAB |
| 6006 | PITCH$INDICATOR TRNG$DEAF |
| 6017 | CENTER TEAM$APPROACH REHAB HH$CHIL |
| 6215 | VISIBLE$SP |
| 6216 | AUDIOMETRIC$EVAL REL HABILITATION REHAB DEAF |
| 6216 | DEAF$REHAB |
| 6304 | COMM$SP$SOUNDS TACTUAL$VOCODER |
| 6415 | INTEGRATION AUD$TRNG LR |
| 6505 | DIAGNOSTIC$REHAB$ASPECTS GERIATRIC$A |
| 6507 | AUD$REHAB HI$BLIND$PERSONS |
| 6615 | COMM$TRNG HI$ADULTS |
| 6615 | MODIFICATION$VOICE DEAF$CHIL |
| 6803 | DIAGNOSTIC-THERAPY$SETTING HI$CHIL |
| 6807 | DESIGN ELECTROACOUS$DEVICE HH$DEAF-MUTE$CHIL |
| 6815 | ADVICE$PARENTS DEAF$CHIL |
| 6815 | MOTHERS$DEAF AID$THERAPY |
| 6816 | TECHNICAL$PHYSIOLOGICAL$PROBLEMS APPLICATION SYNTHETIC $SP AURAL$RE |
| 6816 | VISIBLE$SP$TRANSLATOR |
| 6905 | MILITARY$PATIENT$ATTITUDES AURAL$REHAB |
| 6915 | COMMENTS VERBOTONAL$METHOD |
| 6915 | VERBOTONAL$METHOD |
| 7003 | METRIC EVAL THERAPY HI |
| 7004 | MEAS HNG$HANDICAPPED |
| 7015 | VISIBLE$SP$AID |
| 7015 | VISUAL$SP$DISPLAY |
| 7115 | ADVICE PARENTS DEAF$CHIL |
| 7115 | APPLICATIONS SP$ANALYSIS COMM$AIDS DEAF |
| 7203 | AURAL$REHAB GER |
| 7203 | CRITIQUE SP$RECOGNITION$TESTING HNG$THERAPY |
| 7215 | DEAF HEAR SPEAK |
| 7215 | ORAL$AURAL$PERCEP |
| 7215 | PRESCH VERBOTONAL$INSTRUCTION DEAF$CHIL |
| 7315 | CO-PARENT$PROGRAM HI$CHIL |
| 7405 | REHABILITATIVE$AUD AUDIO RESPONSIBILITIES HABILITATION AUD$HANDICA |
| 7408 | COMPONENTS$VERBOTONAL$INSTRUCTION DEAF$STUDENTS |
| 7408 | SP$LANG$AUDIOLOGICAL$SERVICES |
| 7415 | INTONATION$FEEDBACK DEAF TACTILE$DISPLAY |
| 7503 | ERBER AUDITORY-VISUAL$PERCEPTION SP |
| 7504 | REED IDENTIFICATION DISCRIMINATION VC$SYLLABLES SN $HL |
| 7505 | HULL PROGRAM GERIATRIC$AURAL$REHAB JANUARY |
| 7515 | STRONG SP$AIDS HI |
| 7516 | COMM-BASED EARLY$CHILDHOOD$PROGRAMS DEAF |

7603   BINNIE VISUAL$INTELLIGIBILITY CONSONANTS LR$SCREENING
       $TEST
7615   EISENBERG VERBOTONAL$METHOD AURAL$REHAB
7704   NORTON ANALYTIC$STUDY TADOMA$METHOD
7705   MARGE SERVICE$DELIVERY$SYSTEMS HI
7705   SMITH AUD$REHAB AGED HOSPITAL
7813   GILBERT VOT HI$INDIVIDUALS
7815   LANE ARROW$APPROACH AURAL$REHAB
7816    REHAB$POTIENTIAL HI
7816   REHAB$PROGRAMS
7816   VISUAL$PRODESSING VERBAL$INFO DEAF PEOPLE
7827   BEEBE DEAF$CHIL LEARN HEAR
7827   BENNETT ARTICULATION HNG-IMPAIRED$CHIL DISTINCTIVE
       $FEATURE
7827   HOFFMAN SIMULTANEOUS INTERLEAVED MASKING
7827   MADELL AMPLIFICATION HNG-IMPAIRED$CHIL
7829   BRAINERD COMM$REHAB HI
7833   PURCELL BEFORE AFTER TONOGENESIS


                    0207


5406   HNG$LOSS AIRCRAFT$REPAIR$SHOP$PERSONNEL
5506   PATTERNS$INJURY OVERSTIMULATION$EAR
5606   COMMENTS REL HNG$LOSS NOISE$EXPOSURE
5606   SP$RECEPTION TEMPORARY$HNG$LOSS FUNCTION EXPOSURE
       $HIGH-LEVEL$NOISE
5706   HNG$LOSS AIR$FORCE$FLIGHT-LINE$PERSONNEL
6006   HNG$LOSS GUN$BLAST
6106   NOISE-INDUCED PTS
6111   CHARACTERISTICS HNG$LOSS GUNFIRE STEADY$NOISE
6306   EXPOSURE STEADY-STATE$NOISE HI
6711   HEARING$TEST$PATTERNS NOISE$INDUCED TEMPORARY$HNG
       $LOSS
7406   EFFECTS INTENSE$AUD$STIMULATION HNG$LOSSES INNER$EAR
       $CHANGES CHINC
7406   NOISE-INDUCED$HNG$LOSS CHINCHILLA POSITIVE-RF$TECHNIQUE
7505   YANTIS AUDIO ASSOCIATION OCCUPATIONAL$HRING$CONSERVATION
7506   MILLS NOISE CHILD REVIEW LITERATURE
7511   NERBONNE NOISE$INDUCED$'L TRUCK$DRIVER
7511   NERBONNE NOISE-INDUCED$HEARING$LOSS TRUCK$DRIVER$POPULATION
7603   FINDLAY AUDITORY$DYSFUNCTION NOISE-INDUCED$HNG LOSS
7604   YATES DAMAGE$RISK EVAL EFFECTS DBA$NOISE
7605   MILLER AUDIOLOGIST OCCUPATIONAL$HEARING$CONSERVATION
7606   WILEY LOUDNESS$ADAPTATION LISTENERS NOISE-INDUCED
       $HL

7705   FELDMAN REVIEW REFERRAL INDUSTRIAL$AUDIOGRAMS
7706   JOHNSON MEASUREMENT CONTINUOUS$SOUND$EXPOSURE
7711   HUMES THRES OCTAVE$MASKING$TEST PREDICTOR SUSEPTIBILITY
       NOISE-INDUCEHL
7806   AKAY REVIEW IMPACT$NOISE
7806   BERGER NOISE$INDUCED PTS
7806   UNGAR ESTIMATION PERCENTAGE OVEREXPOSED$WORKERS
7813   WEISS EXPOSURE NEONATES NOISE
7815   JETER NOISE HEARING$HEALTH$HAZARD


                           **0208**

5403   ASPIRATION$LEVELS DEAF$CHIL
5406   NOTE DEFINITION HNG$BC
5415   CHILD$DEAF ADVICE$PARENTS
5415   CHILD$HI
5415   DEAFNESS
5415   RELIGION DEAF$CHIL
5415   SEVERE$DEAFNESS PRE-SPEECH$YEARS
5416   INTERREL TESTS NONLANG$INTELLIGENCE DEAF
5416   QUALITATIVE$ANALYSIS EXPLANATIONS PHYSICAL$CAUSALITY
       DEFECTIVE$HNG
5416   QUALITATIVE$ANALYSIS EXPLANATIONS PHYSICAL$CAUSALITY
       HNG DEFECTIVE
5416   RELIGIOUS$WORK DEAF
5513   DURATION$STEPS DEAF-MUTES
5515   DEAF$ADULTS FOLK$DANCING
5515   DEAF$CHIL HNG$FAMILY
5515   DEAF$CHIL LETTERS$HOME
5515   DEAF$GIRLS
5515   HNG$DIS CHIL
5515   LOSING$HNG
5515   PEDIATRICIAN DEAF$CHILD
5516   RELIGIOUS$WORK DEAF
5516   SP$HNG$PROBLEMS DEAF$CHIL
5603   KERNICTERIC$NUCLEAR$DEAFNESS
5615   DEAF$PERSON$JOB
5615   DEAF$STUDENTS HELP BLIND
5615   DEAFNESS$CHIL
5615   FILMS$FILMSTRIPS DEAFNESS
5616   STUDY INTELLIGENCE DEAF$CHIL COMPARISON PERFORMANCES
       STANDARDIZATI
5703   RECRUITMENT ABRUPT$LOSS$HIGH-FREQ
5715   DEAFNESS FINGER$SURGERY

5716    DEAF
5716    STUDY VISUAL$MEM DEAF$CHIL
5716    STUDY WECHSLER$PERFORMANCE$SCALE KNOX$CUBE$TEST DEAF
        $ADOL
5804    SURVEY HNG$LOSS MIL$PERSONNEL
5806    ENDOLYMPHATIC$HYPOXIA ACOUS$TRAUMA
5815    CHIL TALK DEAF HARD$HNG
5816    ACCOMPLISHMENTS DEAF
5816    DEAF COMM MANUAL$LANG
5816    DEAF$CHIL OTHER$HANDICAPS
5816    FORMATIVE$INFLUENCES DEAF$CHIL DEAF$ADULT
5816    PSYCHOLOGICAL$ASPECTS PROBLEMS EARLY$DEAFNESS
5816    PSYCHOLOGICAL$EVAL VOCATIONAL$ADJUSTMENT
5816    UNDERSTANDING COUNSELING DEAF$ADULT
5904    ERYTHROBLASTOSIS HNG$LOSS
5904    PERFORMANCE HH$PERSONS DAF
5907    RESEARCH$NEEDS SP$PATH$A HNG$PROBLEMS LARGE$GRPS
5907    RESEARCH$NEEDS SP$PATH$A HNG$PROBLEMS ADULTS
5916    ABILITY DEAF$SWIMMERS ORIENT SUBMERGED$WATER
5916    DEAFNESS
5916    STATISTICAL$INFO DEAF$HH USA
6003    CHIL NONORGANIC$HNG$LOSS
6003    SUDDEN$UNILATERAL$HNG$LOSS MUMPS
6004    COLOR-FORM$ATTITUDES DEAF$CHIL
6004    HNG$LEVELS TYPES$HNG$LOSS AIR$FORCE$PERSONNEL
6005    REPORT OCCUPATIONAL$CONDITIONS DEAF
6006    MASKING OCTAVE$BANDS NOISE HI
6011    BINAURAL$HNG HI$ADULTS
6013    SP$LANG$HNG DISORDERS ENCEPHALOPATHY
6015    ACCEPTANCE REJECTION HI
6015    DEAFNESS EQUILIBRIUM
6015    PARENT HI$CHIL
6016    PSYCHOLOGICAL$EFFECTS
6016    RESEARCH$DEPARTMENT CID
6016    RESEARCH$FACILITIES JOHN$TRACY$CLINIC
6016    WORK$POTENTIALS FAMILY$PROBLEMS LITERATE$DEAF$ADOL
        $ADULTS
6103    MECHANISMS$COMPENSATION HNG$LOSS SOVIET$UNION
6104    DEAFNESS EVERYDAY$LIVING
6104    VISUAL$PAIRED-ASSOCIATES$TASK DEAF$CHIL
6115    DEAF$SCOUTS
6115    MARGINAL$DEAFNESS
6203    ANATOMICAL$LOCUS PRESBYCUSIS
6203    APPROACH EMOTIONAL$PROBLEMS HI$CHIL
6203    PSYCHOMETRIC$APPRAISAL DEAF$CHIL COLUMBIA$MENTAL$MATURITY
        $SCALE

6204    PROBLEM-SOLVING$ABILITY DEAF$CHIL
6215    DEAF$CHIL JOB$PROSPECTS
6215    EFFECTS PERCEPTIVE$LOSSES LANG SP$DISCRIM
6215    WISC$PATTERNS DEAF$CHIL
6216    ADULT$DEAF PROFESSIONS
6216    DEAF$CHIL MATURITY PARENTS
6216    MEANING DEAFNESS REPORT WORKSHOP A
6216    OCCUPATIONAL$STATUS DEAF
6216    PSYCHIATRIC$CONSIDERATIONS ADULT$DEAF
6216    PSYCHOLOGICAL$CONSIDERATIONS EARLY$PROFOUND$DEAFNESS
6303    DESCRIPTION PARACUSIS$WILLISIANA HISTORICAL$NOTE
6303    HYPOACUSICS
6303    SUDDEN$DEAFNESS
6304    MAXIMUM$AC$HNG$LOSS
6306    REL HNG$LOSS NOISE$SPECTRUM
6315    PSYCHOLOGICAL$EVAL DEAF STUDIES
6315    ROLE HEREDITY EARLY$TOTAL$DEAFNESS
6315    VOCATIONAL$STATUS ADJUSTMENT DEAF$WOMEN
6316    DEAFNESS GENETIC$FACTOR
6403    FAMILIAL$COINCIDENT$RENAL$DISEASE HNG$LOSS
6403    FUNCTIONAL$HNG$LOSSES
6403    SCALE SELF-ASSESSMENT HNG$HANDICAP
6403    SUDDEN$DEAFNESS CASE
6406    EXPERIMENTAL$STUDY TONE$DEAFNESS
6415    HNG$LOSS INF PRESCH$CHIL
6415    ORAL$DEAF$ADULTS
6415    SOCIAL$EMOTIONAL$ADJUSTMENT DEAF$ADULTS
6415    STUDY EMPLOYMENT$OPPORTUNITIES HI
6415    THOUGHT$PATTERNS DEAF$CHIL
6416    COLLECTION STATISTICS SEVERE$HI USA
6416    PREVALENCE DEAFNESS SCH$AGE$CHIL
6416    STUDY DELAYED$IMMEDIATE$VISUAL$RETENTION DEAF$ADOL
6503    EFFECT CLIMATE INCIDENCE HNG$LOSS
6503    HNG$LOSS POLYCYTHEMIA$VERA
6503    STUDY HNG$LOSS SCH$CHIL INDIA
6504    DIPLACUSIS UNILATERAL$HIGH-FREQ$HNG$LOSS
6504    HNG$LOSS AUD$LATERALIZATION
6506    TTS AUD$DEPRIVATION CONDUCTIVE$HNG$LOSS
6511    FACTORS PERSISTENCE RESOLUTION FUNCTIONAL$HNG$LOSS
6511    MULTIDISCIPLINE$STUDY FUNCTIONAL$HNG$LOSS
6511    SOCIAL$PSYCHOLOGICAL$CHARACTERISTICS VETERANS FUNCTIONAL
        $HNG$LOSS
6515    DEAF$CHIL FAITH
6515    ELECTRICAL$STIMULATION EIGHTH$NERVE$DEAFNESS
6515    PEDIATRICS DIS$COMM SOCIAL$CONSIDERATIONS CARE PRESCH
        $HI$CHIL

6515   TELEPHONE$DEAF
6516   SOCIOMETRIC$INVEST SELF-CONCEPT DEAF$CHIL
6603   PSEUDOHYPACUSIS
6603   RECOVERY AUD$FUNCTION SURGICAL$REMOVAL$CEREBELLAR
       $TUMOR
6603   SUDDEN$HNG$LOSS SPONTANEOUS$RECOVERY
6604   VISUAL$AUD$SEQUENCE$LEARNING HI$CHIL
6615   SOCIAL$ADJUSTMENT HI$ADOL
6615   SOCIAL$ADJUSTMENT HI$CHIL
6616   STUDY RORSCHACH DEAF$ADOL
6617   COUNSELING ADVENTITIOUSLY$HI$ADULTS
6617   NON-ORGANIC$HNG$PROBLEMS SCH$CHIL
6703   COMM$DIS CHIL KERNICTERIC$ATHETOSIS AUD$DIS
6703   COMM$PROBLEMS UNILATERAL$HNG$LOSS
6703   TUBERCULOUS$MENINGITIS DEAFNESS
6704   DESCRIPTIVE$ANALYSIS AUDIOMETRIC$PSYCHOMETRIC$SCORES
       STUDENTS DEAF
6704   PSYCHOACOUS$COMPARISON COCH$EIGHTH$NERVE$DIS
6704   SP$HNG$CHARACTERISTICS FAMILIAL$DYSAUTONOMIA
6706   NORMAL-HNG HIGH-TONE$HI
6711   EFFECT STIMULUS$SENSATION LEVEL DIRECTIONAL$HEARING
       UNILATERALLY$D
6711   HIGH$FREQUENCY$HEARING MENINGITIS
6711   SENSORINEURAL$HNG$IMP MENSTRUAL$CYCLE
6715   CHARACTERISTICS POST-RUBELLA$DEAF$CHIL
6715   DEAF$WORKERS
6715   DEAFNESS$HEREDITARY
6715   INF$HNG$LOSSES
6715   PARENT$ROLE JOB$PLACEMENT DEAF$ADOL
6715   SEMANTICS DEAFNESS
6804   EFFECT SENSORI-NEURAL$HNG$LOSS THR-DURATION$FUNCTIONS
6804   VOWEL$DISCRIM HI$LISTENERS
6806   POLYACUSIS HNG$ANOMALY
6806   RECOVERY TTS CHIL SENSORINEURAL$DEAFNESS
6807   DEV AUD$PERCEP HH$SCH$CHIL
6807   DEV CHIL HNG$DIS
6807   OBJECTIVE$STUDY RESIDUAL$HNG DEAF-MUTE$CHIL
6811   HNG$LOSS PSYCHIATRIC$POPULATION SUBJECT$CHANGE$IN
       $ATTENTION
6815   DEAF$CHIL
6815   DEAFNESS$RESEARCH
6815   NURSES HI$CHIL
6815   RUBELLA CHIL HNG
6815
6816   PERSONALITY$TEST`HI
6816   PRE-MARITAL$COUNSELING DEAF

```
6904   PRACTICE$EFFECTS FREQ$DISCRIM HI$CHIL
6904   SOCIOLOGICAL$PSYCHOLOGICAL$FACTORS HNG$LOSS
6906   REMOTE$MASKING LISTENERS COCH$IMPAIRMENT
6911   CLINICAL$FINDINGS HIGH-FREQ$THR OTOTOXIC$DRUG
6915   AUD$CHARACTERISTICS POST-RUBELLA
6916   DEAFNESS MR$CHIL
6916   PERFORMANCE$SCALE COGNITIVE$CAPACITY DEAF
6916   RAVENS$PROGRESSIVE$MATRICES DEAF
7003   AUDIOMETRIC DEV LEARNING$CHARACTERISTICS RUBELLA$DEAF
       $CHIL
7003   SP$HNG$LANG DE$LANGE$SYNDROME
7004   PERSTIMULATORY$TRACKING PITCH$PERCEP SENSORINEURAL
       $HNG$LOSS
7004   SENSORINEURAL$HNG$LOSS UPWARD$SPREAD$MASKING
7004   SOCIOLOGICAL$PHYSIOLOGICAL$FACTORS HNG$LOSS
7004   USE TOUCH-TONE$TELEPHONE COMM$AID DEAF
7011   EFFECTS SP$INTELLIGIBILITY TIME-COMPRESSED TIME-EXPANDED
       HH GER$MA
7011   HNG$MEAS$SCALE QUESTIONNAIRE ASSESSMENT$AUD$DISABILITY
7011   TEMPORAL$SUMMATION BRIEF$TONES COCH$IMPAIRED$EARS
7015   DEAFNESS FAMILY$PLANNING
7015   ORAL$DEAF$ADULTS
7015   PICTUREPHONE$SERVICE WAY COMM
7015   RESEARCH$DEAFNESS
7016   COMPARISON PROFILES RUBELLA$NON-RUBELLA$DEAF$CHIL
7016   GENETIC$ASPECTS CONGENITAL$HNG$LOSS
7103   PSYCHOLOGICAL$REACTIONS HNG$LOSS
7103   TEMPORAL$INTEGRATION CLINICAL$IMPLICATIONS LAB$STUDY
       DATA HI$SUBJE
7104   DICHOTIC$LISTENING HI$CHIL
7104   SENSORINEURAL$HNG$LOSS UPWARD$SPREAD$MASKING
7104   SENSORINEURAL$LOSS UPWARD$SPREAD$MASKING
7108   SELECTION ACHIEVEMENT$TEST$LEVEL HI$CHIL
7111   INTELLIGENCE$TEST$PERFORMANCE BLACK$CHIL HIGH$FREQ
       $HNG$LOSS
7111   SIMULATED$BILATERAL$HIGH-FREQUENCY$HNG$IMPAIRMENT
7116   PERFORMANCE HI$CHIL NON-VERBAL$PERSONALITY$TEST
7203   SITE$LESION HNG$LOSS RH$INCOMPATABILITY ARGUMENT PERIPHERAL
       $IMPAIR
7203   SP$LANG$HNG$PROBLEMS LAURENCE-MOON-BIEDL$SYNDROME
7211   AL MONAURAL$DEAF
7211   COMMENTS OTITIS$MEDIA RATS
7215   OROSENSORY$PERCEP DEAF
7217   R$TIME EXPANDED$SP PRESBYCUSIC$MALES
7217   R$TIME EXPANDED$SP PRESBYCUSIC$MALES
7304   LOUDNESS$GROWTH MASKING SENSORINEURAL$IMPAIRMENT
```

7306    ANATOMICAL$CORRELATES DEAFNESS
7306    SIGNAL$PROCESSING SP$INTELLIGIBILITY PERCEP$DEAFNESS
7306    TEMPORAL$EFFECTS FREQ$DISCRIM HI$LISTENERS
7311    EFFECTS FREQ$BANDWIDTH SP$DISCRIM HI
7315    DEAF$INF
7315    ORAL$DEAF$ADULT
7315    PARENT DEAF$ADOL
7403    SUBCLINICAL$CONGENITAL$CYTOMEGALOVIRUS$INFECTION HI
7404    AUDIOVISUAL$CONSONANT$RECOGNITION HI$ADULTS
7405    BIBLIOTHERAPY HEARING$HANDICAPPED
7405    RESULTS AUDIOMETRIC$STUDY SENSORINEURALLY$IMPAIRED
        ACUPUNCTURE
7415    PSYCHOLOGICAL$TESTING HI
7415    TEMPORARY$CONDUCTIVE$LOSS STUDENTS SEVERE$SENSORINEURAL
        $DEAFNESS
7415    USHERS$SYNDROME CONGENITAL$DEAFNESS PROGRESSIVE$VISION
        $LOSS
7503    ROESER RECOVERY$AUDITORY$FUNCTION MENINGITIC$DEAFNESS
7503    TAUB SENSORINEURAL$HNG$LOSS
7504    DANAHER MASKING LOW-FREQ$VOWEL$FORMANTS SENSORINEURAL
        $HL
7504    IVEY TYMPANOMETRIC$CURVES OTOSCLEROSIS
7504    MOULTON VERBAL$CODING$STRADEGIES HI
7504    REED IDENTIFICATION DISCRIMINATION VC$SYLLABLES SN
        $HL
7504    RICHARDS MCL PT SP MASKING
7504    ROBINSON DIPLACUSIS BILATERAL$HIGH$FREQ$HL
7504    WALDEN AUD+ADIOVISUAL$FEATURE$TRANSMISSION HI
7504    WILSON NEUROPSYCHOLOGIC$FUNCTION CHILD HNG IMPAIRMENT
7508    GENGEL LISTENLNG$LEVEL SP RECEP HI$CHILD
7511    ARNST VIBROTACTILE$SENSITIVITY TONGUE HNG IMP$SUBJECTS
7511    CARSON STUDY LEARNING DEAF$CHILD
7511    GOETZINGER IMPACT HI PSY$DEV CHILD
7511    GOETZINGER IMPACT HEARING$IMPAIRMENT PSYCHOLOGICAL
        $DEVELOPMENT CHIL
7516    PSYCHOSOCIAL$PROBLEMS DEAF$CHILD FAMILIES
7516    READING$HABITS DEAF$ADULTS
7516    REPORT AD$HOC$COMMITTEE DEFINE DEAF$HARD OF HRING
7524    BLASBERG CHOANAL$ATRESIA
7524    PARADISE ME$PROBLEMS CLEFT$PALATE
7524    SOUDIJN CLEFT$PALATES ME$EFFUSIONS BABIES
7529    MENCHER EARLY$IDENTIFICATION HL A REVIEW
7531    CRANDALL ASSESSMENT READING+WRITING$ADULT$DEAF
7531    MOOREHNG$CHARACTERSTICS IMPLICATIONS AUD$TRNG
7531    SIMS VALIDATION CID$EVERYDAY$SENTENCE$TEST USE HI
7531    SUBTELNY COMMUNICATION NT1D$STUDENTS PLANNING REHAB

7532  GOLDSTEIN AUD$AGNOSIA CORTICAL$DEAFNESS
7605  JETER HEARING$IMPAIRMENT PSYCHIATRIC$PATIENTS
7606  MARGOLIS MONAURAL$LOUDNESS$ADAPT LOW$SL NORMAL + IMPAIRED
      $EARS
7606  PRICE AGE FACTOR SUSCEPTIBILITY HNG$LOSS YOUNG VERSUS
      ADULT$EARS
7611  COMALLI EFFECT STIMULUS$INTENSITY FREQUENCY UNILATERAL
      $HNG$LOSS AL
7611  FRANKLIN ANALYSIS DISCRIM$SCORES CONGENITAL$SN$LOSS
7611  GATEHOUSE AL MONAURAL$SUBJECTS
7611  HARRELL BC$CHANGES STAPEDECTOMY
7611  MCCARTNEY HNG$HANDICAP$SCALE AUDIOMETRIC$MEASURES
      GERIATRIC$POPULATION
7611  TANIGUCHI ACOUSTIC$FAR-FIELD$RESPONSE KANAMYCIN-TREATED
      $GUINEA$PIG
7615  MCELROY ROLE PARENTS SELF-ESTEEM HI CHILD
7616   COGNITIVE$DEV
7616   COMM$CHAR YOUNG$DEAF$ADULTS
7616   EFFECTS HI CHILD FAMILY$BEHAVIOR$PATTERNS
7616   IMPULSIVITY PROFOUND$EARLY$DEAFNESS
7629  TYLER TEMPORAL$INTEGRATION COCHLEAR$HL
7631  HILDRETH SOCIAL$PARTICIPATION FAMILY$LIFE HARD$HNG
      $UNMARRIED$ADULTS
7632  KIMURA IMPAIRMENT NONLINGUISTIC$HAND$MOVEMENTS DEAF
      $APHASIC
7703  BESS WORD$DISCRIM FLAT$HEARING$LOSSES
7705  MARGE SERVICE$DELIVERY$SYSTEMS HI
7711  COZAD SPEECHREADING COMM$DIFFICULTY CHILD ADULTS UNILATERAL
      $HL
7715  MCLEOD USE TELEPHONE ORAL$DEAF
7716   APARTMENT$LIVING PRACTICING REAL$THING
7716   IMAGINATION ORIGINALITY ABSTRACT$THINKING DEAF
7716   OCCUPATIONAL$STEREOTYPES
7716   RECEPTION SENTENCES
7716   WISC-R HISKEY-NEBRASKA$TEST
7732  MANNING LATERAL$CEREBRAL$DIFF DEAF R LING + NONLING
      $STIMULI
7804  KAMM EFFECT SENSORINEURAL$HEARING$LOSS LOUDNESS$DISCOMFORT
      $LEVEL MCL
7805  KATZ CONDUCTIVE$HEARING$LOSS AUDITORY$FUNCTION
7805  POWERS HEARING$PROBLEMS ELDERLY
7806  KRUGER TM$PERFORATIONS CATS CONFIGURATIONS$LOSSES
7806  PROSEN KANAMYMYCIN-INDUCED HL GUINEA$PIG
7806  SILMAN SN$HEARING$LOSS ACOUSTIC$REFLEX GROWTH$FUNCTIONS
7815  MEHTA SEROUS$OTITIS$MEDIA SCHOOL$DEAF
7815  RUBEN SEROUS$OTITIS$MEDIA

7815   RUBIN SEROUS$OTITIS$MEDIA HI$CHIL
7815   RUDNER STANDARD$TESTS HI ITEM$BIAS
7827   BLOOD LISTENERS$IMPRESSIONS HI$CHILD
7827   STREFF HI$YOUNG$ADULTS VERBAL+NONVERBAL$ABILITIES

## 0209

5409   SP DEAF$CHIL
5415   DEAF$CHIL SPEECH$VOCAB
5415   ENRICHING$VOCAB PRIMARY$DEAF
5415   NASALITY
5415   ROLE$LANG SP$TRNG HI$CHIL
5415   SPEECH DEAF$ADULT
5415   SPEECH$LESSON$PLAN
5415   TEACHING VOCABULARY
5415   TEACHING$SP DEAF
5415   TEACHING$SP DIFFERENCES$AGREEMENTS
5415   VOCABULARY$NEEDS PRESCH$DEAF$CHIL
5416   DEV$LANG DAILY$NEWS$PERIOD
5515   TEACHING$SP USE SPONTANEOUS$SP
5515   TEACHING$SP SP$PROGRAM ADVANCED$PUPILS
5515   TEACHING$SP DEV$SP SYNTHETIC$METHOD
5515   TEACHING$SP ASSOCIATION$METHOD$APHASICS APPLICATION
       $DEAF
5515   TEACHING$SP LEXINGTON$SCH
5515   TEACHING$SP TADOMA$METHOD
5516   STUDY WRITTEN$SENTENCE$CONSTRUCTION DEAF$CHIL
5613   ACOUSTIC$ANALYSIS$VOWELS DEAF$CHIL VISIBLE$SP
5615   DEAF$CHIL THINK
5615   EXPRESSIVE$WRITING DEAF
5616   STUDY DEPENDENT$CLAUSE PRIMARY$READING DEAF
5709   ORAL$COMM
5709   TEACHING$LANG DEAF$CHIL
5715   SP$LANG DEAF RUSSIA
5715   SPEECH VISUAL-TACTILE$SYSTEM
5716   FOREIGN$LANG STUDY DEAF$STUDENTS$VOCAB
5716   SUGGESTIONS IMPROVING VOCATIONAL$TRNG
5803   VOICE$QUALITY EMOTIONAL$DEAFNESS
5815   ACOUS$VISUAL$LANG COMM$SYSTEMS
5815   LANG$DEAF
5815   LANG$DEV READING
5815   LANG$DISABILITY CHIL$HI
5815   SP PRESCH$DEAF
5815   VOCAL$EFFECTS DAF IMPLICATIONS TEACHING$SP DEAF

```
5816   DEAF COMM WRITTEN$LANG
5816   SYSTEM SENTENCE$STRUCTURE DEV$LANG DEAF
5904   LANG$SKILLS PROFOUNDLY$DEAF$ADOL
5915   PICTURES$WORDS
5915   TEACH CHIL LANG$GAMES
5918   DEAF$ARTIC
6004   COGNITIVE$ABILITIES DEAF$CHIL
6005   DEAFNESS SP HNG PUBLICATIONS
6016   DEAF$CHIL LANG$ARTS
6016   LANG DEAF$CHIL
6016   LITERALNESS DEAF$STUDENTS
6103   CONCEPT$FORMATION$TEST PRESCH$DEAF
6115   ASSESSMENT VERBAL$LANG$DEV DEAF$CHIL
6115   COMM$SKILLS
6115   ENRICHING LANG DEAF$CHIL PARENT$PART
6115   PARENT$ROLE SPEECH$DEV
6116   COMM$BEHAVIOR DEAF$CHIL ESOTERIC$SYMBOLISM
6203   CORRECTION FALSETTO$VOICE DEAF$ADULT
6205   LANG$DEV CHIL DYSACUSIS
6215   COMPARISON TYPE-TOKEN$RATIO SPOKEN$WRITTEN$LANG DEAF
       $CHIL
6215   DEAF VOICE$QUALITY INVESTIGATION
6215   OBSERVATIONS SP DEAF
6215   PROGRAMMING$LANG DEAF$CHIL
6215   PROGRAMMED$APPROACH WRITTEN$LANG$DEV DEAF$CHIL
6215   REINFORCING$SP$LANG FAMILY
6215   SP DEAF
6215   SP$IMPROVEMENT RESIDENTIAL$SCH DEAF
6216   COMM TEACHING DEAF METHODS
6314   REMARKS ACQUISITION$LANG DEAF$CHIL
6315   LINGUISTIC$DEV MENTAL$GROWTH HI$CHIL
6315   SP$PROBS DEAF
6316   DEV READING$TEST$NORMS DEAF$CHIL
6316   PROGRAMMING$INSTRUCTION WRITTEN$LANG DEAF$CHIL
6403   VOWEL$FORMANTS DEAF$BOYS
6404   ABILITY DEAF$CHIL WORD$CLASSES
6415   EXAMINING LANG$BEHAVIOR DEAF$CHIL
6415   INNER$LANG DEAF DESCRIPTIVE$GRAMMAR
6415   LANG$PROGRAM LEXINGTON$SCH$DEAF
6415   SP$PROGRAM ST.JOSEPH$INSTITUTE$DEAF
6415   STRUCTURAL$LANG
6415   UNDERSTAND LANG$BEHAVIOR
6416   COMPARISON METHODS TEACHING WRITTEN$LANG DEAF$STUDENTS
6416   TEACHING LANG INDIVIDUAL$DEAF$CHIL
6503   NATURE STM$ENCODING DEAF
6511   PICTURE-IDENTIFICATION$TEST HI$CHIL
```

| | |
|---|---|
| 6514 | EFFECT TIME$DISTORTIONS INTELLIGIBILITY DEAF$CHIL $SP |
| 6515 | EMPHASIS READING DEAF$CHIL |
| 6516 | APPROACH TEACHING LANG DEAF$CHIL |
| 6516 | BEFORE$AFTER$CONCEPT DEAF$CHIL |
| 6516 | EVAL VOCAB$DEV DEAF$CHIL |
| 6516 | FOLLOW-UP$STUDY READING$TEST DEAF$CHIL |
| 6516 | RECEPTIVE$LANG USSR NETHERLANDS USA |
| 6603 | USE VISUAL$MEM WRITTEN$LANG$SKILLS DEAF$CHIL |
| 6604 | SPOKEN$SYNTAX HH$DEAF$CHIL |
| 6614 | SP$PROD SPOKEN$LANG DEAF |
| 6615 | ACQUISITION$LANG MULTIPLY$HANDICAPPED$DEAF$CHIL |
| 6615 | EVAL WRITTEN$LANG DEAF$STUDENTS |
| 6615 | LANG$ACQUISITION DEAF$CHIL |
| 6615 | LANG$DEV PARENTS$COUNSELING$GUIDANCE |
| 6615 | LANG$GROWTH DEAF$INF |
| 6615 | LANG$INSTRUCTION DEAF |
| 6615 | RHYTHM LANG DEAF$CHIL |
| 6616 | INFLUENCE EARLY$MANUAL$COMM LINGUISTIC$DEV DEAF$CHIL |
| 6616 | MANUAL$COMM DEAF$ADOL REL ORAL$SKILLS |
| 6704 | ABILITY DEAF$CHIL MORPHOLOGICAL$RULES |
| 6704 | ABILITY DEAF$CHIL MORPHOLOGICAL$RULES |
| 6704 | CLOZE$TECHNIQUE$STUDIES LANG DEAF |
| 6704 | GRAPHEMIC PHONETIC ASSOC$FACTORS VERBAL$BEHAVIOR DEAF |
| 6704 | PHRASE-LEARNING DEAF |
| 6704 | WORD$ASSOC$TEST$PERFORMANCES DEAF |
| 6706 | ANALYSIS PT$AUDIOMETRIC$R REL SP-DEV PROFOUNDLY$DEAF |
| 6714 | LANG HI$CHIL |
| 6715 | BETTER$SP DEAF |
| 6715 | DEAF$VOICE SURVEY$LITERATURE |
| 6716 | ATTAINMENT FIRST-ORDER$CONCEPTS DEAF |
| 6716 | EFFECTS INDUCTION DEDUCTION DEAF |
| 6804 | EMG$STUDY CONSONANT$ARTIC HI$SPEAKERS |
| 6804 | LINGUISTIC$WORD$CLASSES SPOKEN$LANG HH$DEAF$CHIL |
| 6804 | PERCEIVED$NASALITY SP DEAF |
| 6804 | PERCEIVED$NASALITY SP DEAF |
| 6804 | PICTURE-SOUND$ASSOC DEAF$CHIL |
| 6805 | LANG DEV PRESCH$DEAF$CHIL SOVIET$UNION |
| 6807 | SIGNIFICANCE TRNG UNVOICED$HNG DEV PERCEP$ACTIVITY DEAF-MUTE$CHIL |
| 6807 | UTILIZATION RESIDUAL$HNG PRONUNCIATION DEAF-MUTE$CHIL |
| 6815 | DEV COGNITIVE$ABILITIES LANG$DEV DEAF$CHIL SCIENCE |
| 6815 | SP$SCIENCE DEAF |
| 6815 | TEACHING AURAL$LANG |
| 6816 | COMM$FUNCTIONING EARLY$MANUAL$COMM REL DEAF$CHIL |
| 6816 | CORRECTION VOICE$PITCH$LEVEL HH$SUBJECTS |

6816    TEACHING$INTONATION DEAF VISUAL$PATTERN$MATCHING
6816    TEACHING INTONATION DEAF VISUAL$PATTERN$MATCHING
6816    VISUAL$SP$TRAINER VOWEL$SPECTRUM
6816    VISUAL$VIBROTACTILE$AIDS
6816    VOICE$VISUALIZER
6904    INTELLIGIBILITY TIME$COMPRESSED$WORDS FUNCTION AGE
        HNG$LOSS
6907    DEV$STUDIES DEAF$CHIL
6913    CINE$INVEST VELO$FUNCTION DEAF$SPEAKERS
6914    STUDY SYLLABIC$STRESS ENG$WORDS DEAF
6915    DEAF$CHIL EMOTIONAL$CONCEPTS
6915    DESCRIPTIVE$STYLE DEAF$CHIL
6915    SP$PROGRAM DEAF
6916    INVEST VISUAL-SEQUENTIAL$MEM DEAF$CHIL
7004    ARTIC$TRNG DEAF LOW-FREQ$SURROGATE$FRICATIVES
7004    CODING$MEDIUM WORD$RECALL DEAF
7004    PICTURE$IDENTIFICATION$TEST HI$CHIL
7007    DECELERATION INAPPROPRIATE$VOCALS$BEHAVIOR HH$CHIL
7015    MODIFICATIONS VOCAL$FREQ INTENSITY SP DEAF
7016    ANALYSIS COMM$INTERACTION DEAF$CHIL
7016    CONTEXTUAL$CONSTRAINT DEAF$CHIL
7016    EARLY$SP$DEV DEAF$INF
7016    LANG EDUC CHIL EARLY$PROFOUND$DEAFNESS
7016    LANG$MOTHERS DEAF$CHIL
7016    PSYCHOLINGUISTICS DEAFNESS
7017    DIALOG DEAF$MAN
7103    THERAPY REDUCTION CONTINUOUS$PHONATION HH
7103    USE REAL-TIME$VISUAL$DISPLAYS SP TRNG DEAF$NONSPEAKING
        $CHIL
7103    USE REAL-TIME$VISUAL$DISPLAYS SP TRNG DEAF$NONSPEAKING
        $CHIL
7115    TACTILE$PITCH$FEEDBACK DEAF$SPEAKERS
7116    APHASIA LANG$FUNCTIONING DEAF
7116    METHODS$TEACHING$COMM$SKILLS DEAF
7116    MODIFICATION SENTENCE$WRITING DEAF$CHIL
7208    HI$CHIL SP$CLINICIAN INTERDISCIPLINARY$TEAM
7214    TEACHING BA$PA DEAF$CHIL REAL-TIME$SPECTRAL$DISPLAYS
7215    COMM HI
7215    GROUP$COMM DEAF
7215    LANG SOCIAL$ADJUSTMENT HI$CHIL
7215    PLEA COMM
7216    EFFECT PARENT$ORIENTATION SIGN$LANG COMM$SKILLS PRESCH
        $DEAF$CHIL
7216    LANG$UNDERSTANDING DEAF$STUDENTS AUD-VISUAL$STIMULUS
        $CONDITIONS
7303    LANG$TRNG POSTRUBELLA$HNG$IMP$CHIL

7303    PHONOLOGICAL$ANALYSIS SPONTANEOUS$LANG HARD-OF-HEARING
        $CHIL
7304    DEAF$CHIL ACQUISITION$PASSIVE$VOICE
7304    DEAF$CHIL ACQUISITION$PASSIVE$VOICE
7304    DEV$SEMANTIC$ASSOCIATIONS DEAF$CHIL
7304    HI$CHIL COMPREHENSION$PROD$SYNTAX ORAL$LANG
7304    INITIAL$CONSONANT$INTELLIGIBILITY HI$CHIL
7304    OROSENSORY$PERCEP SP$PROD DEAFNESS
7305    EVAL COMM$SKILLS ADULT$DEAF
7311    DISCRIM$VOICING$DISTINCTION HI$CHIL
7315    COMM$NEEDS PRESCH$HI
7315    USE EXPRESSIONS CLASSROOM
7316    EFFECTS CONSEQUENCES CONTINGENT INTELLIGIBLE$SP DEAF
        $CHIL
7316    EXPRESSIVE$SYMBOLIC$REPRESENTATION DEAF
7316    VOICED-VOICELESS$DISTINCTION DEAF$SP
7317    DEAF$CHIL SYNTACTIC$COMPETENCE
7403    PHONOLOGICAL$SUBSITUTION$PROCESSES HARD-OF-HEARING
        $CHIL
7403    SIGNED$ENGLISH MANUAL$APPROACH LANG$DEV
7404    CATEGORICAL$ENCODING SHORT-TERM$MEMORY DEAF$CHIL
7404    COMPREHENSION RELATIVIZED$SENTENCES DEAF
7404    DURATIONAL$ASPECTS VOWEL$PROD SP DEAF$CHIL
7404    GRAMMATICAL$RULE$STRUCTURE DEAF
7404    LINGUISTIC$PERFORMANCES HH$CHIL
7404    PERFORMANCE HI$CHIL BASIC$CONCEPTS
7404    QUESTION$FORMATION LANG DEAF
7414    LINGUISTIC$ANALYSIS MORPHEMIC$SYNTACTIC$STRUCTURES
        HH$CHIL
7415    COMM HI$ADOL PARENTS
7415    INSTRUMENTAL$APPROACH ORAL-NASAL$SP PRESCH$HI
7415    PERFORMANCE DEAF$CHIL LOGICAL$DISCOVERY$PROGRAM
7415    SP$MODEL
7415    SP$PATH HI$CHIL
7415    VISUALLY-ORIENTED$MEDIA MOTIVATE DEV$LANG HI$CHIL
7415
7504    DAVIS STRATEGIES NORMAL-HNG + HI$CHIL COMPREHENSION
        RELATIVE$CLAUSES
7504    JARVELLA DEAF+HEARING$CHILD LANG TEMPORAL$ORDER
7504    MOULTON VERBAL$CODING$STRADEGIES HI
7504    SMITH RESIDUAL$HNG SP$PROD DEAF$CHILD
7504    WILBUR CONJOINED$STRUCTURES LANG DEAF
7512    KLEFFNER TEACHING CHILDREN AUD$PROCESSING LEARNING
        $DISABILITIES
7515    BOOTHROYD COMPUTER-BASED$SYS OF SP$TRNG$AIDS DEAF
7515    CALVERT METHODS DEV$SP

```
7515    EDWARDS PUPPETS NONVERBAL CHILD
7515    MOOG LANG$INSTRUCTION DIAGNOSTIC$OBSERVATION
7515    NICKERSON SP DEAF
7515    ROMNEY DEAF$STUDENTS TELEPHONE
7515    SCHWARTZBERG PARENT$EFFECTIVENESS LANG HOME
7515    STRONG SP$AIDS HI
7515    WILBUR SYNTACTIC STRUCTURES WRITTEN$LANG DEAF$CHILD
7515    WOODWARD MEAS$LANG DEAF CHILD BIB
7516     AUDIOLOGISTS ORALISTS
7516     BSCS,S ME NOW HI$STUDENTS
7516     COMM$PREFERENCE SOCIAL$CONDITIONS
7516     CUED$SP
7516     DEAF$CHILD LANG
7516     ESL$APPROACH TEACHING ENGLISH
7516     HI INSTITUTIONS RETARDED
7516     KNOWLEDGE CONCEPTS DEAF$ADOLESCENTS
7516     LANG$DEV DEAF$CHILD
7516     LITERATURE SIGNS
7516     ROCHESTER$METHOD FLORIDA$SCHOOL
7516     TEACHING SIGN$LANG INTERACTIVE$TELEVISION
7516     TELEVISION TEACHING$TOOL DEAF$STUDENTS
7516     TOTAL$COMM BUFFALO
7516     USE SIGN$LANG TEACHING$ENGLISH
7526    TWENEY SEMANTIC$ORGANIZATION DEAF HRING SS
7527    GREEN SEMANTIC$STRUCTURE DEAF$CHILDREN
7527    SMITH INTERJECTED$SOUNDS DEAF$CHILDREN
7531    JOHNSON COMMUNICATION NTID$STUDENTS
7531    KELLY NTID$TRNG$PROGRAM INTERPERSONAL$COMMUNICATION
7531    MILLER JOB$RELATED$SP+LANG$TRNG
7531    NUTTER DEV PRONUNCIATION$SKILLS
7531    ORLANDO SP+VOICE$TRAINING
7531    SMITH SP+VOICE$THERAPY NTID
7531    STUCKLESS COMMUNICATION WORK INPLICATIONS DEAF$WORKER
7531    SUBTELNY SP$ASSESSMENT DEAF$ADULT
7531    SUBTELNY COMMUNICATION NTID$STUDENTS PLANNING REHAB
7603    DODD PHONOLOGICAL$SYSTEMS DEAF$CHILDREN
7603    NICKERSON COMPUTER-AIDED$SP$TRNG DEAF
7604    MONSEN FORMANT$TRANSITIONS SP DEAF$CHILDREN
7604    QUIGLEY VERB$SYSTEM LANG DEAF
7604    QUIGLEY COMPLEMENT$STRUCTURES LANG DEAF
7604    STEVENS ASSESSMENT NASALIZATION SP DEAF$CHILDREN
7604    WILBUR PRONOMINALIZATION LANG DEAF$STUDENTS
7606    GOLDSTEIN VOCALIZATION PRESCH$DEAF$CHIL VIBROTACTILE
        + VISUAL$DISPLAYS
7606    WHITEHEAD INFLUENCE CONSONANT$ENVIRONMENT DURATION
        VOWELS HI SPEAKERS
```

7615  BELLEFLEUR TTY$COMM
7615  GARRETSON TOTAL$COMM
7615  KRETSCHMER LANG$ACQUISITION
7615  STUCKLESS MANUAL+GRAPHIC COMM
7616   COMM$CHAR YOUNG$DEAF$ADULTS
7616   COMM$TRENDS
7616   COMPARISON LANG$SKILLS
7616   EFFECTS TOTAL$COMM ORALISM
7616   FRAMEWORK SP$DEV
7616   LANG ADAPTIVE$INTERACTION
7616   RECEPTIVE$ABILITIES HI$STUDENTS
7616   ROLE IDIOMATIC$EXPRESSIONS READING
7616   TEACHING LANG MR DEAF$CHILD
7616   VIDEO$TAPES CLASSROOM
7621  MONSEN PHONOLOGICAL$SPACE PROD VOWELS DEAF$ADOLESCENTS
7621  MONSEN PROD ENGLISH$STOP SP DEAF$CHILD
7621  ROTHMAN SPECTROGRAPHIC$INVESTIGATION C-V$TRANSITIONS
      SP DEAF$ADULTS
7627  FLETCHER NASALANCE HI
7703  DAVIS HRN-IMPAIRED$CHILDREN'S RESPONSES ORAL$TOTAL
      $PRESENTATIONS TACL
7704  BRASEL INFLUENCE LANG+COMM$ENVIRONMENTS DEV LANG DEAF
7704  FORNER RESPIRATORY$KINEMATICS PROFOUNDLY$HEARING-IMPAIRED
7706   STANDARDIZATION DEV TECHNICAL$SIGNS
7706  REEDER LOW-FREQUENCY$FORMANT-BASED$SP$CODE SEVERLY
      $HNG$IMPAIRED
7708  RUPP FEASIBILITY$SCALE LANG$ACQUISITION HI$CHILDREN
7715  QUIGLEY LANG$STRUCTURE DEAF$CHIL
7715  STARK SP$AQUISITION DEAF$CHIL
7715  WILBUR DEAF$CHIL DIFFICULTY SYNTACTIC$STRUCTURES
7716   COGNITION+COMM$PATTERNS CLASSROOMS
7716   EARLY$COMM SEMANTIC$FUNCTIONS
7716   LANG HI CHILD
7716   LANG$STORY$METHOD
7716   PEABODY$PICTURE$VOCABULARY$TEST
7716   PROCESSING FINGERSPELLING PRINT BY DEAF
7716   RECEPTION SENTENCES
7721  ROTHMAN ELECTROMYOGRAPHIC$INVEST ARTIC$PHONATION SP
      DEAF$ADULTS
7803  GEERS SYNTACTIC$MATURITY SPONTANEOUS$SP ELICITED$IMITATIONS
      HI$CHILD
7804  CRANDALL INFLECTIONAL$MORPHEMES MANUAL$ENG HRNING-IMPAIRED
      $CHIL MOTHER
7804  MONSEN MEASURING DEAF$CHIL SPEAK
7804  RAFFIN COMPREHENSION INFLECTIONAL$MORPHEMES DEAF$CHIL
      VISUAL$ENGLISH

```
7813   GILBERT VOT HI$INDIVIDUALS
7815   LIEBERTH SP$TRNG AUDITORY$PHONEME$IDENTIFICATION
7815   PRONOVOST COMMUNICATING WORLD-AT-LARGE
7815   PRONOVOST SP-PROCESSING$AIDS DEAF
7815   SCHULTE USE SUPPLEMENTARY$SP$INFO VERBAL$COMM
7815   SCROGGS PITCH$CONTROL SPEAKING$SITUATIONS
7816    DEAF$ADOLESCENTS COMP INFO
7816    SYNTACTIC$DEFICITS CONGENITALLY$DEAF
7816   ASPECTS TOTAL$COMM
7816   CACCAMISE SIGN$LANG SIMULTANEOUS$COMM
7816   CERF ELECTRONIC$MAILBOX COMM$TOOL HI
7816   COMM$INSTRUCTION
7816   DEAF$CHILDS SYMBOLIC$WORLD
7816   EARLY$EDUC HI
7816   LEXICAL$ABILITIES HI CHILD
7816   PERCEP$FEATURES MANUAL$ALPHABET
7816   READING HI
7816   SURVEY MATERIALS PROCEDURES TEACH READING
7816   TELEVISION DEAF
7816   THAYN MEDIA$TECHNOLOGY DEV COMM,SKILLS DEAF
7816   VISUAL$PRODESSING VERBAL$INFO DEAF PEOPLE
7816   WITHROW COMPUTER$ANIMATION LANG$INSTRUCTION
7821   WHITEHEAD VOWEL$ENVIRONMENT DURATION CONSONANTS HEARING-IMPAIRED
7827   BENNETT ARTICULATION HGN-IMPAIRED$CHIL DISTINCTIVE
       $FEATURE
7827   BLOOD LISTENERS$IMPRESSIONS HI$CHILD
7827   LEVITT COMPUTER-ASSISTED$ANALYSIS WRITTEN$LANG DEAF
       $CHIL
7827   LING SP$DEVELOPMENT HGN-IMPAIRED$CHIL
7827   MCGARR PITCH$DEVIANCY INTELLIGIBILITY DEAF$SP
7827   MONSEN VOWEL$ARTICULATION DEAF$CHIL
7827   OLLER PHONOLOGICAL$PROCESSES HNG-IMPAIRED$CHILD
7827   OSBERGER MODEL$SP$TRAINING DEAF$CHIL
7827   PARKHURST EFFECT PROSODIC$ERRORS INTELLIGIBILITY DEAF
       $SP
7827   SLOSBERG COMPUTER$APPLICATION CLINICAL$TRAINING
7827   STOKOE SIGN$CODES LANG
7827   STREFF HI$YOUNG$ADULTS VERBAL+NONVERBAL$ABILITIES
7827   WALTER WORD$KNOWLEDGE WORD$FREQUENCY DEAF$STUDENTS
```

## 0210

```
5503   SPEAKER$DIFFERENCES INTELLIGIBILITY PB$WORD$LISTS
5506   AUD$TESTING VOWEL$ARTIC
```

```
5603   EFFECT PHONIC$TRNG SP$DISCRIM SPELLING
5606   EFFECT REPETITION ARTIC$SCORES PB$WORDS
5706   CONFIRMATION NORMAL$THR$SP CID$AUD$TEST$W-
5803   TEST SOUND$DISCRIM
5806   TEST$PHONEMIC$DIFFERENTIATION RHYME$TEST
6004   SP$DISCRIM$TESTING HI$CHIL
6103   MAP$WORD$LIST
6103   PROGNOSTIC$VALUE IMITATIVE$AUD$DISCRIM$TESTS
6111   RELATIVE$INTELLIGIBILITY ITEMS CID$AUD$TEST$W-
6118   AUD$IMPERCEP
6203   FLAT$SENSORINEURAL$HNG$LOSS PB$SCORES
6203   REVISED$CNC$LISTS AUD$TESTS
6211   CARRIER$PHRASE PB$WORD$TESTING
6211   MEAS INTRA-LIST$STABILITY PAL$WORD$LISTS
6211   RELIABILITY EQUIVALENCY CID$W-
6211   RELIABILITY
6211   SRT DISCRIM METHOD$PRESENTATION FREQ$R
6304   COMPARATIVE$INTELLIGIBILITY WORD$LISTS CONTINUOUS
       $DISCOURSE
6304   PHONEMIC$ANALYSIS HALF-LIST$SP$DISCRIM$TESTS
6304   SP$DISCRIM$TESTS
6403   DERIVATION TWENTY-FIVE$WORD$PB$LISTS
6403   DERIVATION TWENTY-FIVE$WORD$PB$LISTS
6404   COMPARATIVE$EVAL SP$DISCRIM$MEAS
6404   PHONEMIC$ANALYSIS SP$DISCRIM$TESTS
6404   WORD$FAMILIARITY SP$DISCRIM
6406   NOTE PREDICTING SP-DISCRIM$SCORES
6411   ARTIC$FUNCTION SSW$LIST NORMAL$HNG
6411   SUGGESTED$IMPROVEMENTS SP$DISCRIM$TESTING
6504   DISCRIM$TEST WORD$DIFFICULTY
6504   DISCRIM$TEST WORD$DIFFICULTY
6504   INDEX PSEUDO-DISCRIM$LOSS
6504   INDEX PSEUDO-DISCRIM$LOSS
6506   COMPARISONS RHYME$TESTS PB-WORD$INTELLIGIBILITY$TESTS
6511   SP$DISCRIM HI NOISE REL AUDIOMETRIC$A
6511   SP$DISCRIM HI NOISE REL AUDIOMETRIC$PARAMETERS
6604   RELIABILITY VOICE$TESTS SP$DISCRIM
6604   SP$DISCRIM SENSORINEURAL$HNG$LOSS EXPERIMENTS ROLE
       $INTENSITY
6615   COMPARISON CHIL$ABILITY SP$DISCRIM
6711   TASK$ADAPTATION WORD$FAMILIARITY W-
6803   APPROACH SP$AUDIOMETRY
6803   DEVICE RECORDING$SP$AUDIOGRAMS
6804   COMPARISON FAIRBANKS$RHYME$TEST CID$AUD$TEST$W-
6804   DEV CONSTANT$ITEMS SP$DISCRIM$TESTING
6804   TEST SP$DISCRIM
```

6806   STATISTICAL$THEORY SP$DISCRIM$SCORE
6816   COMPARATIVE$MEAS IMPAIRED$DISCRIM SOUND$SPECTRAL$DIFFERENCES
6903   PORTABLE$DIAGNOSTIC$SP$AUDIOMETRY
6904   FACTORS SP$DISCRIM$TEST$DIFFICULTY
6904   IDENTIFICATION VOICELESS$FRICATIVES HIGH$FREQ$HI$LISTENERS
6904   REVALIDATION CLINICAL$TEST$VERSION MODIFIED$RHYME
       $WORDS
6911   EFFECT SP$HNG$LEVEL SP$DISCRIM SENSORINEURAL$HI
6911   SP$DISCRIM MULTIPLE-CHOICE$KEY$WORDS$IN$SENTENCES
7004   COMPARISON SENTENCE$IDENTIFICATION CONVENTIONAL$SP
       $DISCRIM$SCORES
7004   LOW-FREQ$VOWEL$FORMANT$DISCRIM HI$LISTENERS
7004   WRITEDOWN$VS$TALKBACK$SCORING SCORING$BIAS SP$DISCRIM
       $TESTING
7006   REDUCTION OBSERVER$BIAS READING SP$LEVELS VU$METER
7011   PHONEME$DISCRIM HYPACUSICS
7011   SP$DISCRIM AGE HNG$LOSS
7017   SP$DISCRIM$TEST CHIL
7104   AUD$AUDIOVISUAL$RECEPTION WORDS LOW-FREQ$NOISE HI
       $CHIL
7104   AUD$DETECTION SPONDAIC$WORDS WIDE-BAND$NOISE NORMAL
       $HNG$ADULTS HI$
7104   AUDIOMETRIC$CONFIGURATION PREDICTION THR$SPONDEES
7104   AUDIOMETRIC$CONFIGURATION PREDICTION THR$SPONDEES
7104   EVAL MODIFIED$RHYME$TEST HI$LISTENERS
7104   INVEST VOWEL$ITEMS MULTIPLE-CHOICE$SP$DISCRIM$TESTING
7104   ITEM-DIFFICULTY SP$DISCRIM$TEST
7104   SP$DISCRIM NOISE
7104   SP$DISCRIM NOISE
7106   DISCRIM FILTERED/CLIPPED$SP HI$SUBJECTS
7106   NEED STANDARDIZATION MEAS SP$LEVEL
7111   CVC$WORDS TESTS$ITEMS
7111   EVAL KSU$DISCRIM$TEST SENSORINEURAL$HNG$LOSS
7111   SYSTEMATIC$SELECTION
7203   CATEGORICAL$JUDGMENT WEPMAN$TEST$AUD$DISCRIM
7204   AUD$VISUAL$AUD-VISUAL$RECOGNITION CONSONANTS HI$CHIL
7204   CONSONANT$PHONEMIC$ERRORS PT$CONFIGURATIONS HI
7204   RELIABILITY MODIFIED$RHYME$TEST$HNG
7211   PAIRED$PB-
7215   VISUAL$AUD$COMBINED$PRESENTATIONS WIPI$TEST HI$CHIL
7304   EQUIVALENCY CID$REVISED$CID$SENTENCE$LISTS
7304   R$FOILS MODIFIED$RHYME$HNG$TESTS
7304   SAME$DIFFERENT$CONCEPTS CHIL SP$SOUND DISCRIM
7306   EFFECT CLOSED-R$FORMAT MODIFIED$RHYME$TEST
7311   BC$SP$DISCRIM PATHOLOGIES
7311   EVAL NOISE$SUB-TEST GFW$TEST$AUD$DISCRIM

```
7311   REVIEW A$IMPLICATIONS TESTING VOWEL$PERCEP
7403   AUDIO$TAPE$CASSETTS SP$AUDIOMETRY
7403   SPONDEE$RECOGNITION$TEST HI$CHIL
7404   CONSONANTS$CONFUSIONS HNG$LOSS ABOVE$
7404   PERFORMANCE HI$CHIL CLOSED-R$AUDIOMETRY SP$DISCRIM
7404   PT$THR WORD-RECOGNITION$ABILITIES HI$CHIL
7404   VARIABLES PERFORMANCE SP$DISCRIM
7406   STABILITY ACCURACY ADAPTIVE$TESTS SP$DISCRIM
7503   BEATTIE INTELLIGIBILITY CID$SPONDEES MLV
7503   CONN SP$RECEPTION$THRESHOLD PRIOR$FAMILIARIZATION
7503   MARTIN MODIFICATION TILLMAN-OLSEN$METHOD SPEECH$RECEPTION
       $THRESHOLD
7504   DANAHER MASKING LOW-FREQ$VOWEL$FORMANTS SENSORINEURAL
       $HL
7504   FRANKLIN COMBINING$LOW + HIGH-FREQ$PASSBANDS CONSONANT
       $RECOG HI
7504   MOULTON VERBAL$CODING$STRADEGIES HI
7504   REED IDENTIFICATION DISCRININATION VC$SYLLABLES SN
       $HL
7504   WALDEN AUD+ADIOVISUAL$FEATURE$TRANSMISSION HI
7504   WALDEN DIMENSIONS CONSONANT$PERCEP NORMAL+HI
7506   AGRAWAL EFFECT VOICED$SP$PARAMETERS INTELLIGIBILITY
       PB$WORDS
7508   GENGEL LISTENLNG$LEVEL SP RECEP HI$CHILD
7511   GELFAND CARRIER$PHRASE LIVE$VOICE DISCRIM$TESTING
7512   SCHUBERT RELIABILITY GOLDMAN-FRISTOE-WOODCOCK AUD
       $DISCRIM LD CHILDREN
7512   WARYAS PHONOLOGICAL DISCRIM HI$RETARDED CHILDREN
7516    EFFECTS EXPANSIONS COMMS$RATE
7531   RETZINGER GROUP$TESTING HNG$DISCRIMINATION
7531   SIMS VALIDATION CID$EVERYDAY$SENTENCE$TEST USE HI
7603   SANDERSON-LEEPA ARTICULATION$FUNCTIONS TEST-RETEST
       CHIL SP$DISCRIM
7604   BILGER CONSONANT$CONFUSIONS SENSORI-NEURAL$HL
7604   COHEN LOW-PASS$NOISE WORD-RECOGNITION$TESTING
7611   FRANKLIN ANALYSIS DISCRIM$SCORES CONGENITAL$SN$LOSS
7703   BEATTIE COMPARISON AUDITEC$RECORDINGS NU-
7703   BESS WORD$DISCRIM FLAT$HEARING$LOSSES
7703   ERBER STIMULUS$INTENSITY SP$PERCEP DEAF$CHIL
7703   POSNER RELATIONSHIPS COMFORTABLE$LOUDNESS SP SP$DISCRIM
       SN$HNG$LOSS
7703   SCHWARTZ SPLIT-HALF$RELIABILITY DISCRIM$TESTS PRIMARY
       $SECONDARY$RATIO
7704   OWENS DEV CALIFORNIA$CONSONANT$TEST
7704   ZEISER AUD/VIBRATORY$PERCEP SYLLABIC$STRUCTURE HI
       $CHILD
```

7706    MAZOR MODERATE FREQUENCY$COMPRESSION MODERATELY$HNG
        $IMPAIRED
7706    VILLCHUR ELECTRONIC$MODELS SENSORY$DISTORTIONS SP
        $PERCEPTION DEAF
7716     SENTENCE SPONDEE$STIMULI
7721    ROTHMAN ELECTROMYOGRAPHIC$INVEST ARTIC$PHONATION SP
        DEAF$ADULTS
7732    MANNING LATERAL$CEREBRAL$DIFF DEAF R LING + NONLING
        $STIMULI
7803    BARRY PHYSICAL+PSYCHOLOGICAL$CONSTRAINTS BC$SP$AUDIOMETRY
7803    MARTIN SP$THR SPANISH-SPEAKING$CHILD NON-SPANISH$CLINICIANS
7803    STEELE AUD+AISUAL$STIMULI ADAPTIVE$TESTING SP$DISCRIM
7804    THORNTON SP-DISCRIM$SCORES BINOMIAL$VARIABLE
7806    NABELEK PRECEDENCE$EFFECT WORD$ID HI$SUBJECTS
7813    MULLER PHONEME$DISCRIM HEARING$THRESHOLD$LEVEL
7827    LEWIS SEMANTIC$RULES HARD-OF-HEARING$CHILD
7829    BENNETT RELATIONSHIPS SP$DISCRIM COMFORTABLE$LISTENING
        $LEVELS


                            0211


5415    HI$CHIL
5506    LATENT$DAMAGE EAR
5506    TONAL$MONAURAL$DIPLACUSIS
5515    HOSPITAL$CLINICS HI
5515    MOBILIZATION$STAPES
5615    FENESTRATION
5715    ADVANCES EXPERIMENTAL$OTOLOGIC$RESEARCH
5715    MOTHER DOCTOR DEAF$CHIL
5804    STAPEDOLYSIS STAPES$MOBILIZATION NOMOGRAPH$TECHNIC
5815    ADJUSTMENT HI$CHIL
5816    ATTITUDES POPULAR$CONCEPTIONS DEAF
5816    COMMUNITY$OBLIGATIONS DEAF
5906    EXPERIMENTAL$STUDY BC EARS MECHANICAL$IMPAIRMENT OSSICLES
5915    STAPES$SURGERY
5916    HISTORICAL$SKETCH MANUAL$ALPHABET
6016    COMM GESTURES
6016    EXPERIMENTAL$PROGRAM USE TELEPHONE DEAF$HH$CHIL
6017    TEAM$APPROACH REHAB HH$CHIL
6103    HISTORICAL$NOTES STUDY$DEAF
6104    VEIN$PLUG$STAPEDIOPLASTY BC$ACUITY
6111    DIHYDRODESOXY$STREPTOMYCIN$OTOTOXICITY
6111    EFFECTS X-RADIATION$HEAD HNG$RAT
6115    HEREDITARY$ASPECTS DEAFNESS

6116    BRAIN-INJURED$DEAF$CHIL SYMPTOMS CAUSES
6118    AUD$IMPERCEP
6203    OBSERVATIONS MASKING PROGRESSION$AUD$SIGNS ACOUS$NEURINOMA
6205    STAPEDECTOMY A$OTOLOGICAL$EVAL OTOSCLEROTIC$SURGICAL
        $CANDIDATES
6206    MIDDLE-EAR$MECHANICS SURGERY DEAFNESS
6215    ATTITUDES INFORMATION DEAFNESS
6215    HNG$TEAM
6216    CAPTIONED$FILM$PROGRAM DEAF
6315    CAPTIONED$FILMS DEAF
6315    ETIOLOGY$DEAFNESS
6315    OTOLOGIC$RESEARCH
6315    STAPEDECTOMY
6403    AC$RECEIVER$INSERT MASTOID$CAVITY
6403    AC$RECEIVER$INSERT MASTOID$CAVITY
6403    GUIDE PSYCHOLOGICAL$TESTS TESTING$PROCEDURES EVAL
        DEAF$HH$CHIL
6415    GLOSSARY$TERMS CHIL HNG$DIS
6416    INTELLECTIVE$ABILITIES DEAF$CHIL FACTOR$ANALYSES
6419    OTOLOGIC$A$CLINIC
6503    OTO-A$FINDINGS TREACHER$COLLINS$SYNDROME CASE
6504    AUD$PERCEP$THR BRAIN-INJURED$CHIL
6504    EFFECT STAPEDCTOMY LOUDNESS ONES$OWN$VOICE
6511    OTOLARYNGOLOGICAL$MEDICAL$FINDINGS
6513    AUD$AGNOSIA ALTERATION$VOICE PERSONAL$CHARACTER
6515    GENETIC$COUNSELING FAMILIES CONGENITAL$HNG$DEFECT
6515    HI MR BIBLIOGRAPHY
6603    ODE PLASTIC$STAPES
6606    MODEL$LOUDNESS$SUMMATION IMPAIRED$EARS
6615    ADOL$ADJUSTMENT DEAF
6615    CAUSES LATE$RECOGNITION DEAFNESS$CHIL
6615    FAMILY DEAF$CHIL
6615    HEREDITARY$DEAFNESS
6616    CAPTIONED$FILMS DEAF
6616    EMPLOYMENT$PROBLEMS DEAF
6716    COMPARISON MOTOR$BEHAVIOR DEAF$BOYS
6807    HI$CHIL
6815    ADAPTATIONS SCIENTIFIC$METHOD DEAF$CHIL
6815    MOTHERS$ADUL$DEAF
6816    ETHICAL$RELIGIOUS$CONCEPTS DEAF
6904    NUMERICAL$MAGNITUDES$EST LOUDNESS$POST-STAPEDECTOMY
6911    HNG VOCAL$OUTPUT DEAF$INF$MICE
6911    STAPEDECTOMY SP$DISCRIM
6915    ATTITUDES DEAF$ADOL ATTENDANCE$COLLEGE$HNG
6916    PERFORMANCE$SCALE COGNITIVE$CAPACITY DEAF
7003    H1 ADULT$PENAL$INSTITUTION

7011   AUD$DYSFUNCTION SCHIZOPHRENIC$PATIENTS
7011   COMPARISON MIDDLE$EAR$IMPED$NORMS PREDICTORS$OTOSCLEROSIS
7011   DL$INTENSITY CENTRAL$AUD$PATH
7016   BEHAVIOR$THEORY PROBLEMS DEAF
7103   CHARACTERISTICS MANUALLY$COMM DEAF$ADULTS
7111   OTITIS$MEDIA RATS
7116   PERFORMANCE HI$CHIL NON-VERBAL$PERSONALITY$TEST
7203   AUD$DIS BILATERAL$TEMPORAL$LOBE$INSULT CASE$REPORT
7203   BILATERAL$ACOUS$NEUROMAS
7203   GENETIC$HNG$LOSS NO$ABNORMALITIES REVIEW
7204   BEHAVIOR$PROBLEMS DEAF$CHIL DEAF$ADOL FACTOR$ANALYTIC
       $STUDY
7211   FREQ$DISCRIM MASKING PATH$EARS
7211   TINNITUS$AURIUM SCH$CHIL SURVEY
7214   GENERALIZATION SP$DISCRIM$TRNG
7215   HI$CHIL HOSPITAL
7303   DISTURBED$DEAF$CHIL THERAPY BEHAVIOR$SHAPING
7304   SP$CODING SHORT-TERM$MEMORY DEAF
7306   GENETIC$FEATURES DEAFNESS
7306   NOTES ELECTROPHONIC$HNG$EFFECT
7315   HI$CHIL FAMILY$PARENT$PERSPECTIVE
7315   TAX$DEDUCTIONS HANDICAPPED$CHIL
7316   FINGER$SPELLING$INTELLIGIBILITY
7405   ADVOCACY HI
7406   UPPER$LIMIT STAPES$DISPLACEMENT IMPLICATIONS HNG$LOSS
7415   ACUPUNCTURE
7415   ACUPUNCTURE DEAFNESS
7415   ACUPUNCTURE
7415   BEHAVIORAL$CHANGE DEAF-BLIND$MULTIHANDICAPPED$CHIL
7415   CLASSROOM$OBSERVATION SIMULATED$DEAFNESS
7503   JENSEMA CHIL HNG$IMPAIRED MUMPS
7503   SPEAKS CENTRAL$AUDITORY$DEFICITS TEMPORAL-LOBE$LESIONS
7506   SCHELLENG ANOMALY PITCH$PERCEPTION
7511   GOETZINGER IMPACT HEARING$IMPAIRMENT PSYCHOLOGICAL
       $DEVELOPMENT CHIL
7513   GILBERT ORAL NASAL AIRFLOW STOP$CONSONANT$PROD HI
       $SPEAKERS
7513   WEISS LINGUAL$DISCRIM DEAF$CHILDREN
7515   BERRETT PARENTS DISCIPLINE HI CHILD
7515   BOOTHROYD TECHNOLOGY DEAFNESS
7515   CHAPMAN HEALTH$NEEDS HI
7515   HELD ORAL$DEAF$PARENTS COMM DEAF$INFANTS
7515   HINCKLEY HEALTH$CARE HI CHILD
7515   ISRAEL HEALTH$CARE HI
7515   LEIGH HNG$LOSS HEALTH$CARE INFANT CHILD
7515   MARGOLIS  AFFIRMATIVE$ACTION JOB$OPP DEAF INDIV

```
7515   MILLER ADULT ELDERLY HEALTH$CARE HNG$LOSS
7515   NIX TOTAL$COMM
7515   SCHWARTZBERG IMPACT HNG$LOSS
7515   STEWART PROVISION HEALTH$CARE UNDERSERVED
7515   URBAN ID MANAGEMENT HNG IMPAIR
7516    CHILD HL REPORTING DIAGNOSIS
7516    COMM$PREFERENCE SOCIAL$CONDITIONS
7516    EEG REM$SLEEP$STUDIES DEAF$PEOPLE
7516    EXPERIENTIAL$DEPRIVATION IMPOVERISHED$SOCIALIZATION
7516    EXPERIENTIAL$DEPREVATION R
7516    HI INSTITUTIONS RETARDED
7516    HI INSTITUTIONS RETARDED
7516    KNOWLEDGE CONCEPTS DEAF$ADOLESCENTS
7516    LITERATURE SIGNS
7516    SELF-CONCEPT EXPRESSIVE$LANG
7516    SEX$ROLE$ATTITUDES DEAF$ADOLESCENT$WOMEN
7526   KELTER CONCEPT STRUCTURE APHASIC SCHIZOPHRENIC PATIENTS
        SORTING$TASK
7531   CRANDALL ASSESSMENT READING+WRITING$ADULT$DEAF
7531   KELLY NTID$TRNG$PROGRAM INTERPERSONAL$COMMUNICATION
7604   BELMONT REHEARSAL$STRATEGIES DEAF MEMORY$PROCESSING
7604   BILGER CONSONANT$CONFUSIONS SENSORI-NEURAL$HL
7604   JESTEADT TEMPORAL$ACUITY SENSORINEURAL$HL
7604   KELLY INFORMATION$PROCESSING VISUALLY$PRESENTED$STIMULI
        HI$CHILDREN
7605   DOWLING LEGISLATIVE$HORIZONS HEARING$IMPAIRED
7605   JETER HEARING$IMPAIRMENT PSYCHIATRIC$PATIENTS
7605   SMOSKI TTY DEAF
7611   BALDWIN GENERALIZATION VOWEL$DISCRIM$LEARNING HI$CHIL
7615    QUICK LICENSING HRG CLINICIANS TEACHERS HI
7615   FELLENDORF INTERNATIONAL$TRENDS
7615   GLASSCOCK MEDICAL$INTERVENTION
7615   LEVINE PSYCHOLOGICAL$CONTRIBUTIONS
7615   LLOYD SOCIAL+REHAB$SERVICES
7615   NANCE HEREDITARY$DEAFNESS
7616    ADDENDUM INTENSIVE$INTERPRETER$TRAINING
7616    COMPARISON LANG$SKILLS
7616    DEAF$STUDENTS GROUP$PROBLEM$SOLVING$SITUATIONS
7616    GUIDELINES AUDIO$PROGRAMS
7616    INCIDENCE NEUROLOGICAL$PROBLEMS
7616    INTENSIVE INTERPRETER$TRAINING
7616    LANG ADAPTIVE$INTERACTION
7616    MAINSTREAMING COST$ISSUE
7616    ROLE IDIOMATIC$EXPRESSIONS READING
7616    VIDEO$TAPES CLASSROOM
7703   SPARKS TACTUAL$COMMUNICATION$AID HNG$IMPAIRED
```

7704    TOMBLIN SYNTACTIC$ORDER SERIAL-RECALL OF HI
7704    WOOD AUD$REACTION$TIMES HL
7704    ZEISER AUD/VIBRATORY$PERCEP SYLLABIC$STRUCTURE HI
        $CHILD
7705    EGAN HIGH-RISK$REGISTERS
7706    KRUGER MIDDLE$EAR$TRANSMISSION CATS EXPERIMENTALLY
        $INDUCED$TM$PERFS
7706    REEDER LOW-FREQUENCY$FORMANT-BASED$SP$CODE SEVERLY
        $HNG$IMPAIRED
7715    BODNER PERSONALITY HEARING$IMPAIRMENT
7715    CASTLE TELEPHONE$TRNG DEAF
7715    MCCLURE ACAD$ACHIEVEMENT MAINSTREAMED$HI$CHIL RUBELLA
7715    MCLEOD USE TELEPHONE ORAL$DEAF
7715    MURPHY COUNSELING
7715    NORTHCOTT ORAL$INTERPRETER HEARING$IMPAIRED
7715    SCHEIN CURRENT$PRIORITIES DEAFNESS
7716     BEER POT SHOPLIFTING TEENAGE$ABUSES
7716     CHALLENGE PROFESSION
7716     CHAR HI$TEACHERS OF DEAF
7716     COPING$PATTERNS PARENTS DEAF-BLIND$CHILD
7716     DISTINCTIVE$FEATURES$APPROACH ANALYSIS SP
7716     EMPLOYMENT BASIC$SKILLS
7716     HEMISPHERIC$LATERALITY DEAF$CHILD ·
7716     NORTH CAROLINA$LEGISLATURE RESPONDS NEEDS OF DEAF
7716     PSYCHOLOGICAL$SERVICES HI$CHILD
7716     REHEARSAL REACLL$STRATEGIES DEAF+HRING
7716     STANDARDIZATION DEV TECHNICAL$SIGNS
7716     SURVEY MATHMATICS$PROGRAM
7716     USE ADAPTED CLASSICS READING$PROGRAM
7732    MANNING LATERAL$CEREBRAL$DIFF DEAF R LING + NONLING
        $STIMULI
7803    FRANK ACOUSTIC$NEURINOMA CHILD
7803    SILMAN OBSERVATIONS CASE ACOUS$NEUROMA
7804    FINITZO-HIEBER ROOM$ACOUSTICS WORD$DISCRIM HEARING-IMPAIRED
        $CHIL
7804    REED TADOMA$METHOD DISCRIM$ABILITY UNTRAINED$LISTENERS
7804    WANG FILTERING SENSORINEURAL$HEARING$LOSS PATTERNS
        CONSONANT$CONFUSION
7805    CANTERBURY PUBLIC$HEALTH$AUDIOLOGY ALASKA
7805    KRICOS NONTRADITIONAL$SERVICES DEAF SP$HEARING$CENTERS
7815    CARLSON INTELLECTUAL$CAPABILITIES HI$CHIL
7815    COHEN DEAF$ADOLESCENT
7815    FELLENDORF RH$FACTOR
7815    MARKS DEVELOPMENTAL$PROCESSES ADOLESCENCE
7815    PRONOVOST COMMUNICATING WORLD-AT-LARGE
7816     ATTITUDES DEAFNESS

7816   HI DEVOPMENTALLY$DISABLED$PERSONS
7816   MEASUREMENT$ERROR ACHIEVEMENT$TESTS
7816   NEEDS$ASSESSMENT
7816   PARAPROFESSIONAL$TUTORS NOTETAKERS
7816   PSYCHOLOGICAL$SERVICES
7816   SPACIAL+DISTANCING$BEHAVIOR DEAF ADULTS
7816   TV$VIEWING HI$TEENAGERS
7816   USHERS$SYNDROME PERSONAL$SOCIAL$EMOTIONAL$IMPLICATIONS
7816   BELLEFLEUR RADIO/TELETYPE$COMM$SYATEMS CAPTIONS
7816   BRANSFORD COMM$SATELLITES APPLICATIONS HI
7816   CERTIFICATION$REQUIREMENTS TEACHERS DEAF
7816   COMMUNITY$PROGRAMS
7816   EARLEY CAPTIONING WGBH-TV
7816   FUCHS BEH RESOURCES MATERIALS HI
7816   HEALTH$STUDY NEW$ORLEANS
7816   KELLY HEMISPHERIC$SPECIALIZATION DEAF$CHILD
7816   KELLY M
7816   MCLEAN STATUS MEDIA$MATERIALS$CENTER
7816   PERCEP$FEATURES MANUAL$ALPHABET
7816   PROPP MEDIA$DEV$PROJECT HI
7816   REHAB$PROGRAMS
7816   RESEARCH+INFO$PROGRAMS
7816   SELF-CONCEPT$LEVELS POSTSECONDARY$DEAF$ADOLESCENTS
7816   SELF-CONCEPT ADJUSTMENTS$PATTERNS
7816   SEX$EDUCATOR
7816   SILLMAN CLOSED$CAPTIONING TV
7816   TELEVISION DEAF
7816   VOCATIONAL$EVAL$SERVICES HI
7827   ALTSHULER PSYCHOLOGY DEAFNESS
7827   LEVITT ASSESSMENT TRAINING TECHNOLOGY DEAF


## 0301


5406   MEAS HUMAN$CHANNEL$TRANSMISSION$CHARACTERISTICS
5410   VOCAL$FOLD$ACTIVITY SUB-GLOTTIC$AIR$PRESSURE REL VOCAL
       $INTENSITY R
5413   PHYSIOLOGY$VIBRATIONS VOCAL$CORDS
5413   VOCAL$CAVITIES
5418   VELO$SPHINCTER
5506   CALCULATIONS MODEL$VOCAL$TRACT VOWEL LARYNX
5506   TRANSMISSION VOCAL$CAVITIES
5510   TEMPORAL$ASPECTS BREATHING READING$SPEAKING
5513   ROLE LARYNGEAL$VENTRICLE VOICE$PRODUCTION
5515   SOUND$PERCEP BREATH$CONTROL

5613    DIRECT$AND$INDIRECT$DETERMINATION MEAN$SUBGLOTTIC
        $PRESSURE
5706    AIR$RESISTANCE BERNOULLI$EFFECT HUMAN$LARYNX
5713    CHEST$REGISTER MEMBRANE$CUSHION$MODEL VOCAL$CORDS
5804    POSTERIOR$PHARYNGEAL$MOVEMENTS
5804    SOFT$PALATE$MOVEMENT
5806    RELATIVE$INTENSITIES$SOUNDS ANATOMICAL$LOCALES$HEAD
        $NECK
5813    VARIATIONS VIBRATORY$PATTERN NORMAL$LARYNX
5819    REL MANDIBULAR$MOVEMENT INTELLIGIBILITY
5904    RESPIRATORY$MUSCLES SP
5913    ACOUS$MECHANICAL$PROPERTIES VOCAL$FOLDS
6004    LARYNGEAL$CORRELATES VOCAL$PITCH
6004    MEAS VOCAL$FOLDS PITCH$CHANGES
6004    PHYSIOLOGY SP$BREATHING
6004    SEQUENCE$ACTION BREATHING$MUSCLES SP
6004    VOCAL$PITCH$VARIATION REL VOCAL$FOLD$LENGTH
6009    ANATOMY PHYSIOLOGY SP
6013    LARYNGEAL$PHASE DETERMINABLE$FLASH$PHOTOGRAPHY
6113    FUNCTION$VELUM
6113    MOVEMENT TONGUE SOFT$PALATE SINGING$VOWELS
6203    FUNCTIONS$DYSFUNCTIONS VENTRICULAR$FOLDS
6204    INTRALARYNGEAL$REL PITCH$INTENSITY$CHANGES
6204    INVEST MUSCLE$PULSES SP$PROD
6204    INVEST MUSCLE$PULSES SP$PROD
6204    NEONATAL$EKG$R SOUND METHODOLOGY
6204    VELO$CLOSURE VOWELS
6204    VOCAL$FOLD$THICKNESS FUND$FREQ PHONATION
6210    EXPERIMENTS TONGUE-PALATE$CONTACTS
6213    ELEVATION$TILTING VOCAL$FOLDS VOCAL$PITCH
6306    LOUDNESS SOUND$PRESSURE SUBGLOTTAL$PRESSURE SP
6313    EMG$STUDY MOVEMENTS SOFT-PALATE
6314    PHYSIOLOGICAL$PARAMETERS SP
6403    ARTIC PATTERNS PALATOPHARYNGEAL$CLOSURE
6404    EMG$STUDY TONGUE VOWEL$PROD
6406    LONG-TERM LARYNX-EXCITATION$SPECTRA
6414    LIP$POSITIONS AMERICAN$ENG$VOWELS
6507    EMBRYOLOGY ANATOMY GROWTH OROFACIAL$COMPLEX
6510    SEQUENCE RESPIRATORY$MUSCLE$ACTIVITY VOCAL$ATTACK
6513    EVAL TONGUE$PRESSURES$SP
6514    ASPECTS PROD ORAL$NASAL$LABIAL$STOPS
6514    TEMPORAL$PATTERNS COGNITIVE$ACTIVITY BREATH$CONTROL
        SP
6604    INTRAORAL$PRESSURE RATE$FLOW SP
6604    PHYSIOLOGICAL$THEORY PHONETICS
6613    INTRANASAL$SOUND$PRESSURE UTTERANCE$SP

6614 NEUROMUSCULAR$SPECIFICATION LINGUISTIC$UNITS
6614 PLACE$CUES PTK$PHONEMES LOWER$CUT-OFF$FREQ$SHIFTS
CONTIGUOUS$S$PHO
6704 EFFECTS VERBAL$DECISION$BEHAVIOR RESPIRATION SP$PROD
6704 LINGUAL$PRESSURES ALVEOLAR$CONSONANTS
6704 PEAK$INTRAORAL$AIR$PRESSURES SP
6704 TECHNIQUES MEAS INTRAORAL$AIR$PRESSURE RATE AIR$FLOW
6706 DETERMINATION VOCAL-TRACT$SHAPE MEAS FORMANT$FREQ
6706 DETERMINATION GEOMETRY HUMAN$VOCAL$TRACT ACOUS$MEAS
6710 RESPIROMETRIC$STUDY LUNG$FUNCTION UTTERANCE SP$MATERIAL
6713 RESPIROMETRIC$TECHNIQUE EVAL VELO$COMPETENCE SP
6713 VOCAL$INITIATION ACOUS$AERODYNAMIC$INVEST
6717 CHEST-PULSE$THEORY RESEARCH
6804 ELECTRONIC$INTEGRATOR MEAS PARTITIONS LUNG$VOLUME
6804 INSTRUMENTATION MEAS LINGUAL$STRENGTH
6804 LINGUAL$FUNCTION RELATIVE$LENGTH LINGUAL$FRENULUM
6806 MEAS VOCAL$FOLD$MOTION ULTRASONIC$DOPPLER$VELOCITY
$MONITOR
6806 VALIDITY LARYNGEAL$PHOTOSENSOR$MONITORING
6807 METHOD RECORDING FLUCTUATIONS ELECTRICAL$POTENTIALS
SP$MUSCLES
6810 RELATIVE$INTRA-NASAL$INTENSITIES VOWELS
6813 X-RAY$STUDY VOCAL$FOLD$LENGTH
6904 FUNCTION LARYNGEAL$MUSCLES REGULATING FUND$FREQ INTENSITY
$PHONATIO
6904 REL NASAL$SPL PALATOPHARYNGEAL$CLOSURE
6906 GENERATION SP$LIKE$SIGNALS EXCITATION VOCAL$TRACT
LIPS
6906 INTRAORAL$AIR$PRESSURES P$PHONEME ORAL WHISPERED$VOWELS
6906 RESPIRATORY$VOLUMES NORMAL$SP INTRAORAL$PRESSURE DIFFERENCES
6906 TRANSILLUMINATION LARYNX RUNNING$SP
6906 VOCAL-TRACT$CHARACTERISTICS STOP$COGNATES
6910 HYOID$MOVEMENT VOWEL$PROD
6910 ROLE SP EXTRA-SIGNAL$FEEDBACK REGULATION CHIL SENSORIMOTOR
$BEHAVIO
6913 LAMINAGRAPHIC$STUDIES VOCAL$FOLD$THICKNESS
6913 REL INTRAORAL$AIR$PRESSURE ORAL$CAVITY$SIZE
7004 LARYNGEAL$CORRELATES FREQ$CHANGE STROL$STUDY
7004 LATERAL$PHARYNGEAL$WALL$MOVEMENTS SP$PROD
7004 LIP$JAW$COARTICULATION
7004 PHYSIOLOGICAL$DETERMINANTS AUTONOMIC$RESPONSIVITY
SOUND
7004 RELEASED$INFANTILE$ORONEUROMOTOR$ACTIVITY
7006 LENIS-FORTIS$OPPOSITION PHYSIOLOGICAL$PARAMETERS
7006 PROD STOP$COGNATES
7006 SIMULTANEOUS$MEAS INTRAORAL$PRESSURE FORCE LABIAL
$CONTACT LABIAL$E

7007    MODIFICATION ORAL-FACIAL$FUNCTION SP
7007    MUSCULAR$DEV MATURATION DENTOFACIAL$COMPLEX
7007    MUSCULAR$FUNCTIONS DENTOFACIAL$MILIEU SP
7007    NEUROANATOMY SP
7007    PROCESSES$MATURATION MASTICATION DEGLUTITION
7007    TONGUE$ORAL$MORPHOLOGY TONGUE$ACTIVITY SP SWALLOWING
7011    ROLE SENSORY$FEEDBACK TONGUE$CONTROL
7013    INTRAORAL$AIR$PRESSURE PRESSURE TIME$MEAS
7014    SUPRAGLOTTAL$AIR$PRESSURE PROD ENG$STOPS
7103    PRELIMINARY$REPORT MOVEMENT$PATTERNS TONGUE PALATE
        HYPOPHARYNX LAR
7103    TONGUE
7104    HYOID$POSITIONS REPEATED$SYLLABLES
7104    NEUROMUSCULAR$SPINDLES INTRINSIC$MUSCLES HUMAN$LARYNX
7106    ACOUS$LEVEL VOCAL$EFFORT CUES LOUDNESS SP
7106    DETERMINATION VOCAL$TRACT$SHAPE IMPULSE$R LIPS
7106    ELECTROMAGNETIC$METHOD TRANSDUCING JAW$MOVEMENTS SP
7106    FLANAGANS$MODEL VOCAL-CORD$OSCILLATIONS
7106    INVEST TIMING VELAR$MOVEMENTS SP
7106    JAW$MOVEMENTS DAF
7106    LATERALITY$EFFECT LINGUAL-AUD$TRACKING
7107    POSTNATAL$DEV OROFACIAL$MUSCULATURE
7107    RESPIRATION$GROWTH$DEV
7112    LEFT$BRAIN TALKING
7113    ACOUS$ASSESSMENT NASOPHARYNX ANALYSIS RESPIRATORY
        $SOUNDS
7113    ASPECTS SYMMETRY MALE$FEMALE LARYNGEAL$FUNCTION
7113    EFFECT RESPIRATORY$POSTURAL$MECHANISMS VOCAL$CORDS
7203    EFFECT PROLONGED$NASOTRACHEAL$INTUBATION COMM
7204    VELO$ANATOMY
7206    COMPARISON SUBGLOTTAL$AIR$PRESSURE
7206    INFLUENCE UTTERANCE$LENGTH BILABIAL$CLOSURE$DURATION
7206    PRESSURE$MEAS ARTIC ALTERATIONS VOCAL$EFFORT
7206    STUDIES SINGLE$MOTOR$UNITS SP$MUSCULATURE METHODOLOGY
7207    JAW$MOTION SP
7207    SP$MEAS OROFACIAL$FUNCTION
7207    TECHNIQUES MEAS BIOMECHANICAL$EVENTS SP$PROD LAB$EXPERIENCE
7213    RECORDINGS REGISTERED$VARIOUS$POINTS VOCAL$TRACT
7303    VELO$FUNCTION
7304    FORWARD$COARTICULATION VELAR$MOVEMENT MARK$JUNCTURAL
        $BOUNDARIES
7304    INFLUENCE GAMMA$MOTER$SYSTEM JAW$MOVEMENTS SP
7304    INTERPRETATION JAW$ACCELERATION SP MUSCLE$FORCING
        $FUNCTION
7304    KINEMATIC$CHEST$WALL SP$PROD VOLUME$DISPLACEMENTS
7304    LABIAL$MANDIBULAR$DYNAMICS PROD$BILABIAL$CONSONANTS

7304   REL LINGUAL$INTRAORAL$AIR$PRESSURES SYLLABLE$PRODUCTION
7304   RIB-CAGE$ABDOMEN$LUNG
7304   STRAIN$GAGE$TRANSDUCTION$SYSTEM LIPS$JAW$MOTION DESIGN
       $CRITERIA
7306   GLOTTAL-AREA$TIME$FUNCTION SUBGLOTTAL-PRESSURE$VARIATION
7306   MODEL VOCAL$CORD$EXCITATION
7306   ON-LINE$ULTRASONIC$TECHNIQUE MONITORING TONGUE$DISPLACEMENTS
7306   TRANSGLOTTAL$AIRFLOW STOP$CONSONANT$PROD
7313   GLOTTAL$ACTIVITY INTRAORAL$PRESSURE STOP$CONSONANT
7313   LARYNGEAL$CONTROL VOCAL$ATTACK EMG$STUDY
7313   ORAL$AIRFLOW STOP$CONSONANT
7313   SOFT$PALATE$INNERVATION
7313   SP$MECHANISM
7314   ACOUS$FEATURES CHIL VOWELS DEV CHRONOLOGICAL$AGE$VS
       $BONE$AGE
7314   EMG INTRAORAL$AIR-PRESSURE$STUDIES BILABIAL$STOPS
7403   VARIATIONS$VELOPHARYNGEAL$CLOSURE ENDOSCOPY
7404   ELECTROPHYSIOLOGIC$ASSESSMENT HEMISPHERIC$ASYMMETRIES
       SP
7404   EMG$ACTIVITY PHARYNX SP$PRODUCTION
7404   NEURAL$MECHANICAL$R$TIME SP$PROD
7404   VELAR$MOVEMENT TIMING EVALUATION MODEL BINARY$CONTROL
7406   INFLUENCE UTTERANCE$LENGTH BILABIAL$CLOSURE$DURATION
       CHIL
7406   LEFT$HEMISPHERE SP LANG
7406   MODEL WAVE$PROPAGATION LOSSY VOCAL$TRACT
7413   INVEST LARYNGEAL$TRILLS TRANSMISSION$ULTRASOUND LARYNX
7413   LARYNGEAL$MYOTATIC$REFLEXES PHONATION
7413   LARYNGEAL$NEUROMUSCULAR$SPINDLES
7413   LUBRICATION VOCAL$MECHANISM
7413   MORPHOLOGICAL$STRUCTURE$VOCAL$CORD VIBRATOR
7413   PHOTOGLOTTOGRAPHICAL$STUDY FEMALE$VOCAL$FOLDS
7503   SHELTON PANENDOSCOPIC$FEEDBACK VELOPHARYNGEAL$MOVEMENTS
7504   FOLKINS LIP+JAW$MOTOR$CONTROL SP RESISTIVE$LOADING
       JAW
7504   HARDEN GLOTTAL$AREA$CHANGES ULTRA-HIGH-SPEED$PHOTO
       GLOTTOGRAPHS
7504   LEEPER LINGUAL-PALATAL$PRESSURE$MEAS ANALYSIS$TECHNIQUE
7504   SHIPP LARYNGEAL$POSITION VOCAL$FREQ$CHANGE
7504   ZAGZEBSKI ULTRASONIC$MEAS PHARYNGEAL$WALL$MOTION
7506   ALTES CETACEAN$ECHOLOCATION$SIGNALS HUMAN$GLOTTAL
       $PULSE
7506   BELL-BERTI CONTROL PHARYNGEAL$CAVITY$SIZE ENGLISH
7506   COLLIER PHYSIOLOGICAL$CORRELATES INTONATION$PATTERNS
7506   KASPRZYK VOWEL$PERTURBATION FUNCTION TONGUE$HEIGHT
7506   KIRITANI TONGUE-PELLET$TRACKING COMPUTER-CONTROLLED
       $X-RAY MICROBEAMS

7506   SHIPP VOCAL$FREQ VERTICAL$LARYNX$POSITIONING SINGERS
7506   SONDHI MEASUREMENT GLOTTAL$WAVEFORM
7506   TITZE NORMAL$MODES VOCAL$CORD$TISSUES
7511   VENKATAGIRI HEMISPHERIC$ASYMMETRY AUDITORY$FEEDBACK
       $CONTROL SP
7513    KELMAN EMG ACTIVITY ORBICULARIS ORIS
7524   GOSS PALATAL$DEVELOPMENT
7524   KUEHN TOMOGRAPHIC$ASSESSING LATERAL$PHARYNGEAL$WALL
7524   LATHAM VOMER GROWTH PREMAXILLARY$SEGMENT
7524   MOURINO CEPHALOMETRIC VELAR$STRENGTH CHIL
7524   NEIMAN ADENOID$REMOVAL VELOPHARYNGEAL$FUNCTION
7524   SHPRINTZEN MOVEMENT PHARYNGEAL$WALLS VELOPHARYNGEAL
       $CLOSURE
7532   MULFESE BRAIN$LATERALIZATION SP+NONSPEECH
7532   SCHALTENBRAND SP LANG STEREOTACTICAL$STIM THALAMUS
       $CORPUS$CALLOSUM
7532   SUSSMAN HEMISPHERIC$SPECIALIZATION SP
7532   TSUNODA DIFFERENCES CEREBRAL$HEMISPHERES KEY-TAPPING
       $METHOD
7532   VANBUREN THALAMIC$PARTICIPATION SPEECH
7533   NIHALANI AIR$FLOW$RATE STOPS SINDHI
7533   NIHLANI VELOPHARYNGEAL FORMATION VOICED$STOPS SINDHI
7533   PROFFIT TONGUE-LIP$PRESSURES AUSTRALIAN$ABORIGINES
7533   RAPHAEL TONGUE MUSCULATURE TENSION ENGLISH VOWELS
7533   SU LINGUAL$COARTICULATION JUNCTURE$BOUNDARIES
7604   ABBS MOTOR$IMPAIR BLOCKADE INFRAORBITAL$NERVE ANESTHETIZATION
       SP$RES
7604   BELL-BERTI EMG$STUDY VELOPHARYNGEAL$FUNCTION
7604   HIXON DYNAMICS CHEST$WALL SP$PRODUCTION
7604   HIXON MEASURING VELOPHARYNGEAL$ORIFICE VOWEL$PRODUCTION
7604   KENT ANATOMICAL$NEUROMUSCULAR$MATURATION SP$MECHANISM
7606   FLANAGAN DIGITAL$ANALYSIS LARYNGEAL$CONTROL SP$PROD
7606   ISHIZAKA INPUT$ACOUSTIC-IMPEDANCE$MEAS SUBGLOTTAL
       $SYSTEM
7606   KAKITA LARYNGEAL$CONTROL SP THYROMETER
7606   TITZE MECHANICS VOCAL-FOLD$VIBRATION
7613   BUNCH HEAD NECK SUSTAINED$PHONATION COVERED OPEN$QUALITIES
7613   FRITZELL THRYARYTENOID PALATAL$LEVATOR ACTIVATION
7613   KELMAN EMG PLOSIVE /P/ CVC$UTTERANCE
7621   CLUMECK PATTERNS SOFT$PALATE$MOVEMENTS SIX LANG
7621   CONDAX MONITORING$VELIC$ACTION PHOTO-ELECTRIC$NASAL
       $PROBE FRENCH
7621   HADDING FACIAL$MUSCLE$ACTIVITY PROD SWEDISH$VOWELS
       ELECTROMYOGRAPHIC
7621   HAMLET COMPENSATORY$VOWEL$CHAR EXPERIMENTAL$DENTAL
       $PROSTHESES

7621   HANSEN INFLUENCE ACOUSTIC+PHYSIOLOGICAL$FACTORS VOWEL
       $CHANGES DANISH
7621   LEIDNER ARTIC AMERICAN$ENGLISH L GESTURAL$SYNERGY
       ANTAGONISM
7621   LIEBERMAN PHONETIC$FEATURES PHYSIOLOGY
7621   MURRY PEAK$INTRAORAL$AIR$PRESSURES WHISPERED$STOP
7624   KUEHN CINERADIOGRAPHIC VELAR$MOVEMENT
7624   NEWALL FUSION HUMAN$SECONDARY$PALATE
7624   NISHIO MOTOR$NERVE VELOPHARYNGEAL$MUSCLES
7624   NISHIO ROLES NERVES VELOPHARYNGEAL$MOVEMENTS
7624   SHELTON EVALUATION VELO$CLOSURE
7633   HUGHES LABIAL-MANDIBULAR COORDINATION
7633   LINDQVIST-GAUFFIN ACOUSTIC NASAL$TRACT
7633   MRAYATI VOCAL$TRACT ACOUSTIC$CHARACTERISTICS FRENCH
       $VOWELS
7633   PETURSSON ASPIRATION GLOTTAL ACTIVITY CONSONANTS
7704   BAKEN ESTIMATION LUNG$VOLUME$CHANGE TORSO$HEMICIRCUMFERENCES
7704   MCCLEAN AUD$MASKING LIP$MOVEMENTS
7704   SUSSMAN RESPIRATORY$TRACKING TONAL$AMPLITUDES
7704   SUSSMAN RECRUITMENT DISCHARGE$PATTERNS SINGLE$MOTOR
       $UNITS SP
7706   GAY ARTIC$MOVEMENTS VCV$SEQUENCES
7706   HARSHMAN FACTOR$ANALYSIS TONGUE$SHAPES
7706   KRETSCHMAR METHOD MEAS LIP-OPENING$AREA
7706   MCCUTCHEON VIDEO-SCANNING$SYSTEM MEAS LIP+JAW,MOTION
7706   MONSEN VARIATIONS MALE FEMALE$GLOTTAL$WAVE
7706   NAKATANI LOCUS SEGMENTAL$CUES WORD$JUNCTURE
7706   RIORDAN CONTROL VOCAL-TRACT$LENGTH SP
7713   BAKEN ARYTENOID$DISPLACEMENT SIMULATED CONTRACTION
7713   HOLLIEN VOCAL$FOLD PATTERNS PULSE$REGISTER$PHONATION
7721   AMERMAN ASPECTS LINGUAL$COARTIC
7721   BORDEN ELECTROMYOGRAPHIC$CHANGES DAF
7721   HOMBERT DEV TONES VOWEL$HEIGHT
7721   LUBKER INTER-ARTIC$PROGRAMMING
7721   MACNIELAGE DISCHARGE$PATTERNS MOTOR$UNITS SP$MUSCULATURE
7721   NORDSTROM FEMALE+INFANT$VOCAL$TRACTS SIMULATED FROM
       MALE AREA$FUNCTION
7724   AZZAM MUSCULUS$UVULAE
7724   BERKOWITZ OROFACIAL$GROWTH DENTISTRY
7724   BERNTHAL CHANGES VELOPHARYNGEAL$ORIFICE VOWEL$INTENSITY
7724   MAHER PALATAL + OTHER$ARTERIES CLEFT + NON-CLEFT
7724   MAUE-DICKSON ANATOMY PHYSIOLOGY
7724   MAZAHERI SOFT$PALATE NASOPHARYNX SIX$MONTHS SIX$YEARS
7724   NOLL NORMAL$SIX-YEAR$MALES ORAL$MANOMETER
7725   LISHMAN HANDEDNESS CEREBRAL$DOMINANCE LANG
7725   RIZZOLATTI HEMISPHERIC$SUPERIORITY REACTION$TIME FACES
       SEX DIFFERENCE

7729   HANSON SP$PATHOLOGIST ORAL$MYOLOGY
7729   SPEIDEL ROLE TONGUE CLOSURE ANTERIOR$OPEN$BITE
7732   DU BRUL ORIGIN SP$APPARATUS FOSSILS
7732   GATES CEREBRAL$HEMISPHERES MUSIC
7733   FANT LARYNX LANG
7733   KUENZEL VELAR$HEIGHT VOWEL$ARTIC
7803   GAUFFIN PHARYNGEAL$CONSTRICTIONS
7804   BERNTHAL INTRAORAL$AIR$PRESSURE PRODUCTION$/P/ + /B/
7804   FOLKINS STANDARDIZATION LIPS$MUSCLE$NOMENCLATURE
7804   HORII AIR$FLOW VOLUME DURATION ORAL$READING
7804   IZABSKI MINIMAL$REACTION$TIMES PHONATORY$INITIATION
7804   MCCLEAN PERIORAL$REFLEX$AMPLITUDE LIP$MUSCLE$CONTRACTION
7806   ABBS CEPHALOSTAT SP$PHYSIOLOGY$RESEARCH
7806   ATAL ARTIC-TO-ACOUSTIC$TRANSFORMATION VOCAL$TRACT
       COMPUTER
7806   ATKINSON CORRELATION$ANALYSIS PHYSIOLOGICAL$FACTORS
       FF
7806   FLANAGAN COMPUTER$MODEL AIR$VOLUME VOCAL$CORDS
7806   JACKSON ACOUSTIC$INPUT$IMPEDANCE DOG$LUNGS
7806   LASS SPEAKERS HIGHTS WEIGHTS SURFACE$AREAS FF
7813   BENGUEREL FRENCH$STOP$PROD FIBERSCOPIC ACOUSTIC ELECTROMYOGRAPHIC
7813   SAITO OBSERVATION VOCAL$FOLD$VIBRATION
7821   HAMLET COMPENSATORY$ALVEOLAR$CONSONANT$PRODUCTION
       DENTAL$PROSTHESIS
7821   PAINTER IMPLOSIVES INHERENT$PITCH TONOGENESIS LARYNGEAL
       $MECHANISMS
7822   LARSEN REGIONAL$CORTICAL BLOOD$FLOW HEMISHERES AUTOMATIC
       $SP
7833   HIROSE LARYNGEAL$CONTROL VOICING JAPANESE$CONSONANT
7833   PETURSSON JUNCTURE GLOTTAL$LEVEL

## 0302

5403   DYNAMIC$ANALYSIS ACOUS$PHONETICS
5403   VISUAL$TACTILE$SYSTEM PHONETICAL$SYMBOLIZATION
5409   INTRODUCTION GENERAL$AMERICAN$PHONETICS
5409   VOWEL$PHONEMES MEIGRET
5410   PERCEP PHONETIC$VARIABLES
5506   ACOUS$LOCI TRANSITIONAL$CUES CONSONANTS
5506   DEV QUANTITATIVE$DESCRIPTION VOWEL$ARTIC
5506   PHONEMIC$CONFUSION$VECTORS
5509   STUDY PHONETICS
5603   ANALOG$STUDIES NASALIZATION$VOWELS
5606   ACOUS$CUES STOP$CONSONANTS

```
5606    ACOUS$CUES FRICATIVE$CONSONANTS
5606    ELECTRONIC$BINARY$SELECTION$SYSTEM PHONEME$CLASSIFICATION
5606    NATURE VOCAL$CORD$WAVE
5606    PROSODIC$FEATURES WHISPERED$SP
5610    QUANTITATIVE$PHONETICO-SYLLABIC$METHOD DURATION$ANALYSIS
            SP$STREAM
5703    ANALOG$STUDIES NASAL$CONSONANTS
5706    ACOUS$PROPERTIES STOP$CONSONANTS
5706    EFFECTS VOCAL$EFFORT CONSONANT-VOWEL$RATIO SYLLABLE
5706    PROSODIC$FEATURES WHISPERED$SP
5709    OUTLINE ENG$PHONETICS
5709    STUDY SOUNDS
5710    GREEK$ENG$CONSONANTS
5804    PROPERTIES GLOTTAL$SOUND$SOURCE
5804    SYLLABIC$PHONETIC$STRUCTURE INF$WORDS
5806    NASALIZATION$VOWELS REL NASALS
5806    PITCH$RATINGS VOICED$WHISPERED$VOWELS
5809    INTRODUCTION PHONETICS AMERICAN$ENG
5809    PRINCIPLES SP
5809    STRUCTURE AMERICAN$ENG
5810    ORAL$NASAL SPL VOWELS
5814    CUES DISCRIM AMERICAN$ENG$FRICATIVES
5814    CUES DISTINCTION VOICED$VOICELESS$STOPS INITIAL$POSITION
5814    PERCEP COMPOUND$CONSONANTS
5814    REL FUNCTIONAL$BURDENING$PHONEMES FREQ$OCCURRENCE
5904    NONRANDOM$SOURCES$VARIATION VOWEL$QUALITY
5905    CONGRESS IALP
5906    NATURE VOCAL$CORD$WAVE
5906    SOUND$SYSTEMS
5906    VOWEL$AMPLITUDE PHONEMIC$STRESS AMERICAN$ENG
5909    BLOOMFIELD NON-SYLLABIC$CLUSTERS
6004    NASAL$SYLLABICS AMERICAN$ENG
6006    ACOUS$CORRELATES WORD$STRESS AMERICAN$ENG
6006    AMERICAN$ENG$PHONEMES
6009    BLOOMFIELD CLUSTERS
6009    BLOOMFIELD CLUSTERS
6009    PRONUNCIATION AMERICAN$ENG PHONETICS THEORY APPLICATION
            SP$IMPROVE
6014    PERCEP CONSONANT$VOICING NOISE
6014    PERCEP ENG$STOPS ENG$SPEAKERS FOREIGN$SPEAKERS
6014    SPEED$UTTERANCE PHRASE$LENGTH
6014    STATISTICAL$APPROXIMATIONS ENG FRENCH
6014    STRATEGY SPONTANEOUS$UTTERANCE NUMBER$SYMBOLS
6103    MEDIAL$POSITION
6104    ACOUS$THEORY VOWEL$PROD IMPLICATIONS
6104    PARAMETERS VOWEL$QUALITY
```

```
6104   PHONETIC$ELEMENTS PERCEP NASALITY
6106   PHONETIC$TYPEWRITER
6106   PROPERTIES VOICELESS$FRICATIVES
6106   TRANSITIONS GLIDES DIPHTHONGS
6109   PHONETIC-PHONEMIC$SYMBOLIZATION$PROBLEMS
6110   PHONOLOGY NEW$ENGLAND$ENG
6114   DISTRIBUTION PAUSE$DURATIONS SP
6114   HESITATION$PAUSES JUNCTURE$PAUSES SP
6114   PHONEMIC$SIGNIFICANCE
6114   STUDY REPRESENTATION ENG$VOWELS ORTHOGRAPHY
6115   SYSTEM$RECORDING AMERICAN-ENGLISH$SP$SOUNDS
6120   SHAVIAN$APPLICATIONS PHONETICS
6206   ANALYSIS NASAL$CONSONANTS
6210   INITIAL$CLUSTERS
6210   PREDICTION PHONETIC$TRANSCRIPTION$ABILITY
6304   DIMENSION VOWEL$QUALITY
6304   PHONEME-SOUND$GENERALIZATION FUNCTION PHONEME$SIMILARITY
       VERBAL$UN
6306   STATISTICS SPOKEN$ENGLISH
6314   COINCIDENTAL$VARIATION SOURCE CONFUSION EXPERIMENTAL
       $STUDY RATE
6314   REL INDUCED$DYSNOMIA PHONEME$FREQ
6318   SOUND$MINDEDNESS MEAS PHONETIC$ABILITY
6404   AIR$FLOW PROD CONSONANTS
6413   NEONATAL$CRYING
6507   AIR$FLOW AIR$PRESSURE STUDIES
6509   SYLLABIC$N
6510   EFFECTS ASPECTS SENTENCE$STRUCTURE IMMEDIATE$RECALL
6514   ACOUS$CORRELATES STRESS
6514   HESITATION GRAMMATICAL$ENCODING
6604   EFFECTS ABSTRACTNESS MEANINGFULNESS PHONETIC$STRUCTURE
6604   NATURE VOCAL$FRY
6604   PHYSIOLOGICAL$THEORY PHONETICS
6606   SEGMENTATION SP$SOUNDS
6609   SYLLABIC$L
6614   SEQUENTIAL$TEMPORAL$PATTERNS SPONTANEOUS$SP
6614   VARIATIONS VOWEL$INTENS$MEAS
6704   EFFECTS ALTERATIONS PROSODIC$FEATURES SEQUENCING$PERFORMANCE
6706   PHONEME$GROUPING SP$RECOGNITION
6709   ISSUES PHONOLOGICAL$THEORY
6709   PRONUNCIATION ENG RULES
6710   SHORT$U$VOWELS EASTERN$MASSACHUSETTS$SP
6714   EFFECTS CONTEXT VOICE$ONSET$TIME ENG$STOPS
6714   HESITATION$PHENOMENA ENCODING$CHARACTERISTICS SP TYPEWRITING
6804   COARTICULATION LIP$ROUNDING
6810   ADULT$RECONSTRUCTIONS FORM CONTENT CHIL$SP
```

```
6814    DEFINING$JUNCTURE$PAUSES
6814    DIFFERENCES EGOCENTRICITY SPOKEN$WRITTEN$EXPRESSION
        STRESS$CONDITI
6814    SP$PATTERNS PERSONALITY
6814    STRUCTURE NOMINAL$GRP ELABORATEDNESS$CODE
6816    PHONEME$ANALYZER
6906    ACOUS$PROPERTIES VCC$UTTERANCES
6906    ALTERATIONS DURATION PITCH INTENSITY SPOKEN$PASSAGES
        SUCCESSIVELY$
6906    VOICED$VOICELESS$CONSONANTS
6914    COMMENTS VISUAL$PRESENTATION WORD$MATCHING STUDIES
        PHONETIC$SYMBOL
6914    COMPLEX$REGULATING VOICED-VOICELESS$DISTINCTION
6914    DIALECT IDENTIFICATION PERSUASIVE$MESSAGES
7003    ANALYSES PHONETIC$COMPOSITION WORD$FAMILIARITY
7004    POWER$SPECTRAL$DENSITY$MEAS ORAL$WHISPERED$SP
7006    PROD STOP$COGNATES
7007    SP$ARTIC ORAL$MORPHOLOGY
7014    PERCEP$STUDY AMERICAN$ENG$DIPHTHONGS
7017    DATA COMMENTS DESCRIPTIVE$ADEQUACY PHONETIC$RESEARCH
7104    ARTIC FUNCTION CLUSTER WORD$FREQ$OCCURRENCE
7104    ARTIC ORAL$SENSORY$CONTROL
7104    ASSIMILATION DISTANCE
7104    NEWBORN$INF$CRY NONHUMAN$PRIMATE$VOCALIZATION
7106    AIR$CONSUMPTION ORAL$WHISPERED$PLOSIVE-VOWEL$SYLLABLES
7106    AIRFLOW TURBULENCE$NOISE FRICATIVE STOP$CONSONANTS
7106    CLASSIFICATION RUSSIAN$FRICATIVES CV$SYLLABLES SPEAKERS
7106    CLASSIFICATION RUSSIAN$VOWELS
7106    PERCEP$STUCTURE AMERICAN$ENG$VOWELS
7110    INTENSITIES$S$SH ORAL$WHISPERED$VOWELS
7111    CEREBRAL$DOMINANCE VOWEL$SOUNDS LANG
7111    CEREBRAL$HEMISPHERE$DOMINANCE$TEST LOCALIZATION$SP
7114    ALLOPHONIC$PROBLEM AUSTRALIAN$ENG
7114    CLASSIFYING ALLOPHONES
7114    COMPARISON S$Z$PHONEMES ENG$SPEAKER
7114    EFFECTS CONTEXT INTONATION VOICE REACTION$TIME SENTENCES
7114    PERCEPTUAL$REALITY PHONEME HI$CHIL
7114    PHONETIC$SYMBOLISM ADULT$ENG$SPEAKERS
7114    PSYCHOLOGICAL$VARIABLES ABILITY PRONOUNCE SECOND$LANG
7114    SOUND$SYMBOLISM WORDS REL PROXIMITY DISTANCE
7117    ABUTTING$CONSONANTS SENTENCE$ENVIRONMENTS
7203    VOCAL$PARAMETER$MANIPULATION
7203    VOCAL$PARAMETER$MANIPULATION
7204    ARTIC$PROFICIENCY TWINS$SINGLETONS FAMILIES$TWINS
7204    EASE ARTIC
7204    FACOTR$ANALYTIC$STUDY ARTIC ENG$CONSONANTS
```

7204    NATURE GLOTTAL$TONE
7204    PERCEP COARTICULATION ENG$VCV$SYLLABLES
7204    PHONETIC$INTERFERENCE MOTOR$RECALL
7206    BILABIAL$CLOSURE DURATIONS VOICED$WHISPERED$VOWELS
7206    PERCEP$STRUCTURE PREVOCALIC$ENG$CONSONANTS
7206    PHYSICAL$ANALYSIS LINGUISTIC$VOWEL$DURATION
7212    BLACK MCGUFFEY$READERS
7214    ARTIC$GENERALIZATION ARTIC$R
7214    CONSONANTS
7214    PHONETIC$FEATURE VOWEL$LENGTH DUTCH
7214    STRUCTURE ENG$LEXICON HYPOTHESIS
7218    SOUND$SYSTEMS CHIL LANG
7306    ARTIC$MANIFESTATIONS VOWEL$STRESS
7306    CONTINUOUS$SP DATA$BASE MARKED$VOWEL$NASAL$CLASSES
7306    FREQ$ANALYSIS DUTCH$VOWELS MALE$SPEAKERS
7306    VOICING
7309    COMM$MODEL
7310    PHONETIC$TRANSCRIPTION$TEST DESCRIPTION EVAL
7313    ORAL$AIRFLOW STOP$CONSONANT
7314    ACOUS$PARAMETERS STRESS REL SYLLABLE$POSITION SP$LOUDNESS
        SP$RATE
7314    EFFECT REGIONAL$SIMILARITY$DISSIMILARITY COMMUNICATOR
        $CREDIBILITY
7314    PERCEP SUB-PHONEMIC$PHONETIC$DIFFERENCES
7314    PRE-CONSONANTAL$VOWELS
7406    ADAPTATION PHONETIC$ANALYZERS PLACE$ARTIC
7406    AERODYNAMICS ACOUS$STUDY STRESS SENTENCE$PROD
7406    CEPSTRAL$STATIONARITY$ANALYSES FULL-TERM$PREMATURE
        $INF$CRIES
7406    PRIMARY$AUD$STREAM$SEGREGATION REPEATED$CV$SEQUENCES
7406    VOICING$CONTRAST PERCEP$PROD$VOICE$ONSET$TIME$CHARACTERISTICS
        ADUL
7410    INTERPERSONAL$INFORMATION CONTENT VOCAL$ASPECTS SP
7414    HESITATIONS MATERNAL$SP
7414    PHONETIC$SYMBOLISM CZECH$ADULTS
7414    SEX$DIFFERENCES EXTRAVERSION NEUROTICISM REL SP$RATE
        EMOTION$EXPRE
7414    SILENT$INTERVAL STOP$CONSONANTS
7504    KLATT VOT,FRICTION ASPERATION
7504    KLATT VOT FRICTION ASPIRATION CONSONANT$CLUSTERS
7504    LARIVIERE DISTRIBUTION PERCEP$CUES PREVOCALIC$FRICATIVES
7506    BELL-BERTI CONTROL PHARYNGEAL$CAVITY$SIZE ENGLISH
7506    COOPER PERCETUO-MOTOR$ADAPT SP BISYLLABIC$UTTERANCES
        NEURAL$MODEL
7506    DALSTON ACOUSTIC$CHAR ENGLISH$/W,R,L/ CHILD ADULTS
7506    LARIVIERE VOCALIC$TRANSITIONS PERCEP VOICELESS$INITIAL
        $STOPS

7506    OHDE COARTIC$EFFECTS VOICED$STOPS REDUCTION ACOUSTIC
        $VOWEL$TARGETS
7506    UMEDA VOWEL$DURATION AMERICAN$ENGLISH
7521    COKER IMPORTANCE SPECTRAL$DETAIL INITIAL—FINAL$CONTRASTS
        VOICED$STOPS
7521    LEWIS APICAL$COARTIC JUNCTURE$BOUNDARIES
7521    MOSKOWITZ ACQUISITION FRICATIVES PHONETICS PHONOLOGY
7521    ROCA PHONETICS PHONOLOGY
7521    SEMILOFF—ZELASKO ACOUSTIC—PERCEP$STUDY MODERN$HEBREW
7521    STEVENS CONSONANT$PROD$PERCEP RETROFLEX$STOP$CONSONANTS
7521    TIERSMA NATURE F V FRISIAN+MARATHI
7521    WINITZ VARIATIONS VOT ENGLISH INITIAL$STOPS
7523    MENYUK VOT CLUSTER$PRODUCTIONS CHILDREN ADULTS
7527    RATUSNIK BLACK$PRESCH NONSTANDARD$PHONOLOGICAL$GRAMMATICAL
        $PERF
7532    KENT ARTIC$TIMING CONSONANT$SEQUENCES
7533    KRIER PHONOLOGIC$ANALYSE MALTESE
7533    MALECOT GLOTTAL$STOP FRENCH
7604    ZLATIN DEV VOICING$CONTRAST COMPARISON VOT STOP$PERCEP+PROD
7606    BOND ID VOWELS NEUTRAL NASAL$CONTEXTS
7606    MASSARO CONTRIBUTION FF VOT TO /ZI/-/SI/ DISTINCTION
7606    SCOTT TEMPORAL$FACTORS VOWEL$PERCEP
7606    STRANGE CONSONANT$ENVIRONMENT VOWEL$ID
7606    WHITEHEAD INFLUENCE CONSONANT$ENVIRONMENT DURATION
        VOWELS HI SPEAKERS
7621    ANDERSON DESCRIPTION MULTIPLY—ARTICULATED$CONSONANTS
7621    BLADON COARTIC$RESISTANCE ENGLISH
7621    BRASINGTON INHIBITIONS UNIVERSAL$RULES
7621    CONDAX DURATIONS FOUR VOWELS MANUALLY$PRODUCED SYNTHETIC
        $SP
7621    HADDING FACIAL$MUSCLE$ACTIVITY PROD SWEDIISH$VOWELS
        ELECTROMYOGRAPHIC
7621    HAMMARBERG METAPHYSICS COARTIC
7621    HANSEN INFLUENCE ACOUSTIC+PHYSIOLOGICAL$FACTORS VOWEL
        $CHANGES DANISH
7621    LEIDNER ARTIC AMERICAN$ENGLISH L GESTURAL$SYNERGY
        ANTAGONISM
7621    LIEBERMAN PHONETIC$FEATURES PHYSIOLOGY
7621    MIKOS INTONATION QUESTIONS POLISH
7621    MURRY PEAK$INTRAORAL$AIR$PRESSURES WHISPERED$STOP
7621    OSTREICHER COARTIC IDENTIFICATION DELETED$CONSONANT
        $VOWEL
7621    RIODAN ELECTROMYOGRAPHIC$CORRELATES PHONOLOGICAL$DISTINCTION
        FRENCH
7633    HOGAN TEMPORAL$FEATURES EJECTIVE$CONSONANTS
7633    KOHLER WORD—FINAL$ALVEOLAR$PLOSIVES GERMAN

7633   MALECOT ELISION FRENCH$MUTE-E
7633   MALECOT NEUTRALIZATION /E/-/OE/ FRENCH
7633   PIKE STRESS TONE PHONOLOGY DIUXI MIXTEC
7633   PLOTKIN ULTIMATE$PHONOLOGICAL$UNITS
7633   PRIESTLY GLOTTAL$STOP
7706   CARNEY NONCATEGORICAL$PERCEPTION STOP$CONSONANTS DIFFERING
       VOT
7706   COLE PROPERTIES FRICTION$ANALYZERS FOR J
7706   EILERS CONTEXT-SENSITIVE$PERCEPTION CONSONANTS INFANTS
7706   GAY ARTIC$MOVEMENTS VCV$SEQUENCES
7706   SAWUSCH PERIPHERAL$CENTRAL$PROCESSES ADAPT PLACE$ARTIC
       STOP$CONSONANTS
7706   SUMMERFIRLD DISSOCIATION SPECTRAL+TEMPORAL$CUES VOICING
       INITIAL$STOP$C
7706   UMEDA CONSONANT$DURATION AMERICAN ENGLISH
7706   VANDERGIET COMPUTER-CONTROLLED$METHOD MEAS ARTIC$ACTIVITIES
7713   HOLLIEN VOCAL$FOLD PATTERNS PULSE$REGISTER$PHONATION
7721   AMERMAN ASPECTS LINGUAL$COARTIC
7721   BARAN PHONOLOGICAL$CONTRASTIVITY CONVERSATION VOT
7721   BENGUEREL VELAR$COARTIC FRENCH FIBERSCOPIC
7721   BENGUEREL VELAR$COARTIC FRENCH ELECTROMYOGRAPHIC
7721   BLADON VIDEO-FLUOROGRAPHIC$INVESTIGATION$ALVEOLARS
7721   BOND PERCEP ANTICIPATORY$COARTIC CONSONANTS
7721   CLARK PHONOLOGICAL$MARKEDNESS SHORT$TERM$RECALL
7721   CLARKE VARIATION ORAL$NASAL SPL VOWELS
7721   DANILOFF ALTERATION CHILD$ARTIC ORAL$ANESTHESIA
7721   HOMBERT DEV TONES VOWEL$HEIGHT
7721   KENT COARTIC RECENT$SP$PRODS$MODELS
7721   KJELLIN CONSONANT$TYPES TONE TIBETAN
7721   LYBERG TIMING SWEDISH UTTERANCES
7721   PARKER PERCEPTUAL$CUES PHONOLOGICAL$CHANGE
7721   PETURSSON TIMING GLOTTAL$EVENTS PROD ASPIRATION S
7721   ROBINSON PHONOLOGICAL$AMBIGUITY BIUNIQUENESS$CONDITION
7721   RUBACH NASALIZATION POLISH
7721   WILLAIMS VOICING$CONTRAST SPANISH
7721   WILSON INDSCAL$ANALYSIS VOWELS
7721   YENI-KOMSHIAN VOICING LEBANESE$ARABIC
7723   GILBERT TEMPORAL$CONSTRAINTS CONSONANT$CLUSTERS CHILD
       $SP
7723   GILBERT VOICE$ONSET$TIME$ANALYSIS APICAL STOP$PRODUCTION
7723   PRIESTLEY IDIOSYNCRATIC STRATEGY ACQUISITION PHONOLOGY
7724   BERNTHAL CHANGES VELOPHARYNGEAL$ORIFICE VOWEL$INTENSITY
7733   BREEN ANDEGEREBENHA$VOWEL$PHONOLOGY
7733   GLAVE PHONETIC$CLASSIFICATION DAWID$SYSTEM
7733   MACKAY TENSENESS VOWELS
7733   MCCASLAND ENGLISH STOPS AFTER /S/ MEDIAL$WORD-BOUNDARY

7733   WODE L
7806   COLE PERCEP PHONETIC$FEATURES FLUENT$SP
7806   GAY EFFECT SPEAKING$RATE VOWEL$FORMANT$MOVEMENTS
7806   KEATING TRANSITION$LENGTH PERCEP STOP$CONSONANTS
7821   BAILEY SUGGESTIONS TRANSCRIPTION ENGLISH$PHONETIC
       $SEGMENTS
7821   BECKER FEATURE GRAVE
7821   DIXIT PEAK$MAGNITUDES SUPRAGLOTTA $AIR$PRESSURE STOP
       PRODUCTIONS HINDI
7821   ELUGBE WIDER$APPLICATION "TAP"
7821   HAGGARD DEVOICING VOICED$FRICATIVES
7821   MACARI PSYCHOPHYSICAL$EVIDENCE NATURAL$PHOLOGICAL
       $PROCESSESS
7821   O'KANE MANNER VOWEL$TERMINATION PERCEPTUAL$CUE VOICING
7821   PAINTER IMPLOSIVES INHERENT$PITCH TONOGENESIS LARYNGEAL
       $MECHANISMS
7821   ROSSI PERCEPTION INTENSITY$GLIDES VOWELS
7821   WOLF VOICING$CUES ENGLISH$FINAL$STOPS
7826   ZIMMER K/TH ALTERNATION TURKISH
7827   BORDEN LOW$TONGUE$TIPS$/S/
7833   MERLINGEN IMPLOSIVES
7833   PETURSSON JUNCTURE GLOTTAL$LEVEL

                          0303

5403   PITCH$LEVEL NASALITY
5406   IDENTIFICATION$SPEAKERS VOICE
5506   DURATION INTENSITY PHYSICAL$CORRELATES LINGUISTIC
       $STRESS
5506   DURATION INTENSITY PHYSICAL$CORRELATES LINGUISTIC
       $STRESS
5506   EFFECT DURATION PERCEP$VOICING
5506   PARAMETERS PERCEP AM$SIGNALS
5606   BANDWIDTH$CHANNEL$CAPACITY FORMANT$INFO SP
5606   EVAL FORMANT-EXTRACTING$DEVICES
5610   REL VOCAL$CHARACTERISTICS MEN RATINGS VOCAL$CHARACTERISTICS
       OTHER$
5706   EFFECT TIME PITCH$DISCRIM$THR PSYCHOPHYSICAL$PROCEDURES
       COMPARISON
5720   REL VOCAL$HARMONICS FUND$PITCH
5804   VARIABLES PERCEIVED$HARSHNESS
5806   EFFECT THIRD-FORMANT$TRANSITIONS PERCEP$VOICED$STOPS
5806   RELATIVE$INTENSITIES$SOUNDS ANATOMICAL$LOCALES$HEAD
       $NECK

```
5806   VOWEL$DURATION
5903   DOUBLE-SYLLABLE$WORDS
5904   NONRANDOM$SOURCES$VARIATION VOWEL$QUALITY
5904   VOWEL$FORMANT MEAS
5905   IDENTITY IDENTIFICATION
5906   PEAK$VU$DEFLECTION ENERGY MONOSYLLABIC$WORDS
5906   VOWEL$OVERLAP FUNCTION FUND$FREQ DIALECT
5913   PITCH$VARIATION
5914   PRELIMINARY$INVEST INTONATION
5918   DURATION HOMOPHONES
5918   DURATION HOMOPHONES
6004   FORMANT$BAND$WIDTHS VOWEL$PREFERENCE
6006   ANALOG$MEAS SOUND$RADIATION MOUTH
6006   ANALOG$MEAS SOUND$RADIATION MOUTH
6006   DURATION SYLLABLE$NUCLEI ENG
6006   DURATION SYLLABLE$NUCLEI ENG
6014   FREQ$STUDIES ENG$CONSONANTS
6014   MODEL SP$UNIT$DURATION
6104   PARAMETERS VOWEL$QUALITY
6104   PHONETIC$ELEMENTS PERCEP NASALITY
6104   PSYCHOPHYSICAL$INVEST VOWEL$FORMANTS
6106   METHODS MEAS VOWEL$FORMANT$BANDWIDTHS
6106   PITCH$SYNCHRONOUS$ANALYSIS VOICED$SOUNDS
6106   VOWEL$DURATION ENG
6114   REL FUND$FREQ VOCAL$SOUND$PRESSURE RATE$SPEAKING
6204   DIPHTHONG$FORMANTS MOVEMENTS
6204   VOCAL$FOLD$THICKNESS FUND$FREQ PHONATION
6206   FACTORS VOWEL$DURATION CROSS-LINGUISTIC VALIDITY
6206   FUND$FREQ ENVELOPE$AMPLITUDE EMOTIONAL$CONTENT SP
6214   DURATION POST-STRESS$INTERVOCALIC$STOPS PRECEDING
       $VOWELS
6214   DURATION POST-STRESS$INTERVOCALIC$STOPS PRECEDING
       $VOWELS
6214   JUDGMENT VOWEL$COLOR NATURAL$ARTIFICIAL$SOUNDS
6215   SP$SOUND$DURATION SURD-SONANT$ERROR
6304   PERTURBATION VOWEL$ARTIC CONSONANTAL$CONTEXT ACOUS
       $STUDY
6306   FORMANT$PERCEP
6306   FORMANT-AMPLITUDE$MEAS
6306   FORMANT-FREQ$EXTRACTION METHOD MOMENT$CALCULATIONS
6306   PITCH-SYNCHRONOUS TIME-DOMAIN ESTIMATION FORMANT$FREQ
       BANDWIDTHS
6306   R SPECTRUM$ANALYZERS BANK-OF-FILTERS SIGNALS VOWEL
       $SOUNDS
6314   COINCIDENTAL$VARIATION SOURCE CONFUSION EXPERIMENTAL
       $STUDY RATE
```

```
6314   DURATION$EXCERPT
6403   PITCH$CHARACTERISTICS MONGOLOID$BOYS
6406   DISPLAY$FORMAT FLEXIBLE-TIME$INTEGRATOR SPECTRAL-ANALYSIS
6406   EFFECTS SPEAKING$CONDITION PITCH
6406   PERCEPTUAL$BASES SPEAKER$IDENTITY
6406   ROLE TIME$CUES PITCH
6409   CORRELATES LANG$INTENSITY
6413   ACOUS$ANALYSIS FUND$FREQ
6414   FREQ$IMPORTANCE$FUNCTION ISOLATED$WORDS CONVERSATION
       FEMALE$TALKER
6414   TRANSITIONS FRICATIVE$NOISE
6414   VOWEL$DURATION WHISPERED$NORMAL$SP
6506   FORMANT$VOCODERS
6514   FORMANTS FRICATIVE$CONSONANTS
6604   ELECTROPHYSIOLOGICAL$ACOUS$CORRELATES STRESS$PERCEP
6604   PERFORMANCE$INTENSITY$CHARACTERISTICS SYNTHETIC$SENTENCES
6613   INVEST AIR$FLOW SUBGLOTTAL$AIR$PRESSURE REL FUND$FREQ
6613   PARAMETERS AUD$ROUGHNESS
6613   PHYSIOLOGICAL$MODEL INVEST FUND$FREQ
6614   MEAS DURATION$SP
6614   PLACE$CUES PTK$PHONEMES LOWER$CUT-OFF$FREQ$SHIFTS
       CONTIGUOUS$S$PHO
6614   SPEAKING$FUND$FREQ GIRLS
6704   CORRELATES TURBULENT$NOISE$PROD SP
6704   REL NASALITY$SCORE ORAL$NASAL$SPL
6706   DIMENSIONAL$ANALYSIS VOWEL$SPECTRAL
6706   FORMANT$FREQ$REGIONS POLISH$VOWELS
6706   ROLE FORMANT$TRANSITIONS VOWEL$RECOGNITIONS
6706   ROLE FORMANT$TRANSITIONS VOWEL$RECOGNITIONS
6706   VOWEL$QUALITY MUSICAL$TIMBRE FUNCTIONS SPECTRUM$ENVELOPE
       FUND$FREQ
6710   VOCAL$ROUGHNESS STIMULUS$DURATION
6713   SFF MIDDLE-AGED$FEMALES
6714   SECOND$SPECTRAL$PEAK FRONT$VOWELS PERCEP$STUDY ROLE
       SECOND$FORMANT
6804   DEV$STUDY INTONATION$RECOGNITION
6804   PARAMETERS VOICE$PROD MECHANISMS REGULATION$PITCH
6804   REL PROSODIC$VARIATIONS EMOTIONS NORMAL$AMERICAN$ENG
       $UTTERANCES
6806   EFFECT PITCH$AVERAGING QUALITY NATURAL$VOWELS
6806   EFFECT SPEAKING$RATE DIPHTHONG$FORMANT$MOVEMENTS
6806   IDENTIFICATION SPEAKER$SEX ISOLATED$VOICELESS$FRICATIVES
6806   IDENTIFICATION SPEAKER$SEX ISOLATED$WHISPERED$VOWELS
6806   IDENTIFICATION SPEAKER$SEX VOICELESS$FRICATIVES
6806   IDENTIFICATION SPEAKERS NASAL$COARTICULATION
6806   PERCEP$STUDY VOCAL$FRY
```

6806   PERIOD$HISTOGRAM PRODUCT$SPECTRUM METHODS FUND$FREQ
       $MEAS
6810   RELATIVE$INTRA-NASAL$INTENSITIES VOWELS
6813   DEVICE FUND$FREQ$RECORDINGS
6814   PERCEP$TIMING NATURAL$SP COMPENSATION SYLLABLE
6904   VISIBILITY TERMINAL$P1TCH$CONTOUR
6906   ALTERATIONS DURATION PITCH INTENSITY SPOKEN$PASSAGES
       SUCCESSIVELY$
6906   CORRELATION$CHARACTERISTICS DIMENSIONALITY SP$SPECTRA
6906   DETERMINATION RATE$CHANGE FUND$FREQ SUBGLOTTAL$AIR
       $PRESSURE
6906   DISCRIM FREQ$TRANSITIONS
6906   INFLUENCE VOWEL$ENVIRONMENT DURATION
6906   NOTE RANGE ESTIMATES FORMANTS GERMAN ENG CHINESE
6906   PARALLEL$PROCESSING$TECHNIQUES ESTIMATING PITCH$PERIODS
       SP TIME$DO
6906   PERCEIVED$PITCH WHISPERED$VOWELS
6906   PERCEP PITCH WHITE-NOISE$MASK
6913   VOICE$PITCH HOMOSEXUALS
6914   EVAL SFF POST-ADOL$GIRLS
6914   JUDGMENT VOWEL$QUALITY
6919   DEVICE AUTOMATIC$MODIFICATION VOCAL$FREQ$INTENSITY
7004   NORMAL$SIMULATED$ROUGH$VOWELS ADULT$MALES
7006   FORMANT$FREQ$TRAJECTORIES CVC$SYLLABLE$NUCLEI
7006   PARAMETERS PERCEPTIBILITY PITCH
7006   PITCH VOICING$CUE
7006   SYSTEM AUTOMATIC$FORMANT$ANALYSIS VOICED$SP
7011   PITCH$PERTURBATIONS NORMAL$PATHOLOGIC$VOICES
7013   FORMANT$STRUCTURE ARTIC SPOKEN$SUNG$VOWELS
7013   REGISTER$PITCH$INTENSITY$VOICE EMG$INVESTIGATION INTRINSIC
       $LARYNGE
7014   FUND$FREQ$CHARACTERISTICS ADOL$FEMALES
7104   DURATION$PT
7104   MALE$FEMALE$VOICE$QUALITY REL VOWEL$FORMANT$FREQ
7104   MALE$FEMALE$VOICE$QUALITY REL VOWEL$FORMANT$FREQ
7104   PHYSIOLOGIC$CORRELATES VOCAL$FRY
7106   ANALYSIS FUND$FREQ CONTOURS SP
7106   MEAS FUND$FREQ
7106   MODULATION$DATA
7106   NEED STANDARDIZATION MEAS SP$LEVEL
7106   PERCEP COARTICULATED$NASALITY
7114   DURATION FRENCH$VOWELS UNEMPHATIC$STRESS
7114   EFFECTS CONTEXT INTONATION VOICE REACTION$TIME SENTENCES
7204   PHONATIONAL$RANGE MODAL$FALSETTO$REGISTERS
7204   PHONATIONAL$RANGE MODAL$FALSETTO$REGISTERS
7204   SFF CHRONOLOGICAL$AGE MALES

7206    BILABIAL$CLOSURE DURATIONS VOICED$WHISPERED$VOWELS
7206    EMOTIONS SP ACOUS$CORRELATES
7206    IDENTIFICATION PLACE CONSONANT$ARTIC VOWEL$FORMANT
        $TRANSITIONS
7206    VOWEL$DURATION CUE PERCEP VOICING$CHARACTERISTICS
7213    FUND$FREQ
7213    SPECTRAL$CHARACTERISTICS MODAL$FALSETTO$REGISTERS
7214    PAUSES CLAUSES SENTENCES
7304    DISCRIM FORMANT$FREQ$TRANSITIONS SYNTHETIC$VOWELS
7306    DISCRIM FUND$FREQ$CONTOURS SYNTHETIC$SP IMPLICATIONS
        PITCH$PERCEP$
7306    EFFECT POSITION$UTTERANCE SP$SEGMENT$DURATION ENG
7306    INTERACTION FACTORS INFLUENCE VOWEL$DURATION
7306    PERCEP PERSONALITY SP EFFECTS MANIPULATIONS ACOUS
        $PARAMETERS
7313    MODAL$FALSETTO$REGISTERS
7314    MAXIMUM$RATE MINIMAL$DURATION REPEATED$SYLLABLES
7314    ROLE INTONATION RECALL LINGUISTIC$STIMULI
7404    DURATION$S ENGLISH$WORDS
7404    DURATION$S ENGLISH$WORDS
7406    ARTIC$INTERPRETATION SINGING$FORMANT
7406    CEPSTRAL$STATIONARITY$ANALYSES FULL-TERM$PREMATURE
        $INF$CRIES
7406    EFFECT SPEAKING$MODE TEMPORAL$FACTORS SP$VOWEL$DURATION
7406    EFFECT VOWEL$ENVIRONMENT DURATION CONSONANTS SP CHIL
7406    INFLUENCE CONSONANT$ENVIRONMENT DURATION$VOWELS SP
        CHIL
7406    ROLE FORMANT$TRANSITIONS VOICED-VOICELESS$DISTINCTION
        STOPS
7406    ROLE FORMANT$TRANSITIONS VOICED-VOICELESS$DISTINCTION
        STOPS
7406    VARIANCE FUND$FREQ RATINGS PERSONALITY SP
7406    VOICES EFFECTS SIMULTANEOUS$MANIPULATIONS RATE MEAN
        $FUND$FREQ
7413    SP$MELODY ARTIC$MELODY
7414    FORMANT$TRANSITIONS STOP$CONSONANT$PERCEP SYLLABLES
7418    ACOUS$CORRELATES LIES
7504    HORII STATISTICAL$CHAR FF
7504    KLATT VOT FRICTION ASPIRATION CONSONANT$CLUSTERS
7504    LARIVIERE DISTRIBUTION PERCEP$CUES PREVOCALIC$FRICATIVES
7504    RAPHAEL VOWEL + NASAL$DURATION VOICING STOP SPECTROGRAPHIC
        + PERCEP
7504    STEVENS ACCELEROMETER GLOTTAL$WAVEFORMS NASALIZATION
7506    COLLIER PHYSIOLOGICAL$CORRELATES INTONATION$PATTERNS
7506    GLAVE EFFORT$DEPENDENCE SP$LOUDNESS ACOUSTICAL$CUES
7506    HALL ENCODING PITCH$STRENGH COMPLEX$TONES

7506    HOLMER ULTRASONIC$REGISTRATION FUNDAMENTAL$FREQ VOICE
        NORMAL$SP
7506    LISKER VOT FIRST-FORMANT$TRANSITION$DETECTOR
7506    SHIPP VOCAL$FREQ VERTICAL$LARYNX$POSITIONING SINGERS
7506    SONDHI MEASUREMENT GLOTTAL$WAVEFORM
7511    SCHWAB EFFECTS SP$COMPRESSION AFFECTIVE$DIMENSIONS
        DIALOGUE
7521    ALLEN SP$RHYTHM PERFORMANCE$UNIVERSALS ARTIC$TIMING
7521    KLATT VOWEL$LENGTHENING SYNTACTICALLY$DETERMINED CONNECTED
        $DISCOURSE
7521    UMEDA PLACEMENT AUDITORY$BOUNDARIES FLUENT$SP
7527    AUSTIN BASAL$PITCH FREQ$LEVEL VARIATION MALE FEMALE
        CHILDREN
7527    SEYMOUR LOUDNESS$PITCH$RATE MALE$CHILDREN
7532    KENT ARTIC$TIMING CONSONANT$SEQUENCES
7533    BOE LARYNGEAL$FREQ PROSODIC$FACTS FRENCH
7533    KLINGHOLZ SPECTRAL$INTENSITY PHONEME GERMAN
7533    LIBERMAN STRESS ICELANDIC GENERAL$PROSODY
7533    NEWEKLOWSKY DURATION PITCH VOWELS
7533    RIETVELD DURATION VOWEL GERMAN
7533    TEMPORAL$VARIABLES ENGLISH FRENCH
7604    COLEMAN VOICE$CHARACTERISTICS MALENESS FEMALENESS
7606    ATKINSON INTER INTRASPEAKER$VARIABILITY FUND$VOICE
        $FREQ
7606    BURNS NONSPECTRAL$PITCH
7606    GOLDSTEIN SPEAKER-IDENTIFYING$FEATURES FORMANT$TRACKS
7606    LADEFOGED ACOUSTIC$EFFECTS STYLE SP
7606    REPP DICHOTIC$MASKING VOT
7621    KUEHN CINERADIOGRAPHIC VC CV ARTIC$VELOCITIES
7629    HALL SPECTROGRAPHIC INTERSPEAKER$INTRASPEAKER$VARIABILITIES
        STRESS
7633    BROAD ACOUSTIC$PHONATION$EQUIVALENCE VOWELS
7633    HO ACOUSTIC$VARIATION MANDARIN$TONES
7633    HOGAN TEMPORAL$FEATURES EJECTIVE$CONSONANTS
7633    MRAYATI VOCAL$TRACT ACOUSTIC$CHARACTERISTICS FRENCH
        $VOWELS
7633    PAINTER PITCH$CONTROL PHARYNX$WIDTH TWI EMG
7633    VANCE TONE INTONATION CANTONESE
7704    COLEMAN FF SPL PROFILES ADULT$VOICES
7706    BROAD PIECEWISE-PLANNER$REPRESENTATION VOWEL$FORMANT
        $FREQUENCIES
7706    CLEVELAND ACOUS$PROP VOICE$TIMBRE INFLUENCE VOICE
        $CLASSIFICATION
7706    COOPER FUNDAMENTAL$FREQUENCY$CONTOURS SYNTACTIC$BOUNDARIES
7706    HUGGINS SP-QUALITY$TESTING SOME VARIABLE-FRAME-RATE
        LINEAR-PREDICTIVE

7706  POLLACK PITCH$RATINGS HARMONIC$SERIES
7713  MORAVEK TEMPORAL$PATTERN VOCALIZED SILENT SEGMENTS
      LOUD$READING
7721  LUBKER INTER-ARTIC$PROGRAMMING
7721  MILLER AERODYNAMICS STOPS CONTINUOUS$SP
7723  LI ACQUISITION TONE MANDARIN-SPEAKING$CHIL
7724  FLETCHER RESONANCE PHONATION
7733  GANDOUR TONE VOWEL$LENGTH THAI$DIALECTS
7733  HO INTONATION MANDARIN INTERROGATIVE$EXCLAMATORY$DECLARATIVE
7733  MALECOT ACOUSTIC$STATUS MUTE-E FRENCH
7733  PILCH INTONATION FINNISH$ENGLISH$GERMAN
7733  PRABHAKAR EMPHASIS TELUGU
7733  VANCE TONAL$DISTINCTIONS CANTONESE
7804  DEAL WAVEFORM SPECTRAL$FEATURES VOWEL$ROUGHNESS
7804  HORII AIR$FLOW VOLUME DURATION ORAL$READING
7804  MASSARO TEMPORAL$COURSE PERCEIVED$VOWEL$DURATION
7806  ALLEN VOWEL$DURATION RELIABILITY$STUDY
7806  ATKINSON CORRELATION$ANALYSIS PHYSIOLOGICAL$FACTORS
      FF
7806  BRADY RANGE$EFFECT PERCEP VOICING
7806  CHUANG PITCH$BIASES VOWEL$QUALITY INTENSITY$DIFF SEQUENTIAL
      $ORDER
7806  DELGUTTE PERCEPTUAL$INVESTIGATION FF$CONTOURS FRENCH
7806  GAY EFFECT SPEAKING$RATE VOWEL$FORMANT$MOVEMENTS
7806  KEATING FF SP INFANTS CHILD
7806  LADEFOGED GENERATING VOCAL$TRACT$SHAPES FORMANT$FREQUENCIES
7806  LASS SPEAKERS HIGHTS WEIGHTS SURFACE$AREAS FF
7806  LIBERMAN NONSENSE-SYLLABLE$MIMICRY STUDY PROSODIC
      $PHENOMENA
7806  MERMELSTEIN DIFFERENCE$LIMENS FORMANT$FREQ VOWELS
7806  MONSEN INDIRECT$ASSESS SUBGLOTTAL$AIR$PRESSURE VOCAL-FOLD
      $TENSION FF
7806  NAKATANI PROSODIC$CUES WORD$PERCEP
7806  NEUBURG PITCH-DEPENDENT$ALGORITHM SP$RATE$CHANGING
7806  SINGH MULTIDIMENSIONAL$CLASSIFICATION VOICE$QUALITIES
7806  STREETER ACOUSTIC$DETERMINANTS PHASE$BOUNDARY$PERCEPTION
7806  UMEDA OCCURENCE GLOTTAL$STOPS FLUENT$SP
7806  ZAGORSKI NONCOMBINATION PITCH LOUDNESS MULTIDIMENSIONAL
      $SCALING
7813  COLEMAN FUNDAMENTAL$FREQ SPL FEMLAE$SINGERS
7813  EPSTEIN SCALING VOCAL$QUALITY
7813  STONE MINIMUM$INTENSITY VOICE PITCH$RANGE
7821  PETERSEN INTRINSIC$FF DANISH$VOWELS
7821  ROSSI PERCEPTION INTENSITY$GLIDES VOWELS
7821  SMITH TEMPORAL$ASPECTS SP$PRODUCTION
7821  THORSEN ACOUSTICAL$INVESTIGATION DANISH$INTONATION

7821    WHITEHEAD VOWEL$ENVIRONMENT DURATION CONSONANTS HEARING-IMPAIRED
7821    ZEE DURATION INTENSITY CORRELATES FF
7827    BRALLEY VOCAL$PITCH MALE$TRANSSEXUALS
7833    ADAMS CORRELATES STRESS NATIVE NON-NATIVE SPEAKERS
        ENGLISH
7833    ESSER INTONATION GERMAN ENGLISH
7833    HUSS POSTNUCLEAR$&POSITION


## 0304


5803    EFFECT AUD$MASKING OR$RATE
5803    VARIABILITY OR$RATE
5904    EST READING$RATE ARTIC PITCH
6106    EFFECT INSTRUCTIONS RATE$OR
6204    DISTRIBUTION MEAS SYLLABLE$DURATION READING$RATE
6604    PITCH$DURATION$CHARACTERISTICS OR MALES
6614    STUDY PAUSES OR NATIVE$LANG ENG
6704    NOMOGRAM ARTIC$PROD
6704    PERFORMANCE-INTENSITY$CHARACTERISTICS VERBAL$MATERIALS
6706    SYLLABLE$DURATION OR WHISPERED$READING
6804    NOTE OR$RATE
6806    EFFECT MASKING$NOISE SYLLABLE$DURATION OR WHISPERED
        $READING
6814    VOCAL$EMPHASIS EXPERIMENTERS$INSTRUCTION READING DETERMINANT
        SUBJE
6914    RATE$ALTERATIONS OR
7004    SIGNIFICANCE INTRA$INTERSENTENCE$PAUSE$TIMES PERCEP
        $JUDGMENTS OR$R
7112    TEMPORAL$PATTERNS VARIATION$RATES OR
7204    DIADOCH$RATES READING$RATES
7211    STUDY LISTENING$RATE PREFERENCES LISTENERS$OR$RATES
7312    TEMPORAL$PATTERNS REPETITIVE$OR
7314    REL WORDS TONE-OF-VOICE


## 0305


5503    TWO-DIGIT$NUMBER$TRANSMISSION VOLUNTARY$STUTTERING
5606    MEAS FUND$PERIOD SP DELAY$LINE
5606    NATURALNESS DISTORTION SPEECHPROCESSING$DEVICES
5703    USE PALATOGRAPHY
5710    COMPARISON SPEAKING$ABILITY UPPERCLASSMEN
5804    ARTIFICIAL$SP PHONETICS COMM

```
5809   SP VOICE ARTIC
6004   CINE$TECHNIQUES SP$RESEARCH
6006   ANALOG$MEAS SOUND$RADIATION MOUTH
6006   INSTRUMENTS METHODS SP$ANALYSIS
6013   VOCAL$ANALYSIS
6014   ATTITUDINAL$MEANINGS INTONATION$CONTOURS
6104   BILABIAL$STOP NASAL$CONSONANTS MOTION$PICTURE$STUDY
       ACOUS$IMPLICAT
6104   CINE$EQUIPMENT
6104   CINE$SP$RESEARCH
6104   CONCURRENT$REPETITION CONTINUOUS$FLOW$WORDS
6106   REDUCTION SP$SPECTRA ANALYSIS-BY-SYNTHESIS$TECHNIQUES
6115   CINE AID INTELLIGIBLE$SP
6203   ULTRAHIGH$SPEED$PHOTOGRAPHY LARYNGEAL$PHYSIOLOGY
6204   DEV AIDS TECHNIQUES CINE$SP$STUDY
6206   METHOD TIME$NORMALIZATION SP
6213   EXPERIMENTAL$PHONIATRICS
6303   TONGUE$MARKERS CINE$ANALYSIS
6304   CINE$SP$STUDY
6304   USE SURFACE EMG STUDIES SP$BREATHING
6306   EMG ACOUS$STUDY PROD FINAL$CLUSTERS
6306   REDUCED$BLOOD$FLOW
6403   CONTINUOUS$PALATOGRAPHY
6404   EVAL METHODS ESTIMATING SUBGLOTTAL$AIR$PRESSURE
6413   INTRA-ORAL$VOICE$RECORDINGS LARYNGEAL$PHOTOGRAPHY
6503   XERORADIOGRAPHY X-RAY$TECHNIQUE
6506   TECHNIQUES SP$BANDWIDTH$COMPRESSION COMBINATIONS CHANNEL
       $VOCODERS
6507   AIR$FLOW AIR$PRESSURE STUDIES
6507   PHOTOGRAPHIC$RADIOGRAPHIC$PROCEDURES SP$RESEARCH
6603   DETECT ESCAPE NASAL$AIR SP
6604   DEV ROTATIONAL$CINE APPLICATION SP$RESEARCH
6606   SEGMENTATION SP$SOUNDS
6614   SEQUENTIAL$TEMPORAL$PATTERNS SPONTANEOUS$SP
6703   VOICE$CHANGE ADULT$WOMEN VIRILIZING$AGENTS
6704   HIGH$SPEED$PHOTOGRAPHY SP$RESEARCH
6713   CINE$ANALYSIS TONGUE$THRUSTING PARKINSON$PATIENTS
6714   SEQUENTIAL$TEMPORAL$PATTERNS COGNITIVE$PROCESSES SP
6803   ARTIC$RESEARCH
6804   CONSIDERATION KINESTHETIC$FEEDBACK$RESEARCH
6804   PREDICTING CINE$MEAS VELO$OPENING LATERAL$X-RAY$FILMS
6806   LARYNGOSCOPIC$TECHNIQUE USE FIBER$OPTICS
6813   DECAY$ARTIC INFLUENCE ALCOHOL$PARALDEHYDE
6813   SIGNIFICANCE VOCAL$VELOCITY$INDEX
6906   MOTOR$CONTROL COARTICULATION CVC$MONOSYLLABLES
6906   ULTRASONIC$DOPPLER$MONITORING VOCAL$FOLD$VELOCITY
       DISPLACEMENT
```

6906    ULTRASONIC$OBSERVATIONS COARTICULATION PHARYNX
6913    NEOGLOTTIS X-RAY$STUDY
6914    EMG MODEL SP$PROD
7005    SUBVOCAL$SP SP
7006    METHOD OBSERVATION GLOTTAL-SOURCE$WAVE DIGITAL$INVERSE
        $FILTERING
7006    SIMULTANEOUS$MEAS INTRAORAL$PRESSURE FORCE LABIAL
        $CONTACT LABIAL$E
7007    AERODYNAMIC$ULTRASONIC$ASSESSMENT SP-DENTOFACIAL$RESEARCH
7007    ASSESSMENT RADIOGRAPHIC$TECHNIQUES
7007    INTRODUCTION FUNCTIONAL$ANALYSIS SP
7007    PHYSIOLOGICAL$MEAS SP$MOVEMENTS EMG FIBROOPTIC$STUDIES
7013    CINEMATOGRAPHIC$STUDIES NORMAL$SUBJECTS
7013    REGISTER$PITCH$INTENSITY$VOICE EMG$INVESTIGATION INTRINSIC
        $LARYNGE
7104    RECENT$DEV USE EMG SP$RESEARCH
7106    AIR$CONSUMPTION ORAL$WHISPERED$PLOSIVE-VOWEL$SYLLABLES
7106    EFFECT GLOTTAL$PULSE$SHAPE QUALITY NATURAL$VOWELS
7106    ULTRASONIC$SCANS DORSAL$SURFACE TONGUE
7113    DISSOCIATIONS$ELECTROGLOTTOGRAM$PHONOGRAM
7114    SYNTHESIS RULE TOOL PHONOLOGICAL$RESEARCH
7203    CLINICAL$USE TAUB$ORAL$PANENDOSCOPE OBSERVATION VELO
        $FUNCTION
7204    CINE$ANALYSES LINGUAL$CONSONANTS
7204    TIME-BY-COUNT$MEAS DIADOCH$SYLLABLE$RATE
7206    REL ZERO-CROSSING$MEAS SP$ANALYSIS RECOGNITION
7206    TIME-AVERAGED$HOLOGRAPHY
7213    PROCESSING FILM$ANALYSIS
7214    EFFECTS TIME-OUT SPEAKING$RATES DISFLUENCY$RATES NORMAL
        $SPEAKERS
7214    RANDOM$GENERATION SP$RHYTHMS
7215    APPLICATIONS LARYNGOGRAPH
7217    REVIEW METHODS PALATOGRAPHY
7303    SUBMENTOVERTICAL$PROJECTION RADIOGRAPHIC$ANALYSIS
        VELO$DYNAMICS
7304    COMPUTER-ASSISTED$MEAS X-RAY$FILMS VOCAL$TRACT
7306    ARTIC$MODEL STUDY SP$PROD
7306    INVERSE-FILTERING$TECHNIQUE DERIVING GLOTTAL$AIRFLOW
        $WAVEFORM
7403    ORAL$MOTOR$NERVE$BLOCK
7404    BODY$ACOUS$IMMITANCE EAR
7417    CLINICAL$VALIDITY TAUB$ORAL$PANENDOSCOPE
7503    SHELTON PANENDOSCOPIC$FEEDBACK VELOPHARYNGEAL$MOVEMENTS
7504    FLETCHER DYNAMIC$PALATOMETRY
7504    HARDEN GLOTTAL$AREA$CHANGES ULTRA-HIGH-SPEED$PHOTO
        GLOTTOGRAPHS

7504   LEEPER LINGUAL-PALATAL$PRESSURE$MEAS ANALYSIS$TECHNIQUE
7504   PROSEK INTRAORAL$AIR$PRESSURE FEEDBACK CONSONANT$PROD
7506   HALL ENCODING PITCH$STRENGH COMPLEX$TONES
7506   HOLMER ULTRASONIC$REGISTRATION FUNDAMENTAL$FREQ VOICE
       NORMAL$SP
7506   KASPRZYK VOWEL$PERTURBATION FUNCTION TONGUE$HEIGHT
7506   KIRITANI TONGUE-PELLET$TRACKING COMPUTER-CONTROLLED
       $X-RAY MICROBEAMS
7513   GOULD ANESTHESIA SUPERIOR LARYNGEAL NERVE PHONATION
7513   KOTHY PERCUTANEOUS LARYNGEAL ELECTROMYOGRAPHY
7513   LECLUSE ELECTROGLOTTOGRAPHY GLOTTAL$ACTIVITY
7513   TANABE HIGH-SPEED$MOTION$PICTURES VOCAL$FOLDS
7519   SEWELL SPEECH$SILENCE AUTHENTICITY
7521   ALLEN SP$RHYTHM PERFORMANCE$UNIVERSALS ARTIC$TIMING
7521   BARRY CO-ARTIC AIRFLOW$CHAR INTERVOCALIC$VOICELESS
       $PLOSIVES
7521   CLARKE MEAS ORAL NASAL SOUND$PRESSURE$LEVELS SP
7521   COKER IMPORTANCE SPECTRAL$DETAIL INITIAL-FINAL$CONTRASTS
       VOICED$STOPS
7521   HART INTEGRATING$DIFFERENT$LEVELS INTONATION$ANALYSIS
7521   KLATT VOWEL$LENGTHENING SYNTACTICALLY$DETERMINED CONNECTED
       $DISCOURSE
7521   LOFQVIST SUBGLOTTAL$PRESSURE PROD SWEDISH$STOPS
7524   KUEHN TOMOGRAPHIC$ASSESSING LATERAL$PHARYNGEAL$WALL
7524   MIYAZAKI FIBERSCOPIC$ASSESSMENT VELOPHARYNGEAL$CLOSURE
7524   MOURINO CEPHALOMETRIC VELAR$STRENGTH CHIL
7526   BARON CHILD$ERRORS PRONOUNS
7526   MISHLER DISCOURSE$INITIATED SUSTAINED$THROUGH$QUESTIONING
7526   SALTER LATENCY GENERATION
7527   DANILOFF VERBALIZABLE$KNOWLEDGE SP$ARTIC
7527   MCNUTT ASYMMETRY TWO-POINT$DISCRIM TONGUES ADULTS
       CHILDREN
7527   WINITZ PHONETIC$INTERFERENCE VARYING$CONDITIONS PHONETIC
       $FACILITATION
7604   ABBS MOTOR$IMPAIR BLOCKADE INFRAORBITAL$NERVE ANESTHETIZATION
       SP$RES
7604   BELL-BERTI EMG$STUDY VELOPHARYNGEAL$FUNCTION
7604   HIXON MEASURING VELOPHARYNGEAL$ORIFICE VOWEL$PRODUCTION
7604   KENT ANATOMICAL$NEUROMUSCULAR$MATURATION SP$MECHANISM
7604   PUTMAN CINERADIOGRAPHIC$STUDY ARTIC ORAL$SENSORY$DEPRIVATION
7606   BROWN COMFORTABLE$EFFORT$LEVEL
7606   FLANAGAN DIGITAL$ANALYSIS LARYNGEAL$CONTROL SP$PROD
7606   KAKITA LARYNGEAL$CONTROL SP THYROMETER
7606   LASS INVESTIGATION SPEAKER$HEIGHT$WEIGHT$ID
7613   KELMAN EMG PLOSIVE /P/ CVC$UTTERANCE
7620   MOTLEY STAGE$FRIGHT$MANIPULATION

7621    BUTCHER ELECTROMYOGRAPHIC COARTIC VCV$SEQUENCES
7621    CONDAX DURATIONS FOUR VOWELS MANUALLY$PRODUCED SYNTHETIC
        $SP
7621    CONDAX MONITORING$VELIC$ACTION PHOTO-ELECTRIC$NASAL
        $PROBE FRENCH
7621    HADDING FACIAL$MUSCLE$ACTIVITY PROD SWEDIISH$VOWELS
        ELECTROMYOGRAPHIC
7621    HAMLET COMPENSATORY$VOWEL$CHAR EXPERIMENTAL$DENTAL
        $PROSTHESES
7621    KUEHN CINERADIOGRAPHIC VC CV ARTIC$VELOCITIES
7621    LEIDNER ARTIC AMERICAN$ENGLISH L GESTURAL$SYNERGY
        ANTAGONISM
7621    MURRY PEAK$INTRAORAL$AIR$PRESSURES WHISPERED$STOP
7621    RIODAN ELECTROMYOGRAPHIC$CORRELATES PHONOLOGICAL$DISTINCTION
        FRENCH
7624    HOLLIEN INSTRUMENTATION CRANIOFACIAL$RESEARCH
7624    KUEHN CINERADIOGRAPHIC VELAR$MOVEMENT
7624    RYAN ULTRASONIC$MEASUREMENT PHARYNGEAL$WALL$MOVEMENT
        VELO$PORT
7629    HALL SPECTROGRAPHIC INTERSPEAKER$INTRASPEAKER$VARIABILITIES
        STRESS
7633    GANDOUR LARYNX MOVEMENT THAI
7706    KRETSCHMAR METHOD MEAS LIP-OPENING$AREA
7706    MCCUTCHEON VIDEO-SCANNING$SYSTEM MEAS LIP+JAW,MOTION
7706    ROTHENBERG FILTERING$TECHNIQUE ESTIMATING GLOTTAL-AREA
        $WAVEFORM
7706    VANDERGIET COMPUTER-CONTROLLED$METHOD MEAS ARTIC$ACTIVITIES
7713    MULLER READING TIME ARTIC MASKING$NOISE ALTERED ORAL
        $CAVITY
7713    PEDERSEN ELECTROGLOTTOGRAPHY STROBOSCOPY NORMAL$PHONATION
7716    DISTINCTIVE$FEATURES$APPROACH ANALYSIS SP
7720    ANDREWS AEEECTS ALCOHOL SP (SUMMER
7721    BARAN PHONOLOGICAL$CONTRASTIVITY CONVERSATION VOT
7721    BENGUEREL VELAR$COARTIC FRENCH ELECTROMYOGRAPHIC
7721    BENGUEREL VELAR$COARTIC FRENCH FIBERSCOPIC
7721    BLADON VIDEO-FLUOROGRAPHIC$INVESTIGATION$ALVEOLARS
7721    CLARK PHONOLOGICAL$MARKEDNESS SHORT$TERM$RECALL
7721    CLARKE VARIATION ORAL$NASAL SPL VOWELS
7721    COLEMAN ORAL$MUZZLE$PRESSURE UNDERWATER$COMM
7721    DANILOFF ALTERATION CHILD$ARTIC ORAL$ANESTHESIA
7721    DEBROCK ACOUSTIC$CORRELATE FORCE ARTIC
7721    MILLER AERODYNAMICS STOPS CONTINUOUS$SP
7721    NORDSTROM FEMALE+INFANT$VOCAL$TRACTS SIMULATED FROM
        MALE AREA$FUNCTION
7723    GILBERT VOICE$ONSET$TIME$ANALYSIS APICAL STOP$PRODUCTIONS
7724    NOLL NORMAL$SIX-YEAR$MALES ORAL$MANOMETER

7724  SKOLNICK RADIOLOGICAL$STUDY VELOPHARYNGEAL$PORTAL
7733  KUENZEL VELAR$HEIGHT VOWEL$ARTIC
7803  NETSELL NONINVASIVE$METHOD ESTIMATING$SUBGLOTTAL$AIR
      $PRESSURE
7804  CHUANG USE OPTICAL$DISTANCE-SENSING TRACK$TONGUE$MOTION
7804  WATKIN ULTRASONCI-EMG$TRANSDUCER BIODYNAMIC$RESEARCH
7806  ABBS CEPHALOSTAT SP$PHYSIOLOGY$RESEARCH
7806  YEGNANARAYANA FORMANT$EXTRACTION LINEAR-PREDICTION
      $PHASE$SPECTRA
7809  CRAIG COGNITIVE$SCIENCE
7813  BASTIAN AERODYNAMICS$EVAL FEMALE$VOICE
7813  BENGUEREL FRENCH$STOP$PROD FIBERSCOPIC ACOUSTIC ELECTROMYOGRAPHIC
7813  BRUNNER INFLUENCE VOCAL STRESS VIENNA$BOYS$CHOIR
7813  JENTZSCH ELECTROGLOTTOGRAPHIC VOCAL$INITIATION CONTINUAL
      $SP
7813  SAITO OBSERVATION VOCAL$FOLD$VIBRATION
7818  BEHNKE SP$ANXIETY PREDICTOR TREMBLING
7819  BEATTY EFFECTS COMPRESSED$SP LEARNER$ANXIETY
7821  HAMLET COMPENSATORY$ALVEOLAR$CONSONANT$PRODUCTION
      DENTAL$PROSTHESIS
7821  KUENZEL REPRODUCIBILITY EMG + VELOGRAPHIC$MEAS VELO
      $CLOSURE$MECH
7821  LASS SPEAKER$HEIGHT WEIGHT$IDENTIFICATION DIRECT$ESTIMATIONS
7821  MACARI PSYCHOPHYSICAL$EVIDENCE NATURAL$PHOLOGICAL
      $PROCESSESS
7821  SMITH TEMPROAL$ASPECTS SP$PRODUCTION

## 0306

7513  LECLUSE ELECTROGLOTTOGRAPHY GLOTTAL$ACTIVITY
7613  BUNCH HEAD NECK SUSTAINED$PHONATION COVERED OPEN$QUALITIES
7633  FONAGY RADIOLOGICAL$ASPECTS EMOTIVE$SP
7633  PAINTER PITCH$CONTROL PHARYNX$WIDTH TWI EMG

## 0307

5606  AUTOMATIC$EXTRACTION FORMANT$FREQ CONTINUOUS$SP
5703  PLASTIC-TAPE$SPECTROGRAPH
5804  ESTIMATION FORMANT$BAND$WIDTHS MEAS TRANSIENT$R VOCAL
      $TRACT
5914  PHONEME VOICE$IDENTIFICATION STUDIES JAPAENSE$VOWELS
6014  SPECTRA FRICATIVE$NOISE SP

6206    AMPLITUDE$CONTOUR$DISPLAY SOUND$SPECTROGRAMS
6206    LAB$SET-UP OBTAINING SOUND$SPECTROGRAMS
6206    PRINTOUT$SYSTEM AUTOMATIC$RECORDING SPECTRAL$ANALYSIS
        SPOKEN$SYLLA
6306    ANALYSIS-SYNTHESIS CONNECTED$SP ORTHOGONALIZED EXPONENTIALLY
6306    DISPLAY SOUND$SPECTROGRAPHS REAL$TIME
6306    INSTRUMENTATION SPECTROGRAPHIC$PICTURES SP
6306    SPECTROGRAPHIC$STUDY VOWEL$REDUCTION
6406    AUTOMATIC$REDUCTION VOWEL$SPECTRA ANALYSIS-BY-SYNTHESIS
        $METHOD EVA
6406    SONOGRAPH TECHNIQUES
6410    LENGTHS$SILENCE INTIAL$S-PLOSIVE$BLENDS
6414    SPECTRAL$ANALYSIS FLUCTUATIONS SOUND$ENERGY INSECTS
        HUMANS
6506    EXAMINATION FORMANT-ESTIMATION$TECHNIQUES
6506    MEAS SP$SPECTRA RECORDED CLOSE-TALKING$MICROPHONE
6514    SPECTROGRAPHIC$INVEST STRUCTURAL$STATUS UEBERLAENGE
        GERMAN$VOWELS
6606    COARTIC VCV$UTTERANCES SPECTROGRAPHIC$MEAS
6606    HIGH-SPEED$SOUND$SPECTROGRAPH
6704    PHYSICAL$PSYCHOLOGICAL$CORRELATES SPEAKER$RECOGNITION
6709    ACOUS$PARAMETERS INTERNAL$OPEN$JUNCTURE
6806    SPECTROGRAPHIC$ANALYSIS DIVERS$SP DECOMPRESSION
6814    SPECTRAL$FORM$DURATION CUES RECOGNITION ENG$GERMAN
        $VOWELS
6814    SPECTROGRAPHIC$INVEST AUSTRALIAN$VOWELS
6816    PERCEP VISUAL$TRANSFORMS SP
6907    LAB$STUDIES EFFECTS DURATION$SPECTRAL$COMPLEXITY
6913    SPECTRAL$FEATURES ROUGH$VOWELS
6914    SPECTROGRAPHIC$INVEST DIPHTHONGAL$PHONEMES AUSTRALIAN
        $ENG
7004    SPECTRAL$NOISE$LEVELS ROUGHNESS$SEVERITY$RATINGS
7004    SPECTRAL$NOISE$LEVELS ROUGHNESS$SEVERITY$RATINGS SIMULATED
        $ROUGH$V
7006    FORMANT$CONCENTRATION$POSITIONS SP CHIL LEVELS LINGUISTIC
        $DEV
7006    VOWEL$SPECTRA VOWEL$SPACES VOWEL$IDENTIFICATION
7104    NEWBORN$INF$CRY NONHUMAN$PRIMATE$VOCALIZATION
7106    AUTOMATIC$FORMANT$TRACKING NEWTON-RAPHSON$TECHNIQUE
7106    VOICE$SPECTROGRAMS FUNCTION AGE VOICE DISGUISE VOICE
        $IMITATION
7206    IDENTIFICATION STOPS VOWELS BURST$PORTION CONVERSATIONAL
        $SP
7313    SPECTRAL$NOISE ROUGHNESS$RATINGS$VOWELS MALES$FEMALES
7406    TALKER$DIFFERENCES CORRELATION$MATRICES CONTINUOUS
        $SP$SPECTRA

7406   VOICEPRINTS
7414   ACOUS$MEAS DISTINCTIVE$VOWEL$QUANTITY MALAYALAM
7414   COMPARISON METHODS ESTIMATING$TRANSITION$PROBABILITY
       SP
7414   IDENTIFICATION CONSONANTS FORMANT$TRANSITIONS FORWARD
       $BACKWARD
7504   KLATT VOT FRICTION ASPIRATION CONSONANT$CLUSTERS
7504   RAPHAEL VOWEL + NASAL$DURATION VOICING STOP SPECTROGRAPHIC
       + PERCEP
7506   INGEMANN SP$RECOGNITION SPECTROGRAM$MATCHING
7506   STRONG COMPUTER-BASED$SOUND$SPECTROGRAPH$SYSTEM
7527   FITCH ELECTROACOUSTIC CONTINGENCY MANAGEMENT ACOUSTIC
       $SPECTRA SP
7533   EMERIT LOCUS$THEORY
7533   LAREVIERE FUNDAMENTAL$FREQ FORMANT$FREQ SPEAKER$IDENTIFICATION
7613   SIRVIO CRY ANALYSIS INFANTS
7633   EMERIT LOCUS$THEORY INDIVIDUALITY TONE$SHAPES
7813   TARDY-RENUCCI SONAGRAPHIC$ANALYSIS NEWLY-BORNS
7813   WEDIN EVAL VOICE$TRAINING SPECTRAL$ANALYSIS LISTENERS
       $JUDGEMENTS


                              0308


7533   GILES CINEFLUOROGRAPHIC STUDY ALLOPHONES ENGLISH /L/


                              0309


5409   SP SCH$CHIL
5515   DEV$SP CHIL
5709   CHIL$SP
5803   PERSONAL$EXPERIENCE SP
5804   INF$SP CONSISTENCY AGE
5815   REL SP$LANG$DEV INTELLIGENCE SOCIO-ECONOMIC$STATUS
5903   SP$STIMULATION PRESCH$CHIL
5915   DEV SP$PATTERNS
6104   CHIL$ARTIC SOUND$LEARNING$ABILITY
6104   INF$VOCAL$LEARNING
6107   REPETITIONS VOCALIZATIONS SP CHIL INF
6213   VOCALIZATION$INF
6303   OBSERVATIONS TONGUE-THRUST$SWALLOW PRESCH$CHIL
6313   DEV FREQ$RANGE VOICE$CHIL
6404   FACTOR$ANALYSIS ORAL$COMM CHIL

6413    NEONATAL$CRYING
6414    FACTOR$ANALYSIS CONSONANT$ARTIC CHIL
6514    HESITATIONS CHIL$SP
6610    VOCAL$PITCH INF
6804    ACQUISITION V$WORDS FUNCTION CONSISTENCY V$ERRORS
6804    DISCRIM$LEARNING CHIL$ACQUISITION$PHONOLOGY
6804    ROLE DISTINCTIVE$FEATURES CHIL ACQUISITION$PHONOLOGY
6903    PHONOLOGICAL$MODEL CHIL$ARTIC
6904    CHIL$IDENTIFICATION$REPROD
7004    USE CONTRASTIVE$STRESS PRESCH$CHIL
7007    DEV NEUROMUSCULAR$SYSTEMS SP$PROD
7007    PROCESSES$MATURATION MASTICATION DEGLUTITION
7103    CHIL SPONTANEOUS$SP
7104    NEWBORN$INF$CRY NONHUMAN$PRIMATE$VOCALIZATION
7107    HUMAN$PRENATAL$ACTIVITY FACIAL$REGION REL POSTNATAL
        $DEV
7114    VOCAB PRONUNCIATION$ACQUISITION BILINGUALS$MONOLINGUALS
7203    SP$SOUNDS LEARNED
7207    SP$MATURATION
7208    LONGITUDINAL$STUDY ARTIC$CHANGE
7213    STUDY$PHONES CHIL
7218    SOUND$SYSTEMS CHIL LANG
7304    CHIL$PHONETIC$LEARNING
7304    GLOTTAL$CUES PARENT$JUDGMENT EMOTIONAL$ASPECT INF
        $VOCALIZATIONS
7306    ACQUISITION PHONOLOGICAL$CONTRAST STOP$CONSONANTS
7310    COMM$PATTERNS SEX LENGTH$VERBALIZATION SP$CHIL
7313    CHIL$SP HEREDITARY$SEX$DIFFERENCES
7314    ACOUS$FEATURES CHIL VOWELS DEV CHRONOLOGICAL$AGE$VS
        $BONE$AGE
7314    REFERENTIAL$EFFECTS ARTIC$LEARNING
7403    FEATURE$DEVELOPMENT
7414    UNIDENTIFIABLE$UTTERANCES CHIL$SP
7503    PRATHER ARTICULATION$DEVELOPMENT CHIL
7504    GALLAGHER ARTICULATORY$INCONSISTENCIES SP NORMAL$CHILD
7504    GALLAGHER CONTEXTUAL$VARIABLES S+Z$PROD SP CHILD
7504    ZLATIN VOICING$CONTRAST PERCEP STOP$CONSONANTS
7506    PRESCOTT INFANT$CRY$SOUND DEV FEATURES
7523    STARK FEATURES INFANT$SOUNDS
7526    BARON CHILD$ERRORS PRONOUNS
7526    FRASER MOTHERS$SP CHILD
7526    MOERK PROCESSES PRODUCTS IMITATION
7526    RUDER EFFECTS VERBAL$IMITATION COMP$TRAINING VERBAL
        $PROD
7526    SNOW MOTHER$SP THREE$SOCIAL$CLASSES
7526    STEINGART PSYCHOLOGICAL$DIFFERENTIATION LANG$BEHAVIOR

7604  ZLATIN DEV VOICING$CONTRAST COMPARISON VOT STOP$PERCEP+PROD
7621  BUTCHER ELECTROMYOGRAPHIC COARTIC VCV$SEQUENCES
7623  EILERS ROLE SP$DISCRIM DEVELOPMENTAL$SOUND$SUBSTITUTIONS
7704  GALLAGHER REVISION$BEHAVIORS SP NORMAL$CHILD
7708  BRALLEY DEV ARTIC$PROFICIENCY SCHOOL$CHILDREN
7721  ROSENHOUSE ANALYSIS TYPES BABY'S$CRIES
7723  GILBERT TEMPORAL$CONSTRAINTS CONSONANT$CLUSTERS CHILD
      $SP
7723  GILBERT VOICE$ONSET$TIME$ANALYSIS APICAL STOP$PRODUCTION
7723  LI ACQUISITION TONE MANDARIN-SPEAKING$CHIL
7723  PRIESTLEY IDIOSYNCRATIC STRATEGY ACQUISITION PHONOLOGY
7803  MOWRER R$BIAS CHILD$PHONOLOGICAL$SYSTEMS
7806  SIMON CROSS-LANG$STUDY SP-PATTERN$LEARNING
7812  HODSON FEATURE$COMPETENCIES FOUR-YEAR-OLDS
7823  LEONARD ASPECTS CHILD$PHONOLOGY IMITATIVE SPONTANEOUS
      $SP
7823  STARK FEATURES INFANT$SOUNDS EMERGENCE COOING

## 0310

5413  ORIGIN VOCAL$PERIOD
5503  MECHANISMS$PHONATION$RESPIRATION$GLUTINATION
5513  PSYCHOLOGICAL$REL ONE'S$OWN$VOICE
5603  EFFECT VOICE$QUALITY COMM
5606  NATURE VOCAL$CORD$WAVE
5706  AIR$RESISTANCE BERNOULLI$EFFECT HUMAN$LARYNX
5804  MYOELASTIC—AERODYNAMIC$THEORY VOICE$PROD
5806  PHONATION$VOWELS
5809  VOICE ARTIC
5810  BASIS ASSOCIATION VOICE$CHARACTERISTICS PERSONALITY
      $TRAITS
5904  ESTIMATES INTRAGLOTTAL$PRESSURE PHONATION
5904  OPTIMAL$VOCAL$FREQ
5906  NATURE VOCAL$CORD$WAVE
5913  PITCH$VARIATION
5914  JOSHUA$STEELE SP$MELODY
5914  VOCAL$BEHAVIOR DURATION SP$UNITS
6004  LAMINAGRAPHIC$STUDY VOCAL$PITCH
6106  CONSIDERATIONS ANALYSIS INTONATION
6106  PITCH$SYNCHRONOUS$ANALYSIS VOICED$SOUNDS
6110  PITCH$CHANGE COMPREHENSION
6114  STUDIES INTONATION
6204  ACOUS$STUDY NASALITY
6214  METHOD EVAL LISTENERS$TRANSCRIPTION$INTONATION INSTRUMENTAL
      $DATA

| | |
|---|---|
| 6303 | MAXIMUM$DURATION$PHONATION |
| 6306 | ANALOGIES PITCH LATERLIZATION$PHENOMENA |
| 6404 | AIR$FLOW PROD CONSONANTS |
| 6404 | REGULATORY$MECHANISMS VOICE$INTENSITY$VARIATION |
| 6406 | CHANNEL$VOCODER DIGITAL PITCH$EXTRACTOR |
| 6413 | EXPERIMENT NASAL$RESONANCE SINGING |
| 6507 | AIR$FLOW AIR$PRESSURE STUDIES |
| 6510 | ADOL$VOICE$CHANGES SOUTHERN$WHITE$MALES |
| 6604 | AGE$RECOGNITION VOICE |
| 6613 | PHONATION RESPIRATION |
| 6614 | EXPERIMENTAL$ANALYSIS RELATIVE$IMPORTANCE PITCH QUALITY INTENSITY |
| 6704 | EFFECTS ALTERATIONS PROSODIC$FEATURES SEQUENCING$PERFORMANCE |
| 6710 | EVAL CROSS-SECTIONAL$STUDIES ADOL$VOICE$CHANGES MALES |
| 6710 | RESPIROMETRIC$STUDY LUNG$FUNCTION UTTERANCE SP$MATERIAL |
| 6713 | REGULATION SUSTAINED$PHONATION |
| 6713 | RESPIRATION$PHONATION |
| 6713 | RESPIROMETRIC$TECHNIQUE EVAL VELO$COMPETENCE SP |
| 6713 | VARIABLES LARYNGEAL$TONE |
| 6713 | VOCAL$INTENSITY SUBGLOTTIC$PRESSURE AIR$FLOW$REL SINGERS |
| 6813 | PHONATION$TIME AIR$USAGE PHONATION |
| 6813 | X-RAY$STUDY PHONATION |
| 6903 | VOCAL$CONDITIONING INF |
| 6903 | VOCAL$CONDITIONING INF |
| 6906 | IDENTIFICATION SHIFT VOCAL$REGISTERS |
| 6906 | SUSTAINED$PHONATION |
| 6906 | VOCAL$LOUDNESS EFFORT CONTINUOUS$SP |
| 6913 | CONSTANCY INTRAORAL$AIR$PRESSURE |
| 6913 | REL INTRAORAL$AIR$PRESSURE ORAL$CAVITY$SIZE |
| 6913 | SUBGOLTTAL$PRESSURE PHONATION |
| 7006 | PITCH VOICING$CUE |
| 7006 | SP$PROD |
| 7006 | SP$PROD |
| 7014 | DESCRIPTION PERCEP FREQ$BREAKS ADOL$FEMALES |
| 7104 | EFFECTS DRUGS PHONATION |
| 7104 | PHONATIONAL$FREQ$RANGES ADULTS |
| 7106 | ACOUS$CONSEQUENCES LIP$TONGUE$JAW$LARYNX$MOVEMENT |
| 7106 | AIRFLOW TURBULENCE$NOISE FRICATIVE STOP$CONSONANTS |
| 7106 | EFFECT GLOTTAL$PULSE$SHAPE QUALITY NATURAL$VOWELS |
| 7106 | SPEAKER$SEX$RECOGNITION CHIL$VOICES |
| 7106 | SWEEP-TONE$MEAS VOCAL$TRACT$CHARACTERISTICS |
| 7113 | AERODYNAMIC$STUDY VIBRATO STRAIGHT$TONE$SINGING |
| 7113 | DISSOCIATIONS$ELECTROGLOTTOGRAM$PHONOGRAM |
| 7204 | NATURE GLOTTAL$TONE |
| 7204 | PHONATIONAL$RANGE MODAL$FALSETTO$REGISTERS |
| 7204 | PHONATIONAL$RANGE MODAL$FALSETTO$REGISTERS |

7213    VOCAL ACTIVITY
7214    LOCATION RHYTHMIC$STRESS$BEATS ENG EXPERIMENTAL$STUDY
7219    VOICE PERSONALITY
7304    REL LINGUAL$INTRAORAL$AIR$PRESSURES SYLLABLE$PRODUCTION
7304    SPEAKING$RATE EFFECTS CHIL$COMPREHENSION NORMAL$SP
7306    VOICING
7311    PHONATION$TIME$RATIO
7312    MEANINGFUL$MEANINGLESS$EMOTIONALLY$TONED$SENTENCES
7313    ACOUS$PARAMETERS PERCEP MODAL$FALSETTO$VOICE
7313    ACOUS$STUDY REGISTER$EQUALIZATION SINGING
7313    JUDGMENTS VOCAL$ROUGHNESS RATE$EXTENT$VIBRATO
7313    VOCAL$INTENSITY MODAL$FALSETTO$REGISTERS
7313    VOCAL$INTENSITY SUBGLOTTIC$PRESSURE AIR$FLOW$REL SINGERS
7504    FOLKINS RHYTHM+SYLLABLE$TRAINING PHRASE-LEVEL$STRESS
        $PATTERNING
7521    MOSKOWITZ ACQUISITION FRICATIVES PHONETICS PHONOLOGY
7533    LIBERMAN STRESS ICELANDIC GENERAL$PROSODY
7604    ADAMS STUTTERERS + NONSTUTTERERS PHONATION VOWEL
7604    COLEMAN VOICE$CHARACTERISTICS MALENESS FEMALENESS
7627    LEEPER VOICE$INITIATION NORMAL$CHILDREN CHILDREN$VOCAL
        $NODULES
7633    BHATIA PREDICTIVE$ROLE THEORIES ASPIRATION
7703    BLOOD CHILDREN'S$PERCEP NASAL$RESONANCE
7704    BAKEN ESTIMATION LUNG$VOLUME$CHANGE TORSO$HEMICIRCUMFERENCES
7704    ROTHENBERG MEAS AIRFLOW SP
7721    PETURSSON TIMING GLOTTAL$EVENTS PROD ASPIRATION S
7721    ROSENHOUSE ANALYSIS TYPES BABY'S$CRIES
7733    HAAG AIRFLOW GERMAN$STOP$CONSONANTS
7733    MARCHAL VOT BOUROUCHASKI
7803    HASKELL SELF-PERCEP SPEAKING$PITCH$LEVELS
7806    FLANAGAN COMPUTER$MODEL AIR$VOLUME VOCAL$CORDS
7806    SINGH MULTIDIMENSIONAL$CLASSIFICATION VOICE$QUALITIES
7813    ACKERMANN VOCAL$CHANGES YOUNG$PEOPLE
7813    MALLARD CONTROL FUNDAMENTAL$FREQ
7813    SAITO OBSERVATION VOCAL$FOLD$VIBRATION
7821    PAINTER IMPLOSIVES INHERENT$PITCH TONOGENESIS LARYNGEAL
        $MECHANISMS
7827    HUTCHINSON PATTERNS NASALANCE GERONTOLOGIC$SUBJECTS
7829    MUELLER LISTENER$ID SPEAKER$SEX CHILD

                    0311

5904    PITCH DURATION OLDER$MALES
6010    COMM$PROBLEMS GER$PATIENT

6205    PROGRAM GERIATRIC$PATIENT
6404    VOCAL$PITCH GER$WOMEN
6503    CENTENARIAN$AUDIOGRAMS PT
6604    PHONATORY$RELATED$CHANGES ADVANCED$AGE
6604    R GER$MALES TIME-ALTERED$SP
6904    SP$DISCRIM GER$POPULATION
6911    SP$DISCRIM GER
7104    PHONEME$DISCRIM GER VARYING$S/N$CONDITIONS
7207    CHANGES COMM AGING
7618    CARMICHAEL COMM GERONTOLOGY
7729    NEELLEY COMM$PROBLEMS ELDERLY
7820    BARTON MEDIA AGING COMM$RESEARCH
7827    HUTCHINSON PATTERNS NASALANCE GERONTOLOGIC$SUBJECTS


                                  0312


5403    ASPECTS PERSONALITY VOCAL$EFFECTS DSF
5503    EFFECT FILTERING SIDE-TONE INTELLIGIBILITY
5506    LISTENING FILTERED$COMPETING$VOICE$MESSAGES
5506    RELATIVE$INTELLIGIBILITY SP RECORDED$SIMULTANEOUSLY
        $EAR$MOUTH
5606    INTELLIGIBILITY DIPHASIC$SP
5606    NATURALNESS DISTORTION SPEECHPROCESSING$DEVICES
5606    SP-BAND$COMPRESSION
5703    TIME$COMPRESSION COMPREHENSION CONNECTED$SP
5706    WORD$INTELLIGIBILITY FUNCTION TIME$COMPRESSION
5804    LISTENER$EVALS SP$INTERRUPTIONS
5806    CONFIDENCE$RATING MESSAGE$RECEPTION FILTERED$SP
5806    INTERAURAL$EFFECTS SP$INTELLIGIBILITY HIGH$NOISE$LEVELS
5806    POWER CLIPPING$SP AUDIO$BAND
5906    EFFECT SAMPLE DURATION ARTIC CLIPPED$SP
5906    INTELLIGIBILITY PEAK-CLIPPED$SP HIGH$NOISE$LEVELS
6004    SP$COMPRESSION$DEVICES
6104    INTELLIGIBILITY SLOW-PLAYED$SP
6304    EFFECTS TACTILE$AUD$ALTERATIONS SP$OUTPUT
6306    HELIUM$SP
6306    INTERRUPTED$SP POSSIBILITY INCREASING COMM$EFFICIENCY
6306    PITCH-INDUCED SPECTRAL$DISTORTION CHANNEL$VOCODERS
6306    R SPECTRUM$ANALYZERS BANK-OF-FILTERS SIGNALS VOWEL
        $SOUNDS
6406    BANDPASS$COMPRESSOR TYPE SP-COMPRESSION$DEVICE
6406    DISTORTION TEMPURAL$PATTERN SP INTERRUPTION ALTERNATION
6406    INTELLIGIBILITY FM$SP
6411    PREDICTION EFFECTS COMBINED$DETERRENTS INTELLIGIBILTY

6414  GATING$TECHNIQUE AID SP$ANALYSIS
6504  DETERMINING$PERCEP$SPACES QUALITY FILTERED$SP
6506  PITCH$SHIFTS LOW-PASS HIGH-PASS NOISE$BANDS
6510  EFFECT PRACTICE COMPREHENSION TIME-COMPRESSED$SP
6604  R GER$MALES TIME-ALTERED$SP
6606  ANALYSIS$SP HELIUM-OXYGEN$MIXTURE PRESSURE
6606  CONDITIONS$DISTORTION
6606  EFFECTS BANDPASS-FILTERED$NOISE INTELLIGIBILITY FILTERED
      $SP
6606  IMPROVING NATURALNESS INTELLIGIBILITY HELIUM-OXYGEN
      $SP VOCODERS$TEC
6606  INTELLIGIBILITY SP RIGHT$LEFT$EAR BINAURAL$NOISE
6606  SP$INTELLIGIBILITY SPACE$VEHICLES NITROGEN HELIUM
      INERT$GAS
6609  EFFECT HIGH$LOW$PASS$FILTERING VOCAL$QUALITY MALE
      $FEMALE$SPEAKERS
6703  REMOVING$SEGMENTS SP$SAMPLE
6704  INTELLIGIBILITY FILTERED$SYNTHETIC$SENTENCES
6706  INFLUENCE COMPRESSOR$ACTION SP$INTELLIGIBILITY
6706  RELATIVE$INTELLIGIBILITY TRANSFORMS CLIPPED$SP
6706  TECHNIQUE CORRECTING HELIUM-SP$DISTORTION
6714  DISTORTION TEMPORAL$PATTERN SP SYLLABLE-TIED$ALTERNATION
6714  EFFECTS INTERRUPTION INTERAURAL$ALTERNATION SP$INTELLIGIBILITY
6804  DIFFICULTY LISTENING TIME-COMPRESSED$SP
6806  INTELLIGIBILITY VOWELS ALTERED DURATION FREQ
6806  REL INTELLIGIBILITY$SCORES TEST$METHODS SP$DISTORTION
6806  REL INTELLIGIBILITY$SCORES TEST$METHODS SP$DISTORTION
6806  SPECTROGRAPHIC$ANALYSIS DIVERS$SP DECOMPRESSION
6906  PERCEP CONSONANTS CLIPPED$SP
6911  EFFECT NOISE$BACKGROUND SP$FUNCTION
7006  EFFECTS FILTERING VOWEL$ENVIRONMENT CONSONANT$PERCEP
7011  MENTAL$ATTITUDE COMPREHENSION TIME-COMPRESSED$LISTENING
7104  ARTIC STRESS/JUNCTURE$PROD ORAL$ANESTHETIZATION MASKING
7106  CONTRAST DETECTION GATED$NOISE
7106  EFFECT SMOOTHING QUANTIZING PARAMETERS FORMANT-CODED
      $VOICED$SP
7106  PERCEP VOWELS CLIPPED$SP
7106  PHONOLOGICAL$OPPOSITIONS CHIL PERCEP$STUDY
7106  SP$SYNCHRONIZED PERIODIC$INTERAURAL$SWITCHING SP
7111  REACTION$TIME AUDITORY$IDENTIFICATION SEGMENTS SYLLABLES
7114  INTELLIGIBILITY INTERAURAL$ALTERNATED$SP NOISE WORDS
      NONSENSE
7114  PERCEP ELECTRONICALLY$GATED$SP
7204  COMMENT ARTIC STRESS/JUNCTURE$PROD ORAL$ANESTHETIZATION
      MASKING
7204  COMMENT ARTIC STRESS/JUNCTURE$PROD ORAL$ANESTHETIZATION
      MASKING

```
7204    INTELLIGIBILITY TIME$COMPRESSED$CNC$MONOSYLLABLES
7206    EFFECT FRINGE MASKING$LEVEL$DIFFERENCE GATING
7211    PERCEP TIME-COMPRESSED$CNC$MONOSYLLABLES
7304    ACOUS$CHARACTERISTICS SP$PRODUCED$WITHOUT$ORAL$SENSATION
7304    PHONEMIC$CONTENT BACKWARD-REPRODUCED$SP
7306    INTELLIGIBILITY TEMPORALLY$INTERRUPTED$SP
7311    EFFECT OR$SKILL COMPREHENSION TIME-COMPRESSED$SP
7311    EFFECTS LISTENING COMPRESSED$SP INTELLECTIVE$PROCESSES
        CHIL
7406    AERODYNAMIC$ASPECT SENSORY$DEPRIVED$SP
7406    INTERAURAL$ALTERNATION SP$INTELLIGIBILITY
7414    ACOUS$DISTORTED$SP
7414    EXPERIMENTAL$STUDY INTERFERENCE RECEPTIVE$PROD$PROCESSES
        REL
7504    WINGFIELD ACOUS$REDUNDANCY PERCEP TIME-COMPRESSED
        $SP
7506    GUPTA PERCEPTION HINDU$CONSONANTS CLIPPED$SP
7511    SCHAWB EFFECTS SP$COMPRESSION AFFECTIVE$DIMENSIONS
        DIALOGIE
7511    SCHWAB EFFECTS SP$COMPRESSION AFFECTIVE$DIMENSIONS
        DIALOGUE
7527    CHANG-YIT RELIABILITY SIDETONE$AMP EFFECT VOCAL$INTENSITY
7603    BEASLEY CHILDREN'S$PERCEP TIME-COMPRESSED$SP SP$DISCRIM
7611    REINSCHE DISCRIM TIME-COMPRESSED$CNC$MONOSYLLABLES
        NORMAL$LISTENERS
7706    HOLLIEN SPEAKER$IDEN LONG-TERM$SPECTRA DISTORTED$SP
7706    POWERS INTELLIGIBILITY TEMPORALLY$INTERRUPTED$SP INTERVENING
        $NOISE
7713    BROWN SEX$IDENTIFICATION CONSTANT$LARYNGEAL$SOURCE
7721    COLEMAN ORAL$MUZZLE$PRESSURE UNDERWATER$COMM
7721    DANILOFF ALTERATION CHILD$ARTIC ORAL$ANESTHESIA
7732    WINGFIELD PERCEP ALTERNATED$SP
7804    DOWNS PROCESSING$DEMANDS AUD$LEARNING DEGRADED$LISTENING
7806    MAKHOUL MIXED-SOURCE$MODEL SP$COMPRESSION SYNTHESIS
7819    BEATTY EFFECTS COMPRESSED$SP LEARNER$ANXIETY
7821    DOHERTY MULTIPLE-FACTOR$SPEAKER$IDENTIFICATION NORMAL
        DISTORTED$SP
7821    HAMLET COMPENSATORY$ALVEOLAR$CONSONANT$PRODUCTION
        DENTAL$PROSTHESIS
```

## 0313

```
5506    ANALYSIS PERCEP$CONFUSIONS ENG$CONSONANTS
5606    PROSODIC$FEATURES WHISPERED$SP
```

5706  PROSODIC$FEATURES WHISPERED$SP
5906  DIFFERENCE$SOUNDS
6506  ACOUS$CUES SYNTHESIS N-D$DISTINCTION
6606  CROSSLANGUAGE$STUDY PERCEP$CONFUSION PLOSIVE-PHONEMES
6614  CUES PHONEMIC$DISTINCTIONS SWEDISH
6704  EFFECT DISTINCTIVE$FEATURE$PRETRNG PHONEME$DISCRIM
      $LEARNING
6709  PROSODIC$FEATURES HAWAIIAN$ENG
7014  NUCLEUS$COMPONENT DURATION
7204  COMPARISON FEATURE$SYSTEMS DATA PSYCHOPHYSICAL$METHODS
7204  COMPARISON PHONEMIC$GRAPHEMIC$FEATURES ENG$CONSONANTS
      AUD$VISUAL$M
7206  ALTERNATIVE MD-SCAL$ANALYSIS GRAHAM$HOUSE$DATA
7206  COMMENT ALTERNATIVE MD-SCAL$ANALYSIS GRAHAM$HOUSE
      $DATA
7211  CONSONANT$DISCRIM FUNCTION DISTINCTIVE$FEATURE$DIFFERENCES
7211  MINIMAL-CONTRASTS$CLOSED-R$SP$TEST
7214  PHONETIC$FEATURE VOWEL$LENGTH DUTCH
7214  R$LATENCY$DIFFERENCES SP$SHADOWING INDICATOR DISTINCTIVE
      $FEATURES
7306  CONSONANT$CONFUSIONS NOISE STUDY PERCEP$FEATURES
7306  EFFECT POSITION$UTTERANCE SP$SEGMENT$DURATION ENG
7306  MULTIDIMENSIONAL$CODING TEMPORAL$MICROSTRUCTURE AUD
      $DISPLAYS
7306  MULTIDIMENSIONAL$ENCODING TEMPORAL$MICROSTRUCTURE
      AUD$DISPLAYS
7312  INTERCONSONANTAL$DISTANCES REL IMMEDIATE$RECALL
7403  COMPARISON LINGUISTIC$FEATURE$SYSTEMS
7403  DISTINCTIVE$FEATURE$SYSTEMS
7404  CONCEPTUAL$REALITY DISTINCTIVE$FEATURES
7404  DISTINCTIVE$PHONETIC$FEATURES SP$DISCRIM$LEARNING
7414  DISTINCTIVE$FEATURE$CONFUSIONS PROD DISCRIM CONSONANTS
7506  BELL-BERTI CONTROL PHARYNGEAL$CAVITY$SIZE ENGLISH
7526  LEONARD CHILD$JUDGMENTS LINGUISTIC$FEATURES
7533  GANDOUR FEATURES LARYNX N-ARY$BINARY
7533  LOFQVIST INTRINSIC EXTRINSIC F0 VARIATIONS SWEDISH
7533  NIHALANI AIR$FLOW$RATE STOPS SINDHI
7533  RAPHAEL TONGUE MUSCULATURE TENSION ENGLISH VOWELS
7606  RICHMAN VOCAL$DISTINCTIVE$FEATURES GELADA$MONKEYS
7621  HAMMARBERG METAPHYSICS COARTIC
7633  BHATIA PREDICTIVE$ROLE THEORIES ASPIRATION
7633  PETURSSON ASPIRATION GLOTTAL ACTIVITY CONSONANTS
7633  PIKE STRESS TONE PHONOLOGY DIUXI MIXTEC
7633  VANCE TONE INTONATION CANTONESE
7706  PARKER DISTINCTIVE$FEATURES ACOUSTIC$CUES
7721  KENT COARTIC RECENT$SP$PROD$MODELS

7733   PILCH PHONOLOGY BASEL$GERMAN
7733   VANCE TONAL$DISTINCTIONS CANTONESE
7806   KEATING TRANSITION$LENGTH PERCEP STOP$CONSONANTS
7806   SPARKS MULTIPOINT$ELECTROTACTILE$SP$AID SEGMENTAL
       $FEATURES
7809   COLE PERCEP PHONETIC$FEATURES FLUENT$SP
7821   BECKER FEATURE GRAVE
7821   CUTLER PHONEME-MONITORING CONTEXT PHONETIC$SEQUENCES
7821   DIXIT PEAK$MAGNITUDES SUPRAGLOTTAL$AIR$PRESSURE STOP
       PRODUCTIONS HINDI
7821   HAGGARD DEVOICING VOICED$FRICATIVES
7821   HIGGS PHONOLOGICAL$PERCEPTION OBSTRUENT$COGNATES
7821   MADDIESON TONE$EFFECTS CONSONANTS
7821   O'KANE MANNER VOWEL$TERMINATION PERCEPTUAL$CUE VOICING
7821   ODEN INTEGRATION PLACE + VOICING$INFO IDEN SYN$STOP
7821   WOLF VOICING$CUES ENGLISH$FINAL$STOPS


                              0314


5403   EXPERIMENTAL$STUDY ERRORS SP SPELLING
5403   INFORMATION SOUNDS PHONETIC$DIGRAMS ONE$AND$TWO-SYLLABLE
       $WORDS
5606   RUSSIAN$SENTENCE$INTONATION LINGUISTIC$STRUCTURE
5609   SP ELEMENTARY$CLASSROOM
5609   VARIETIES INDIV$SP
5706   INFORMATION VOWELS
5709   FUNDAMENTALS FORMS SP
6103   INVOLUNTARY$VOCALIZATION
6111   HUMMING SOUND SYMBOL
6206   ISOPREFERENCE$METHOD EVAL SP$TRANSMISSION$CIRCUITS
6206   PITCH$RESIDUE
6211   INFLUENCE VIBRATIONS SP
6214   LINGUISTIC$CODES HESITATION$PHENOMENA INTELLIGENCE
6314   ANTAGONISTIC$FUNCTIONS VERBAL$PAUSES
6414   CROSS$CULTURAL$STUDY SP$RATE
6606   VOCAL$R BULLFROG NATURAL$SYNTHETIC$MATING$CALLS
6613   TURBULEMT$NOISE$SOURCES SP
6704   EFFECTS VERBAL$PUNISHERS DISFLUENCIES NORMAL$SPEAKERS
6704   EFFECTS VERBAL$PUNISHERS DISFLUENCIES NORMAL$SPEAKERS
6709   PRONUNCIATION ENG RULES
6914   EXPERIMENTAL$INVEST FUNCTION FILLED$PAUSES SP
7003   REL OROSENSORY$DISCRIM ARTIC$ASPECTS SP$PROD
7004   TEMPORAL$PATTERNS SP SAMPLE$SIZE
7114   SYNTACTIC$LOCATION HESITATION$PAUSES

7204    FLUENT$HESITATION$PAUSES FUNCTION SYNTACTIC$COMPLEXITY
7206    TIMING UTTERANCES LINGUISTIC$BOUNDARIES
7306    INTERRUPTIBILITY SP
7309    SP$CHARACTERISTICS EMPLOYABILITY
7406    TEMPORAL$INTERACTION PHRASE$SENTENCE$CONTEXT
7414    ELABORATED$SP HESITATION$PHENOMENA
7414    FILLED$PAUSES SYNTACTIC$COMPLEXITY
7414    TIME$PATTERNS SPONTANEOUS$SP
7505    CUTTING REL SP LANG AUGUST
7505    MUSSEN COMM DEV PROSOCIAL$BEHAVIOR MAY
7506    SINNOTT REGULATION VOICE$AMPLITUDE MONKEY
7511    VENKATAGIRL HEMISPHERIC$ASYMMETRY AUD$FEEDBACK$CONTROL
        SP
7606    RICHMAN VOCAL$DISTINCTIVE$FEATURES GELADA$MONKEYS
7627    BRADAC VERBAL$BEHAVIOR INTERVIEWEES
7627    SOKOLOFF REFINEMENT CONCEPT$RETICENCE
7633    KOHLER WORD-FINAL$ALVEOLAR$PLOSIVES GERMAN
7706    CLEVELAND ACOUS$PROP VOICE$TIMBRE INFLUENCE VOICE
        $CLASSIFICATION
7706    HARSHMAN FACTOR$ANALYAIS TONGUE$SHAPES
7706    JENNINGS REPRODUCTION FAMILIAR$MELODIES PERCEPTION
        TONAL$SEQUENCES
7721    CLARK PHONOLOGICAL$MARKEDNESS SHORT$TERM$RECALL
7721    KENT COARTIC RECENT$SP$PROD$MODELS
7721    ROSENHOUSE ANALYSIS TYPES BABY'S$CRIES
7724    BERKOWITZ OROFACIAL$GROWTH DENTISTRY
7803    MOWRER EFFECT LISPING AUDIENCE$EVAL MALE$SPEAKERS
7804    HOROVITZ STAPEDIAL$REFLEX ANXIETY DISFLUENT$SPEAKERS
7804    MANNING RIGHT-EAR$EFFECT AUDITORY$FEEDBACK$CONTROL
        ChIL$PHONEMES
7804    WINITZ INTERFERENCE PERSISTENCE ARTICULATORY$RESPONSES
7806    ATAL LINEAR$PREDICTION$ANALYSIS SP
7818    BEHNKE SP$ANXIETY PREDICTOR TREMBLING
7821    BAILEY SUGGESTIONS TRANSCRIPTION ENGLISH$PHONETIC
        $SEGMENTS
7821    VANLANCKER CERBRAL$DOMINANCE PITCH$CONTRASTS TONE
        $LANG$SPEAKERS
7825    GORDON HEMISPHERE$DOM RHYTHM DICHOTICALLY-PRESENTED
        $MELODIES
7825    HICKS HANDEDNESS ANXIETY
7825    MCFARLAND BRAIN$LATERALIZATION FUNCTION MANUAL$SKILL
7825    MCGLONE SEX$DIFFERENCES FUNCTIONAL$BRAIN$ASYMMETRY


                          0315


5506    ACOUS$LOCI TRANSITIONAL$CUES CONSONANTS

5506  VOWEL$SYNTHESIS RESONANT$CIRCUITS
5606  NOISE$DURATION CUE DISTINGUISHING FRICATIVE$AFFRICATE
      $STOP$CONSONA
5606  SP$ANALYSIS$SYNTHESIS
5606  SP$SOUND$CODER
5806  DYNAMIC$ANALOG$SP$SYNTHESIZER
5806  SEGMENTS$INVENTORY SP$SYNTHESIS
5806  SEGMENTATION SP$SYNTHESIS
5806  SOUND$SYNTHESIZER OPTICAL$CONTROL
5814  SYNTHESIS ENG$VOWELS
5904  NONRANDOM$SOURCES$VARIATION VOWEL$QUALITY
5906  MINIMAL$RULES SYNTHESIZING$SP
5906  SYNTHESIS PERCEP NASAL$CONSONANTS
6014  OBJECTIVES TECHNIQUES SP$SYNTHESIS
6106  SP$SYNTHESIS PRERECORDED$SYLLABLES$WORDS
6114  IDENTIFICATION DISCRIM SYNTHETIC$VOWELS
6114  PERCEP VOWEL$COLOR FORMANTLESS$COMPLEX$SOUNDS
6114  SEGMENT$INVENTORIES SP$SYNTHESIS
6206  SP$SYNTHESIZER
6206  STUDIES NASAL$CONSONANTS ARTIC SP$SYNTHESIZER
6206  VOWEL$FORMANTS BANDWIDTHS SYNTHETIC$VOWELS
6214  JUDGMENT VOWEL$COLOR NATURAL$ARTIFICIAL$SOUNDS
6306  PITCH-INDUCED SPECTRAL$DISTORTION CHANNEL$VOCODERS
6306  PITCH-SYNCHRONOUS TIME-DOMAIN ESTIMATION FORMANT$FREQ
      BANDWIDTHS
6306  REDUCED$BLOOD$FLOW
6410  VARIATIONS VERBAL$BEHAVIOR SECOND$SPEAKER
6414  SP$SYNTHESIS RULE
6414  SP$SYNTHESIS
6506  VOCAL-R$SYNTHESIZER
6604  PERFORMANCE$INTENSITY$CHARACTERISTICS SYNTHETIC$SENTENCES
6606  ACOUS$DESCRIPTION SYLLABIC$NUCLEI INTERPRETATION DYNAMIC
      $MODEL$ART
6614  SYNTHESIS RULE PROSODIC$FEATURES
6704  EFFECT COMPETING$MESSAGE SYNTHETIC$SENTENCE$IDENTIFICATION
6704  EFFECT NOISE SYNTHETIC$IDENTIFICATION
6704  SYNTHETIC$SENTENCE$IDENTIFICATION ROC
6706  MACHINE-AIDED FORMANT$DETERMINATION SP$SYNTHESIS
6706  TIME$ADJUSTMENT SP$SYNTHESIS
6711  TRANSPOSITION$HIGH$FREQUENCY$SOUNDS PARTIAL$VOCODING
      SP$SPECTRUM
6714  CATEGORICAL$R SYNTHETIC$VOCALIC$STIMULI SPEAKERS VARIOUS
      $LANGS
6714  PHONEME$CATEGORIZATION SYNTHETIC$VOCALIC$STIMULI FOREIGN
      $SPEAKERS
6714  SECOND$SPECTRAL$PEAK FRONT$VOWELS PERCEP$STUDY ROLE
      SECOND$FORMANT

6806    DIGITAL-FORMANT$SYNTHESIZER SP-SYNTHESIZER STUDIES
6806    FORMANT$TRANSITIONS PERCEP SYNTHETIC$SEMIVOWELS
6806    SIMULATION SECONDARY$RESIDUE$EFFECT DIGITAL$COMPUTER
6814    PERCEP STOP$CONSONANTS SYNTHETIC$CV$SYLLABLES
6814    PERCEP$CATEGORIZATION SYNTHETIC$VOWELS TOOL DIALECTOLOGY
        TYPOLOGY
6816    FUND$STUDIES SP$ANALYSIS$SYNTHESIS
6904    VELO$ORIFICE$AREA REPLICATION ANALOG$EXPERIMENTATION
6906    EXCITATION VOCAL-TRACT$SYNTHESIZERS
6906    INFLUENCE FUND$FREQ CUES PERCEP SYNTHETIC$INTONATION
        $CONTOURS
6906    INVEST STRESS$PATTERNS SP$SYNTHESIS RULE
7004    NORMAL$SIMULATED$ROUGH$VOWELS ADULT$MALES
7004    SPECTRAL$NOISE$LEVELS ROUGHNESS$SEVERITY$RATINGS SIMULATED
        $ROUGH$V
7006    INPUT$GENERATORS DIGITAL$SOUND$SYNTHESIS
7014    CONTEXTUAL$EFFECTS PERCEP SYNTHETIC$VOWELS
7106    SP$ANALYSIS SYNTHESIS LINEAR$PREDICTION SP$WAVE
7114    METHODOLOGY EXPERIMENTS PERCEP SYNTHETIC$VOWELS
7114    SYNTHETIC$VOWEL$CATEGORIZATION DIALECTOLOGY
7204    SYNTHETIC$VOWEL$CATEGORIZATION$TESTS DIALECTOLOGY
7206    COMMENTS SP$ANALYSIS SYNTHESIS LINEAR$PREDICTION SP
        $WAVE
7206    DURATION CUE RECOGNITION SYNTHETIC$VOWELS
7214    EFFECT FORMANT$AMPLITUDE IDENTITY SYNTHETIC$VOWELS
7306    PATTERN-TRANSFORMATION$MODEL PITCH
7314    VOWEL SPEAKER$IDENTIFICATION NATURAL$SP SYNTHETIC
        $SP
7404    AUD-MOTOR$FORMANT$TRACKING SP$IMITATION
7414    INFLUENCE PRECURSIVE$SEQUENCES PERCEP SYNTHESIZED
        $VOWELS
7506    OLIVE FF$RULES SYNTHESIS SIMPLE$SENTENCES
7506    PATISAUL TIME-FREQ$RESOLUTION SP$ANALYSIS+SYNTHESIS
7526    TORRANS ORAL$STEREOGNOSIS VARYING$FORM ANSWER$TYPE
        RETENTION TIME
7533    LAUFER SYNTHESIZING HEBREW SPEECH
7606    MOORE R COCHLEAR-NUCLEUS$NEURONS SYNTHETIC$SP
7606    OLIVE SP$RESYNTHESIS PHONEME-RELATED$PARAMETERS
7706    ROTHENBERG VIBROTACTILE$FREQUENCY ENCODING SP$PARAMETER
7721    SCHOUTEN IMITATION SYNTHETIC$VOWELS BILINGUALS
7806    ERBER VOICE/MOUTH$SYNTHESIS TACTUAL/VISUAL$PERCEPTION
7806    KENT IMITATION SYNTHESIZED$VOWELS PRESCHOOL$CHILD
7806    KUHL SP$PERCEP CHINCHILLA VOT$STIMULI
7806    MAKHOUL MIXED-SOURCE$MODEL SP$COMPRESSION SYNTHESIS
7821    ODEN INTEGRATION PLACE + VOICING$INFO IDEN SYN$STOP

0316

5716    TACTILE$PERCEP RHYTHMIC$PATTERNS BLIND DEAF APHASIC
        CHIL

5819   RELATIVE$CONTRIBUTION AUD$TACTILE$CUES SP
5919   EFFECTS DISRUPTED$TACTILE$CUES PROD$CONSONANTS
6106   PITCH$SENSATION REL PERIODICITY STIMULUS HNG SKIN
       $VIBRATIONS
6111   VIGILANCE CUTANEOUS$AUD$SIGNALS
6206   INVESTIGATION PARAMETERS CUTANEOUS$THR VIBRATION
6306   EFFECT CONTACTOR$AREA VIBROTACTILE$THR
6504   ORAL$PERCEP TWO-POINT$DISCRIM
6506   MULTIPLE$CUTANEOUS$STIMULATION DISCRIM VIBRATORY$PATTERNS
6506   TEMPORAL$SUMMATION VIBROTACTILE$SENSITIVITY
6704   ORAL$PERCEP TEXTURE$DISCRIM
6704   ORAL$PERCEP MANDIBULAR$KINESTHESIA
6903   ASSESSMENT LINGUAL$TACTILE$SENSATION$PERCEP
7004   ORAL$ASSESSMENT OBJECT$SIZE
7007   ORAL$SENSATION$PERCEP REVIEW
7011   ROLE SENSORY$FEEDBACK TONGUE$CONTROL
7104   ARTIC ORAL$SENSORY$CONTROL
7106   TWO-FREQ$STIMULATION CUTANEOUS$MECHANORECEPTOR
7117   VIBRATION TOOL
7120   ORAL$TACTILE$PERCEP
7204   DURATION$EFFECTS SUPRALIMINAL$ELECTRICAL$STIMULI TONGUE
7204   ORAL$VIBROTACTILE$SENSATION EVAL DEFECTIVE$SPEAKERS
7304   ACOUS$CHARACTERISTICS SP$PRODUCED$WITHOUT$ORAL$SENSATION
7406   TACTILE$PERCEP COMPUTER-DERIVED FORMANT$PATTERNS VOICED
       $SP
7417   EFFECTS VIBROTACTILE$THR TONGUE
7506   LOPATER FREQ$STIMULATION TACTILE$RECEPTORS
7511   ARNST VIBROTACTILE$SENSITIVITY TONGUE HEARING-IMPAIRED
7513   JENSEN ORAL$SENSORY-PERCEP STUTTERERS
7521   HARDCASTLE SP$PROD ORAL$ANAESTHESIA AUD$MASKING
7529   BEASLEY INTRA-ORAL$DURATION INTERVAL$MEAS ORAL$STEREOGNOSIS
7618   HANLEY ORAL$STEREOGNOSIS CHILD
7706   YENI-KOMSHIAN ID SP$SOUNDS DISPLAYED VIBROTACTILE
       $VOCODER
7806   ERBER VOICE/MOUTH$SYNTHESIS TACTUAL/VISUAL$PERCEPTION
7806   SPARKS MULTIPOINT$ELECTROTACTILE$SP$AID SEGMENTAL
       $FEATURES
7827   GIVENS DISCRIM SP$INTENSITY VIBROTACTILE$STIMULATION


                              0317


5419   SOUTHERN$AMERICAN DIPHTHONG
5503   NATIVE$AMERICAN$LISTENERS$ADAPTATION UNDERSTANDING
       $SPEAKERS$FOREIG

```
5509  FIELD$MATERIALS DETERMINATION DIALECT$GRPS
5509  RELATIVE$INTELLIGIBILITY LANG$GRPS
5609  COMPARATIVE$ANALYSIS U$VARIANTS SAN$FRANCISCO LOS
      $ANGELES
5710  EFFECTS LANG$TRNG$PROGRAM FOREIGN$SOUNDINGNESS
5906  VOWEL$OVERLAP FUNCTION FUND$FREQ DIALECT
6014  PERCEP ENG$STOPS ENG$SPEAKERS FOREIGN$SPEAKERS
6019  SP$OCRACOKE NORTH$CAROLINA
6105  SP$PROBLEMS FOREIGN$STUDENTS SURVEY$LITERATURE
6110  PHONOLOGY NEW$ENGLAND$ENG
6114  LISTENER$COMPREHENSION SPEAKERS STATUS$GRPS
6306  FOREIGN$ACCENT SP$DISTORTION
6504  SP AURAL$COMPREHENSION FOREIGN$STUDENTS
6514  CLOZE$PROCEDURES TECHNIQUE INVEST SOCIAL$CLASS$DIFFERENCES
      LANG$US
6514  ELABORATED$CODE WORKING$CLASS$LANG
6604  SELF-ADMINISTERED$PROCEDURES CHANGING$PRONUNCIATION
      $DIALECT
6606  STUDY INTERVOCALIC$CONSONANTS SPOKEN RECOGNIZED LANG
      $GRPS
6610  PERCEP FOREIGN$ACCENT JAPANESE$ENG AMERICAN$BRITISH
      $JAPANESE$LISTE
6709  PROSODIC$FEATURES HAWAIIAN$ENG
6710  STUDY FOREIGN$ACCENT JAPANESE$ENG
6714  PHONEME$CATEGORIZATION SYNTHETIC$VOCALIC$STIMULI FOREIGN
      $SPEAKERS
6810  ORIGIN NYC$PATHOGNOMIC$DIPHTHONG HYPOTHESIS
6905  LANG$COGNITIVE$ASSESSMENTS NEGRO$CHIL
6919  NORTH$CAROLINA$ACCENTS
7004  PSYCHOLOGICAL$CORRELATES SP$CHARACTERISTICS SOUNDING
      $DISADVANTAGED
7005  BLACK$CHIL WHITE$DIALECT
7012  BLACK$ENG
7012  CHIL STANDARD$ENG
7014  NEGRO$CHIL$SP SOCIAL$CLASS$DIFFERENCES WORD$PREDICTABILITY
7103  DIALECTAL$DIFFERENCES PROFESSIONAL$CLINICAL$IMPLICATIONS
7105  ETHNOGRAPHIC$FRAMEWORK INVEST COMM$BEHAVIOR
7109  DIALECT$PERCEP REVIEW RE-EVAL
7110  CHIL$COMPREHENSION STANDARD$NEGRO$NONSTANDARD$ENG
7112  BLACK$ENG
7112  DIALECT$RESEARCH CLASSROOM
7112  NEGRO$SP
7114  RACIAL$DIFFERENCES ASSOCIATIVE$STYLE
7114  SYNTHETIC$VOWEL$CATEGORIZATION DIALECTOLOGY
7117  RACE$IDENTIFICATION BASIS BIASED$SP$SAMPLES
7119  NONVERBAL$ASPECTS BLACK$ENG
```

7120    NEGRO$DIALECT
7120    REGIONAL$VARIATIONS TEACHER$ATTITUDES CHIL LANG
7204    SYNTHETIC$VOWEL$CATEGORIZATION$TESTS DIALECTOLOGY
7208    ROLE SCH$SP$CLINICIAN INNER-CITY$CHIL
7214    EFFECT STIMULUS$MILDNESS-BROADNESS EVAL ACCENTS
7214    LEVELS$ANALYSIS SOCIAL$CLASS$DIFFERENCES LANG
7214    PHONEME$USE PERCEP MEANING CHIL HAWAII
7217    INVEST PHONOLOGICAL$VARIATIONS SCH$BLACK$CHIL
7220    EFFECTS SOCIAL$STATUS SOCIAL$DIALECT LISTENER$R
7304    DIALECT$PROFICIENCY AUD$COMPREHENSION BLACK$NONSTANDARD
        $ENG
7306    FRENCH-ENGLISH$BILINGUALS
7311    LOWER$SOCIO-ECONOMIC$STATUS
7314    INTELLIGIBILITY BLACK$SPEAKERS BLACK$WHITE$LISTENERS
7314    INTONATION$PATTERNS AUSTRALIAN$ENG
7317    SPANISH-SPEAKING$CHIL
7408    EVALUATING$ENGLISH$ARTICULATION NONNATIVE$SPEAKERS
7409    EFFECTS PHONOLOGICAL$SP FOREIGNESS ATTITUDE AMERICAN
        $LISTENERS
7414    EVAL REACTIONS COLLEGE$STUDENTS DIALECT$DIFFERENCES
        ENG MEX-AMERIC
7510    FISHER MEXICAN$AMERICANS$EVALUATIONS SPANISH$ENGLISH
7510    MILLER DIALECT ETHNICITY$EFFECTIVENESS
7510    MILLER EFFECT DIALECT ETHNICITY COMM EFFECTIVENESS
7510    MULAC EVAL SP$DIALECT ATTITUDINAL$SCALE
7512    REY BLACK WHITE CUBAN$TEACHERS'$ATTITUDES SPANISH
        ACCENTED ENGLISH
7520    CONNOLLY PERSONAL$SPACE BLACK WHITE AMERICANS (SPRING
7520    DELIA REGIONAL$DIALECT PERCEP SPEAKER (FALL
7521    LOFQVIST SUBGLOTTAL$PRESSURE PROD SWEDISH$STOPS
7521    SEMILOFF-ZELASKO ACOUSTIC-PERCEP$STUDY MODERN$HEBREW
7523    MENYUK VOT CLUSTER$PRODUCTIONS CHILDREN ADULTS
7526    CREMONA ATTITUDES$TOWARD$DIALECT ITALIAN$CHILD
7526    JAMES BLACK$CHILD$PERCEP BLACK$ENGLISH
7533    HAMEYER DIALECT LOW-GERMAN$
7533    HUSS NEUTRALIZING ENGLISH ACCENT
7533    SAVITT COGNATE$RECOGNITION DIALECTS
7534    BOCK LEVELS BLACK DIALECT PERCEIVED SPEAKER IMAGE
7534    HARPOLE NONSTANDARD SP
7603    ARNOLD GRAMMATIC$CLOSURE ITPA BLACK CHILDREN
7604    BARAN PHONOLOGICAL$RULES BLACK$ENGLISH DISCRIM WORD
        $PAIRS
7604    STEPHENS IMITATION ENGLISH$DIALECTS HEAD$START$CHILDREN
7605    PICKERING BILINGUAL+BICULTURAL$EDUCATION SP$PATHOLOGIST
7606    STREETER EFFECTS LEARNING$ENG SECOND$LANG ACQUI PHONEMIC
        $CONTRAST

```
7610  GILES VOICE RACIAL$CATEGORIZATION BRITAIN
7610  MULAC SP$DIALECT$ATTITUDINAL$SCALE
7610  MULAC SP$DIALECT$ATTITUDINAL$SCALE
7621  CLUMECK PATTERNS SOFT$PALATE$MOVEMENTS SIX LANG
7621  CONDAX MONITORING$VELIC$ACTION PHOTO-ELECTRIC$NASAL
      $PROBE FRENCH
7621  HANSEN INFLUENCE ACOUSTIC+PHYSIOLOGICAL$FACTORS VOWEL
      $CHANGES DANISH
7621  MIKOS INTONATION QUESTIONS POLISH
7703  SEYMOUR THERAPEUTIC$MODEL COMMUNICATIVE$DISORDERS
      CHIL BLACK$ENGLISH
7704  BOUNTRESS APPROXIMATIONS STANDARD$ENGLISH SPEAKERS
      BLACK$ENGLISH
7706  ELMAN PERCEPTUAL$SWITCHING BILINGUALS
7706  HOUSE IDENTIFICATION LANG UTTERANCE
7708  BASKERVILL SP-LANG$PATHOLOGIST STANDARD$ENGLISH
7708  DUCHAN R BLACK$CHILDREN GRAMMATIC$CLOSURE ITPA
7708  RATUSNIK BIRACIAL$TESTING CLINICIANS'$INFLUENCE CHILDREN'S
      $PERF
7721  BENGUEREL VELAR$COARTIC FRENCH ELECTROMYOGRAPHIC
7721  BENGUEREL VELAR$COARTIC FRENCH FIBERSCOPIC
7721  KJELLIN CONSONANT$TYPES TONE TIBETAN
7721  LYBERG TIMING SWEDISH UTTERANCES
7721  MAJEWSKI ACOUSTIC$COMPARISONS AMERICAN$ENGLISH POLISH
7721  RUBACH NASALIZATION POLISH
7721  SCHOUTEN IMITATION SYNTHETIC$VOWELS BILINGUALS
7721  WILLAIMS VOICING$CONTRAST SPANISH
7721  YENI-KOMSHIAN VOICING LEBANESE$ARABIC
7723  BLOUNT FEATURES PARENT-CHILD$SP ENGLISH SPANISH
7723  EDELSKY SPANISH$LANG$ACQUI AGE SCHOOL CONTEXT R 'DILE'
      $'PREGUNTALE'
7804  BOUNTRESS COMPREHENSION PRONOMINAL$REFERENCE BLACK
      $ENGLISH
7812  REY TEACHERS$ATTITUDES SPANISH$ACCANTED$ENGLISH
7827  NELSON COMPREHENSION STANDARD$ENGLISH SPEAKING$RATES
      BLACK$ENGLISH
```

## 0318

```
5409  HANDBOOK VOICE$TRNG DICTION
5409  TEACHING$SP ADOL
5609  SP ELEMENTARY$CLASSROOM
5709  ESTABLISHING MAINTAINING STANDARD$SP
5709  VOICE$TRNG SP
```

5809   PRINCIPLES SP
6009   PRONUNCIATION AMERICAN$ENG PHONETICS THEORY APPLICATION
       SP$IMPROVE
6319   APPROACH TEACHING VOICE$DICTION
6604   SELF-ADMINISTERED$PROCEDURES CHANGING$PRONUNCIATION
       $DIALECT
6814   FACTORS EFFECTIVE$COMM
7003   REVIEW PROCEDURES INCREASE$VERBAL$IMITATION$SKILLS
       FUNCTIONAL$SP
7104   CHANGES RELIANCE AUD$FEEDBACK$CUES FUNCTION ORAL$PRACTICE
7114   EFFECT GERMAN-LANG$COURSE ENG
7408   SP$IMPROVEMENT$SYSTEM TAPED$PROGRAM REMEDIATION

## 0319

5406   METHOD$REPROD IDENTIFICATION AUD$DISPLAYS
5803   PERSONAL$EXPERIENCE SP
5806   PHONATION$VOWELS
5906   REPROD IDENTIFICATION ELEMENTS AUD$DISPLAYS
6106   PERTURBATIONS VOCAL$PITCH
6204   SP ELEMENT ORGANIZATION MOTOR$R
6304   PERTURBATION VOWEL$ARTIC CONSONANTAL$CONTEXT ACOUS
       $STUDY
6314   EFFECT SUBJECT SEX VERBAL$INTERACTION SP$DISRUPTION
6604   ORAL$COPYING HEARD$PHRASES
6614   PREDICTABILITY DISRUPTION SPONTANEOUS$SP
6704   PERFORMANCE-INTENSITY$CHARACTERISTICS VERBAL$MATERIALS
6806   STUDY SYSTEM MINIMAL$SP$REPRODUCING$UNITS ITALIAN
       $SP
6904   EFFECTS RANDOM$R$CONTINGENT$NOISE DISFLUENCY NORMAL
       $SPEAKERS
6904   EFFECTS RANDOM$R$CONTINGENT$NOISE DISFLUENCY NORMAL
       $SPEAKERS
6906   MOTOR$CONTROL COARTICULATION CVC$MONOSYLLABLES
6913   PITCH$PERTURBATION FUNCTION SUBJECTIVE$VOCAL$CONSTRICTION
6914   SP$RATES FUNCTION INTERVIEWER$BEHAVIOR
7003   REVIEW PROCEDURES INCREASE$VERBAL$IMITATION$SKILLS
       FUNCTIONAL$SP
7007   STUDY REPRODUCE UNFAMILIAR$SOUNDS PRESENTED$ORALLY
7104   CHANGES RELIANCE AUD$FEEDBACK$CUES FUNCTION ORAL$PRACTICE
7114   SPOKEN$DISAMBIGUATION SUPERFICIALLY$AMBIGUOUS$SENTENCES
7210   VOWEL-R$SYMBOLIZATION
7314   SP$IMITATION SIMULATED$DEAFNESS VISUAL$CUES RECODED
       $AUD$INFORMATIO

```
7406   AUD$FEEDBACK REGULATION$VOICE
7406   MYNAH$BIRD IMITATE HUMAN$SP
7504   PROSEK INTRAORAL$AIR$PRESSURE FEEDBACK CONSONANT$PROD
7526   DRAPER R$CONTINGENT$CONSEQUATION ARTIC$R
7526   KEARSLEY QUESTIONS VERBAL$DISCOURSE
7526   LINDSLEY PROD$SIMPLE$UTTERANCES PLANNING$PROCESS
7526   RUDER EFFECTS VERBAL$IMITATION COMP$TRAINING VERBAL
       $PROD
7621   HAMLET COMPENSATORY$VOWEL$CHAR EXPERIMENTAL$DENTAL
       $PROSTHESES
7704   CECCONI READING$LEVEL$DIFFICULTY DISFLUENCIES NORMAL
       $CHILD
7721   BORDEN ELECTROMYOGRAPHIC$CHANGES DAF
7721   SCHOUTEN IMITATION SYNTHETIC$VOWELS BILINGUALS
7810   GOURAN BEHAVORIAL$CORRELATES PERCEPTIONS QUALITY DECISION-MAKING
7813   MALLARD CONTROL FUNDAMENTAL$FREQ
7818   BEHNKE SP$ANXIETY PREDICTOR TREMBLING
7820   INFANTE PREDICTORS SP$ANXIETY
```

### 0320

```
5403   EFFECT DST LEVEL RATE OR
5403   MECHANICAL$ADAPTER DST
5403   VOCAL$EFFECTS READING TIME$DELAYS DSF
5410   LOUDNESS SIDE-TONE
5503   PERSISTENCE EFFECTS DST
5503   VOCAL$EFFECTS DAF
5603   ADAPTATION DST
5606   EXPERIMENTS BINAURAL$TIME$DELAY INTELLIGIBILITY
5606   INTELLIGIBILITY AIRBORNE$SIDE-TONE
5703   PITCH SIDE-TONE
5703   PITCH SIDE-TONE
5706   FACTORAL$ANALYSIS DSF
5803   DAF REPETITION$SP$SOUNDS
5804   EFFECTS DAF ARTIC
5903   ADAPTATION DST
5904   BIBLIOGRAPHY DAF
5904   EFFECTS LOUDNESS$RECRUITMENT DSF
5904   EXPERIMENTAL$BLOCKAGE PHONATION DISTORTED$SIDETONE
5920   EFFECTS VOCAL$PITCH FREQ MODULATED$AUD$FEEDBACK
6106   CONTEXTUAL$CONSTRAINTS DISRUPTIONS READING DAF
6106   VOICE$LEVEL AUTOPHONIC$SCALE PERCEIVED$LOUDNESS EFFECTS
       SIDETONE
6110   EFFECT DST READING$RATE WHISPERED$SP
```

6111   CONTROLLED$READING$RATE DSF
6204   DST AUD$FLUTTER
6204   EFFECTS FREQ$FILTERING DST VOCAL$R
6204   EFFECTS SIMULTANEOUS$DAF UNDELAYED$AUD$FEEDBACK SP
6204   EFFECTS SIMULTANEOUS$DAF UNDELAYED$AUD$FEEDBACK SP
6204   NO-INFORMATION$DAF PERFORMANCE SKILLED$TYPISTS
6204   VOCAL$R DAF CONGENITALLY$BLIND$ADULTS
6206   DELAYS SIDETONE PATHWAYS
6304   EFFECTS DAF PALMAR$SWEATING HEART$RATE PULSE$PRESSURE
6404   DAF DELAY$TIMES EAR
6514   STUDY NONSENSE$SYLLABLES LANG$GRPS SIDETONE READING
       RATE
6519   ADAPTATION DAF
6604   EFFECT DAF SP AMERICAN$FOREIGN$STUDENTS
6604   EFFECTS DAF PRONOUNCEABILITY IMMEDIATE$RECALL KEY
       $PRESSING
6704   VISUALLY$AUD$PACED$KEYTAPPING SYNCHRONOUS$DECREASED
       $DAF
6711   DAF BREATHING$NOISE
6804   DEV AUD$FEEDBACK$MONITORING DAF INF$CRY
6804   DEV AUD$FEEDBACK$MONITORING DAF$STUDIES SP CHIL$PRESCH
6804   DIFFERENTIAL$SENSITIVITY DAF$INTERVALS PRELIMINARY
       $STUDY
6804   PERCEP DAF SUBJECTIVE$EST DELAY$MAGNITUDE
6806   METAMORPHOSIS CRITICAL$INTERVAL AGE-LINKED$CHANGES
       DAF DISRUPTION$
6811   VISUALLY$KEYTAPPING SYNCHRONOUS$DECREASED$DELAYED
       $AUD$FEEDBACK
6911   ATTENTIONAL$FACTORS DELAYED$VOCAL$AUD$FEEDBACK EFFECTS
6911   EFFECT SIMULTANEOUS$DICHOTIC$PRESENTATION DAF OR$TIME
7010   DURATIONAL$DIFFERENCES SP$PROD DAF
7013   EXPERIMENTAL$INTERFERENCE AUD$FEEDBACK
7104   DSF AGE
7111   EFFECTS DIFFICULTY$READING$MATERIAL SP DELAYED$FEEDBACK
7211   PASSAGE$FOR$TESTING$CHIL DSF
7304   DEVELOPMENT$AUD$FEEDBACK$MONITORING DAF VOCALIZATIONS
       INF
7314   EFFECT DAF READING FUNCTION SYLLABIC$LENGTH WORDS
7413   LONGTIME$EFFECT DAF
7526   SALTER TRANSFORMATIONS DAF SENTENCE$GENERATION
7527   BURKE SUSCEPTIBILITY DAF DEPENDENCE AUD$ORAL$SENSORY
       $FEEDBACK
7604   GARBER MASKING LOMBARD SIDETONE$AMP
7721   BORDEN ELECTROMYOGRAPHIC$CHANGES DAF


                        0321


5706   OUTPUT MECHANICAL$SP$RECOGNIZER

5806  AUTOMATIC$RECOGNITION PHONETIC$PATTERNS SP
5814  ANALYSIS STRUCTURED$CONTENT APPLICATION ELECTRONIC
      $COMPUTER$RESEAR
5814  SOLUTION FUNDAMENTAL$PROBLEMS MECHANICAL$SP$RECOGNITION
5906  RESULTS VOWEL$RECOGNITION COMPUTER$PROGRAM
5914  EXPERIMENT VOICE$RECOGNITION
6014  OBJECTIVES TECHNIQUES SP$SYNTHESIS
6106  COMPUTER$IDENTIFICATION VOWEL$TYPES
6106  RECOGNITION SP COMPUTER$PROGRAM SIMULATE HUMAN$VISUAL
      $PATTERN$PERC
6114  AUTOMATIC$SP$RECOGNITION PROCEDURES
6206  COMPUTER$PROGRAM PITCH$EXTRACTION
6206  DEMONSTRATION SP$PROCESSING$SYSTEM SP$ANALYZER TRANSLATOR
      TYPER
6206  PHONEME SELECTION STUDIES AUTOMATIC$SP$RECOGNITION
6306  COMPUTER$TECHNIQUE HIGH-SPEECH EXTRACTION SP$PARAMETERS
6306  DIGITAL$COMPUTER$SIMULATION SAMPLED-DATA VOICE-EXCITED
      VOCODER
6306  PATTERN-MATCHING$PROCEDURE AUTOMATIC TALKER$RECOGNITION
6306  PITCH$EXTRACTION COMPUTER$PROCESSING HIGH-RESOLUTION
      FOURIER$ANALY
6306  USE NONACOUS$MEAS COMPUTER$RECOGNITION SPOKEN$DIGITS
6314  RECOGNITION SPEAKER$IDENTITY
6406  CHANNEL$VOCODER DIGITAL PITCH$EXTRACTOR
6406  SHORT-TIME$SPECTRUM CEPSTRUM$TECHNIQUES VOCAL-PITCH
      $DETECTION
6406  TALKER-RECOGNITION$PROCEDURE ANALYSIS$VARIANCE
6506  COMPUTER$RECOGNITION SPOKEN$DIGITS NONACOUS$MEAS
6506  DIGITIZED VOICE-EXCITED$VOCODER TELEPHONE-QUALITY
      INPUTS USING
6606  COMPUTERIZED$INVESTIGATION THR-DECISION PHENOMENON
6606  CORRELATION$VOCODER
6606  EFFECTS STIMULUS$CONTENT DURATION TALKER$IDENTIFICATION
6606  EXPERIMENTAL$STUDIES SPEAKER$VERIFICATION ADAPTIVE
      $SYSTEM
6706  COMPUTER$RECOGNITION CONNECTED$SP
6715  DEV VISUAL$DISPLAYS SP$INFORMATION
6806  SIMILARITY$MEAS AUTOMATIC$SP SPEAKER$RECOGNITION
6806  SIMULTANEOUS$DETECTION-RECOGNITION$TASK
6806  SP$RECOGNITION FUNCTION CHANNEL$CAPACITY DISCRETE
      $SET$CHANNELS
6806  SPEAKER$AUTHENTICATION$IDENTIFICATION COMPARISON SPECTROGRAPHIC
6806  SPEAKER$IDENTIFICATION NASAL$PHONATION
6816  PHONEME$ANALYZER
6904  COMPARISON TECHNIQUES DISCRIM TALKERS
6904  COMPARISON TECHNIQUES DISCRIM TALKERS

6906   AUTOMATIC$SPEAKER$VERIFICATION CEPSTRAL$MEAS
6906   SP$RECOGNITION
7006   SP$RECOGNITION
7006   SPEAKER$IDENTIFICATION SP$SPECTROGRAMS LEGAL$PURPOSES
7106   ON-LINE$RECOGNITION$SYSTEM SPOKEN$DIGITS
7106   SP$ANALYSIS SYNTHESIS LINEAR$PREDICTION SP$WAVE
7107   SPEAKER$RECOGNITION
7112   COMPUTER$APPLICATION HUMAN$COMM
7206   ACOUS$PARAMETERS SPEAKER$RECOGNITION
7206   AUTOMATIC$SPEAKER$RECOGNITION PITCH$CONTOURS
7206   COMMENTS SP$ANALYSIS SYNTHESIS LINEAR$PREDICTION SP
       $WAVE
7206   COMPUTER$RELIABILITY DEPENDENT$INDEPENDENT$CONDITIONS
7206   EXPERIMENT VOICE$IDENTIFICATION
7206   REL ZERO-CROSSING$MEAS SP$ANALYSIS RECOGNITION
7214   COMPUTER$APPROACH ANALYSIS SP$PATTERNS
7306   EFFECTS PHONETIC$CONTEXTS SPECTROGRAPHIC SPEAKER$IDENTIFICATION
7306   INFLUENCE HUMAN$FACTORS PERFORMANCE REAL-TIME$SP$RECOGNITION
       $SYSTE
7306   SPEAKER$IDENTIFICATION ABSENCE INTER-SUBJECT$DIFFERENCES
       GLOTTAL$S
7306   SPEAKER$IDENTIFICATION SP$SPECTROGRAMS OBSERVATIONS
7406   AUTOMATIC$SPEAKER$IDENTIFICATION$VERIFICATION
7506   MERMELSTEIN AUTOMATIC$SEGMENTATION SP SYLLABIC$UNITS
7513   LAREVIERE FUNDAMENTAL$FREQ FORMANT$FREQ SPEAKER$IDENTIFICATION
7523   MURRY PERCEPTUAL$RESPONSE INFANT$CRYING MATERNAL$RECOGNITION
       SEX$JUDGE
7606   GOLDSTEIN SPEAKER-IDENTIFYING$FEATURES FORMANT$TRACKS
7606   LASS INVESTIGATION SPEAKER$HEIGHT$WEIGHT$ID
7606   LASS SPEAKER$PHONOGRAPH$ID
7606   LASS SPEAKER$SEX$IDENTIFICATION ISOLATED$SYLLABLES
7621   CONDAX DURATIONS FOUR VOWELS MANUALLY$PRODUCED SYNTHETIC
       $SP
7621   DOHERTY EVAL ACOUSTIC$PARAMETERS SPAEKER$IDENTIFICATION
7706   HOLLIEN SPEAKER$IDEN LONG-TERM$SPECTRA DISTORTED$SP
7706   HOUSE IDENTIFICATION LANG UTTERANCE
7806   KENT IMITATION SYNTHESIZED$VOWELS PRESCHOOL$CHILD
7821   DOHERTY MULTIPLE-FACTOR$SPEAKER$IDENTIFICATION NORMAL
       DISTORTED$SP
7821   LASS SPEAKER$HEIGHT WEITHT$IDENTIFICATION DIRECT$ESTIMATIONS
7821   PARNELL SPEAKER$AGE PERCEPTUAL$CUE$DISTRIBUTION


                        0322


5403   SIGNAL$RECEPTION INTELLIGIBILITY SIDE-TONE

5406   INTELLIGIBILITY SP$MATERIALS
5415   FARMAN-PHILLIPS SP$INTELLIGIBILITY DIAGNOSTIC$TEST
5506   EFFECTS TRNG LISTENERS INTELLIGIBILITY$STUDIES
5603   EFFECT ACOUS$ENVIRONMENT SPEAKER$INTELLIGIBILITY
5603   PREDICTING$INTELLIGIBILITY$SP ACOUS$MEAS
5606   EFFECT VISUAL$FACTORS SP$INTELLIGIBILITY
5606   INTELLIGIBILITY UHF$VHF$TRANSMISSIONS AIR$TRAFFIC
       $CONTROL$TOWERS
5606   UNDERWATER$COMM
5703   EFFECTS DURATION ARTIC$CHANGES INTELLIGIBILITY WORD
       $RECEPTION
5703   INTELLIGIBILITY WHISPERING TONE$LANG
5703   MULTIPLE-CHOICE$INTELLIGIBILITY$TESTS
5703   RECOGNITION INTELLIGIBILITY$TEST$MATERIALS
5806   INTELLIGIBILITY MESSAGE-SETS
5806   STEREOPHONIC$LISTENING SP$INTELLIGIBILITY VOICE$BABBLE
5906   INTELLIGIBILITY REITERATED$SP
5906   INTELLIGIBILITY MESSAGE$SETS
5906   LINGUISTIC$CONSIDERATIONS STUDY SP$INTELLIGIBILITY
5906   LOW-FREQ$NOISE METHODS CALCULATING SP$INTELLIGIBILITY
5906   NUMBER AXIS$CROSSINGS INTELLIGIBILITY$SP
5906   NUMBER AXIS$CROSSINGS INTELLIGIBILITY$SP
5914   WORD$LENGTH INTELLIGIBILITY
5915   TEST SP$INTELLIGIBILITY
6004   REL PHONETIC$STRUCTURE INTELLIGIBILITY WORDS RECORDED
       $LIPS$EAR
6006   EXPERIMENTAL$STUDY RELATIVE$INTELLIGIBILITY ALPHABET
       $LETTERS
6006   INTELLIGIBILITY$TESTS
6013   PREDICTING$INTELLIGIBILITY WORDS
6104   INTELLIGIBILITY WORDS FAMILIARITY
6106   NOISE-BAND$MASKING APPLICATION PREDICTION SP$INTELLIGIBILITY
6110   PITCH$CHANGE COMPREHENSION
6111   REL SP$INTELLIGIBILITY ELECTRO-ACOUS$CHARACTERISTICS
       LOW$FIDELITY
6114   SIGNIFICANCE CHANGES RATE$ARTIC
6206   METHODS CALCULATION USE ARTIC$INDEX
6206   VALIDATION ARTIC$INDEX
6303   MULTIPLE-CHOICE$INTELLIGIBILITY$TESTS
6314   INTELLIGIBILITY EXCERPTS$FLUENT$SP EFFECTS RATE$UTTERANCE
6314   INTELLIGIBILITY EXCERPTS$FLUENT$SP EFFECTS RATE$UTTERANCE
       DURATION
6314   INTELLIGIBILITY EXCERPTS CONVERSATION
6318   STAGE$INTELLIGIBILITY STUDENT$ACTORS
6403   MATERIALS SELF-ADMINISTERED$TRNG INTELLIGIBILITY
6506   EVERYDAY-SP$INTELLIGIBILITY

6506   PT$ACUITY INTELLIGIBILITY EVERYDAY$SP
6511   SPEAKING LISTENING HEAD SP$INTELLIGIBILITY QUIET$RECORDED
       POSITION
6606   MEAS REACTION$TIME INTELLIGIBILITY$TESTS
6706   USE SEQUENTIAL$STRATEGY INTELLIGIBILITY$TESTING
6810   EFFECT INFLECTION VOWEL$INTELLIGIBILITY
6814   PERCEP$VERBAL$DISCRIM ELABORATED$RESTRICTED$CODE$USERS
6904   CHIL$IDENTIFICATION$REPROD
6904   EFFECT SPATIALLY$SEPARATED$SOUND$SOURCES SP$INTELLIGIBILITY
6920   SEX$AGE$DIFFERENCES SPEAKER$INTELLIGIBILITY
7003   CNC$INTELLIGIBILITY$WORD$LISTS
7006   EFFECT FORWARD$BACKWARD$MASKING SP$INTELLIGIBILITY
7111   CARRIER$PHRASE SP$INTELLIGIBILITY SCORE
7116   EFFECT CLASSROOM$LISTENING$CONDITIONS SP$INTELLIGIBILITY
7204   INTELLIGIBILITY CONNECTED$DISCOURSE
7211   SENTENCE$INTELLIGIBILITY$TEST
7404   SENTENCE$INTELLIGIBILITY KEY$WORD$SELECTION
7506   WINGFIELD INTERNAL$ALTERATION INFO$LOAD SP$INTELLIGIBILITY

## 0323

5703   MULTIPLE-CHOICE$INTELLIGIBILITY$TESTS
5710   COMPARISON SPEAKING$ABILITY UPPERCLASSMEN
6103   SELF-JUDGMENTS SP$ADEQUACY JUDGMENTS TRAINED$OBSERVERS
6210   PREDICTION PHONETIC$TRANSCRIPTION$ABILITY
6303   MULTIPLE-CHOICE$INTELLIGIBILITY$TESTS
6706   EFFECTS CONTEXT TALKER$IDENTIFICATION
6803   SP$LANG$SCREENING SUMMER$HEADSTART
6806   ISOPREFERENCE$METHOD SP$EVAL
6809   EFFECT PERCEIVED$MISPRONUNCIATION SP$EFFECTIVENESS
       $RATINGS RETENTI
6904   COMPARISON TECHNIQUES DISCRIM TALKERS
6904   COMPARISON TECHNIQUES DISCRIM TALKERS
6906   COMMENTS LEARNING ARTIC$TESTING MISTUNED$SINGLE-SIDEBAND
       $LINKS
7106   EFFECTS AUD$MASKING VOCAL$INTEN INTRAORAL$AIR$PRESSURE
       SENTENCE$PR
7112   VERBAL$TESTING BILINGUAL$SOCIETIES
7204   PERCEP$EFFECTS FORWARD$COARTICULATION
7204   SPEAKING$TASK
7206   PRESSURE$MEAS ARTIC ALTERATIONS VOCAL$EFFORT
7211   PASSAGE$FOR$TESTING$CHIL DSF
7306   TEST SP$COMM$QUALITY
7403   SP$LANG$SCREENING PRESCH$CHIL

7513    KELMAN ASSESSMENT VOCAL$FUNCTION AIR-FLOW$MEAS
7613    GATEHOUSE EMG ORBICULARIS$ORIS DIFFERENT ELECTRODE
        CONFIGURATIONS
7629    STARR RELIABILITY VOICE$PROFILING$SYSTEM
7810    DALY ASSESSMENT ANXIETY SELF-REPORTS
7825    MAZZOCHI COMPUTER$TOMOGRAPHY NEUROPSYCH$RES LESION
        $MAPPING
7827    MANNING COMPETING$SP ESTIMATE ARTICULATORY$AUTOMATIZATION
        CHIL

## 0401

5403    LINGUISTICS RECOVERY APHASIA
5403    SPELLING$ABILITY DYSPHASICS
5409    GRP$THERAPY METHOD$RETRNG APHASICS
5503    ABSTRACT$CONCRETE$BEHAVIOR DYSPHASIC$PATIENTS
5503    AUD$DEDIFFERENTIATION DYSPHASIC
5503    CLINICAL$TREATMENT APHASIA
5509    APHASIA
5509    APHASIA$THERAPEUTICS
5513    CEREBRAL$LANG$DISORDERS
5515    DEV APHASIC$CHIL
5515    TRNG APHASIC$CHIL
5603    APHASIA KERNICTERUS
5603    LANG BEHAVIORAL$PROBLEMS RH$APHASIC$CHIL
5603    SOCIO-PSYCHOTHERAPEUTIC$APPROACH TREATMENT$APHASIC
5603    STUDY APHASIA ANOMIA
5615    TEACHING APHASIC$CHIL
5616    LANG$TRNG COMPARISON CHIL$APHASIA DEAFNESS
5703    HNG$LOSS APHASIA
5703    SOCIAL$EMOTIONAL$ASPECTS APHASIA
5715    APHASIA$CHIL
5803    AGRAMMATISM APHASIA
5803    LINGUIST APHASIA CHIL
5803    REL SELF-CORRECTION RECOVERY APHASIA
5814    BRAIN$DIS LANG$ANALYSIS
5814    PECULIARITIES$THOUGHT SENSORY$APHASIA
5815    IMPLICATIONS STATE$LEGIS APHASIC$CHIL
5815    TEACHING$SP$LANG APHASIC$CHIL
5816    MASSACHUSETTS$LAW EDUC$APHASICS
5903    COMM$SKILLS INTELLIGENCE HEMIPLEGICS
5903    LANG$R APHASIA
5903    MULTI-EVAL$STUDY APHASIC$NONAPHASIA RIGHT$HEMIPLEGIC
        $PATIENTS

```
5904   DYSPHASIC$SP$R VISUAL$WORD$STIMULI
5907   RESEARCH$NEEDS SP$PATH$A APHASIA
5914   PHONEMIC$SUBSTITUTIONS APHASIA
5916   ASSESSMENT TEACHING APHASIC$CHIL CID
5918   APHASIA$EVAL
5918   PHYSIOLOGIC$PHYSICAL$ASPECTS APHASIA
6003   A$EVAL APHASICS
6003   STUDIES APHASIA BACKGROUND THEORETICAL$FORMULATIONS
6004   AUD$DISCRIM$LEARNING APHASIC$CHIL
6004   MOTIVATING$INSTRUCTIONS LANG$PERFORMANCE DYSPHASIC
6004   VISUAL-SPATIAL$MEM APHASIC$CHIL
6013   POLYGLOT$APHASICS
6103   APHASIC$CHIL
6103   HNG SP LEFT$HEMISPHERECTOMY
6104   DIMENSIONS LANG$PERFORMANCE APHASIA
6104   REL AUD$COMPREHENSION WORD$FREQ APHASIA
6105   CLINICAL$PSYCHOLOGIST EVAL APHASIA$REHAB
6114   LANG INTELLECTUAL$MODIFICATIONS RIGHT$CEREBRAL$DAMAGE
6114   LINGUISTIC$FEATURES SP APHASICS
6203   RATIONALE GRP$TREATMENT APHASICS
6203   RECONDITIONING CONSONANT$DISCRIM APHASIC EXPERIMENTAL
       $CASE$HISTORY
6204   APHASICS REPEATING$COMMON$WORDS REPEATING$RARELY$USED
       $WORDS
6204   FACTOR$ANALYSIS MINNESOTA$TEST$DIFFERENTIAL$DIAGNOSIS
       $APHASIA
6204   PRELIMINARY$STUDY NONVERBAL$LEARNING APHASIA
6213   DYSPHATIC$STUTTERING
6303   BLACK$LIGHT$BOX REDUCING$ATTENTION$SCATTER APHASOID
       $CASES
6303   FILMSTRIPS LANG$THERAPY APHASIA
6303   PERSONAL$ACCOUNT DYSPHASIA
6303   PERSONAL$ACCOUNT DYSPHASIA
6304   REL PSYCHOLOGICAL$LANG$TEST$SCORES AUTOPSY$FINDINGS
       APHASIA
6304   STUDIES NONVERBAL$LEARNING APHASIA
6304   WORD$LENGTH FREQ SIMILARITY DISCRIM$BEHAVIOR APHASICS
6313   APHASIC$LANG$MODIFICATION DISRUPTION$CULTURAL$VERBAL
       $HABITS
6313   AUSCULTATION HEAD CONGENITAL APHASOID
6314   CLASSIFICATION PARTS$OF$SP CHARACTERIZATION APHASIA
6315   CHILDHOOD$APHASIA
6403   ACRONYMIC$ELEMENTS APHASIC$SP
6403   ACRONYMIC$ELEMENTS APHASIC$SP
6403   APHASIA BILINGUAL$POLYGLOT$PATIENTS NEUROLOGICAL$PSYCHOLOGICAL
       $STU
```

```
6403   AUD$THR$CONSISTENCY DIFFERENTIAL$DIAGNOSIS APHASIA
       CHIL
6403   AUD$THR$CONSISTENCY DIFFERENTIAL$DIAGNOSIS APHASIA
       CHIL
6403   CASE APHASIA
6403   SEQUENCE$LEARNING APHASIC$CHIL DEAF$CHIL
6404   EFFECT WORD$LENGTH APHASIC$SPELLING$ERRORS
6404   PERFORMANCE APHASICS AUTOMATED$PERCEP$DISCRIM$PROGRAMS
6404   WORD$LENGTH DISCRIM APHASICS
6404   WORD$LENGTH DISCRIM APHASICS
6413   ACQUIRED$APHASIA CHIL
6413   DYSPHASIA DYSLEXIA SCH$CHIL
6414   ORAL$R APHASICS SYNTACTICAL$CONDITIONS
6504   AUTOMATED$TRNG MATCHING-TO-SAMPLE$TASK APHASIA
6504   AUTOMATED$MULTIPLE$R$ALTERNATIVE$TRNG$PROGRAM APHASICS
6504   EFFECT MEPROBAMATE RECOVERY$APHASIA
6504   PERFORMANCE APHASICS AUTOMATED$VISUO-PERCEP$DISCRIM
6504   TEMPORAL$DISCRIM APHASOID$CHIL
6504   TEST$R PREDICTORS FREE-SP$CHARACTERISTICS APHASICS
6510   PHONETIC-LINGUISTIC$VIEW READING$CONTROVERSY
6603   METHOD ELICITING$NAMING$BEHAVIOR APHASIC$PATIENTS
6603   RE-EVAL SHORT$EXAM APHASIA
6604   OPERANT$CONDITIONING INVEST SP$DISCRIM APHASIC$CHIL
6604   REL WORD$ASSOC GRAMMATICAL$CLASSES APHASIA
6614   LEXICAL$GRAMMATICAL$IMPAIRMENT DYSPHASIA
6615   HOME$TRNG DYSACUSIC$AND$APHASIC$CHIL
6617   GRP$THERAPY APHASICS
6617   PROGRAM SP$LANG$THERAPY STROKE$PATIENT
6703   A$REPORT PATIENT LEFT$HEMISPHERECTOMY
6703   SELF-GENERATED$CUES APHASIC
6703   USE SPECIFIC$ELECTRIC$BOARD REHAB$APHASICS
6704   APHASIC$CHIL
6704   EFFECT METHYLPHENIDATE VERBAL$PROD CHIL CEREBRAL$DYSFUNCTION
6704   PROSODIC$FACTORS GRAMMAR-EVIDENCE APHASIA
6704   SP$DISCRIM APHASICS INTERSOUND$INTERVAL$VARIED
6705   FAMILY$COUNSELING RELATIVES APHASIC$PATIENTS
6709   CHIL$APHASIA BRAIN$DAMAGE DIFFERENTIAL$DIAGNOSIS
6711   PERCEP$BINAURAL$BEATS BRAIN$DAMAGED$ADULTS
6713   PROGRAMMED$INSTRUCTION PICTURE-SOUND$ASSOC APHASIC
6713   RE-EDUC$SP$APHASIA
6803   CHIL$AUD$AGNOSIA
6803   CHIL$AUD$AGNOSIA
6803   DEV$APHASIA THERAPEUTIC$IMPLICATIONS
6803   NATURE RECEPTIVE$EXPRESSIVE$IMPAIRMENTS APHASIA
6804   APHASICS
6804   PHONIC$TRENDS WRITING APHASICS
```

```
6804    PSYCHOLINGUISTIC$ASPECTS APHASIA
6804    SENSORY$MODALITY OBJECT-NAMING APHASIA
6804    VISUAL$DISCRIM R$REVERSAL$LEARNING APHASIC
6804    VISUAL$DISCRIM R$REVERSAL$LEARNING APHASIC
6807    EFFECT STATE$CEREBRAL$CORTEX MOTOR$APHASIA$SYNDROME
6807    HIGHER$NERVOUS$ACTIVITY MOTOR$APHASIA
6807    PATHOPHYSIOLOGY APHASIC$DIS VASCULAR$DISEASES BRAIN
6807    PROBLEM TRANSCORTICAL$SENSORY$APHASIA
6807    RESTORATIVE$THERAPY APHASIA VASCULAR$ORIGIN
6813    RETRNG AGNOSIC$ALEXIA
6903    APHASIA APHASIC
6903    EXPRESSED$ATTITUDES FAMILIES APHASICS
6904    PROBABILITY$LEARNING APHASIC
6904    PROBABILITY$LEARNING APHASIC
6904    PSYCHOLINGUISTIC$APPROACH STUDY LANG$DEFICIT APHASIA
6904    SPONTANEOUS$RECOVERY APHASIA
6904    VISUAL$SEQUENCING APHASIC$CHIL
6911    RELIABILITY CONVENTIONAL$AUDIOMETRY APHASIC
6914    PHONOLOGICAL$GRAMMATICAL$ASPECTS JARGON APHASICS CASE
        $STUDY
6915    A$FINDINGS TESTING APHASIC$CHIL
6916    PROVISIONS APHASIC$CHIL PUBLIC$RESIDENTIAL$SCH$DEAF
        USA
6917    GESTURAL$COMM APHASICS DYADIC$SITUATION
6917    PSYCHOLINGUISTIC$CONSIDERATIONS COMPREHENSION ADULT
        $APHASICS
7003    CASE$STUDIES APHASIA$REHAB PROGRAMMED$INSTRUCTION
7003    ROLE-PLAYING$ACTIVITIES APHASIC$PATIENTS
7004    ABILITY APHASICS JUDGE DURATION INTENSITY PT
7004    DIMENSIONS AUD$LANG$COMPREHENSION APHASIA
7004    SP$THERAPY LANG$RECOVERY APHASIA
7012    BREAKDOWN SYMBOL$PROCESSING BRAIN$DAMAGE
7017    APHASIA$REHAB MULTIDIMENSIONAL$APPROACH
7017    CLINICAL$IMPLICATIONS APHASIA$RESEARCH$THEORY
7017    PROCESSES NONDOMINANT$HEMISPHERE$LESIONS
7103    IMPORTANCE SELF-TEACHING$TECHNIQUES ADULT$APHASIA
7103    INDICES SEVERITY CHRONIC$APHASIA STROKE$PATIENTS
7103    INDICES SEVERITY CHRONIC$APHASIA STROKE$PATIENTS
7104    APHASIC$WORD$IDENTIFICATION FUNCTION LOGICAL$REL ASSOC
        $STRENGTH
7104    APHASICS
7104    AUD$PERCEP SEQUENCED$WORDS APRAXIA$SP
7104    MULTIDIMENSIONAL$SCORING APHASIC$TESTING
7104    STM$RECOGNITION$SEARCH APHASICS
7112    SYNTACTIC$GENERALIZATION APHASICS FUNCTION RELEARNING
        $SENTENCE
```

```
7203   APHASIA HYPERCALCEMIA
7203   APHASIA$THERAPY
7203   AUD$AGNOSIA TREATMENT
7203   COMPARISON TESTS AUD$COMPREHENSION ADULT$APHASICS
7203   EFFICACY LANG$REHAB APHASIA
7203   PERCEP STRESS SEMANTIC$CUE APHASIA
7203   RECOVERY APHASIA AER$AUDIOMETRY
7203   SCALING APHASICS$ERROR$R
7203   USE BASELINE$PROBE$TECHNIQUE MONITOR TEST$R APHASIC
       $PATIENTS
7204   APRAXIA$SP
7204   EFFECT HYPERBARIC$OXYGEN COMM APHASIC$ADULTS STROKE
7204   EFFECTS TASK$DIFFICULTY NAMING$PERFORMANCES APHASICS
7204   EFFECTS TASK$DIFFICULTY NAMING$PERFORMANCES APHASICS
7204   PERCEP$LEVEL$FUNCTIONING DYSPHASIC$CHIL
7212   CHIL$APHASIA
7214   EFFECTS UNISENSORY$MULTISENSORY$PRESENTATION$STIMULI
       NAMING APHASI
7303   APRAXIA$SP ADULTS
7303   CHIL$VERBAL$APRAXIA TREATMENT
7304   ACOUS$CUE$DISCRIM ADULT$APHASIA
7304   APHASIC COMPREHENSION TIME$SPACING
7304   EFFECTS FATIGUE ISOKINETIC$EXERCISE COMM$ABILITY APHASIC
       $ADULTS
7304   ORAL$SENSATION$PERCEP APRAXIA$SP APHASIA
7304   USE LEITER$INTERNATIONAL$PERFORMANCE$SCALE APHASIC
       $CHIL
7311   PERFORMANCE APHASIA DICHOTIC$LISTENING$TASK
7312   IDENTIFICATION APHASIC
7314   MEAS LEXICAL$DIVERSITY APHASIC$LANG
7314   PSYCHOLINGUISTIC$ANALYSIS APHASIC$LANG
7317   DIAGNOSIS AUD$DISTURBANCES CHIL MTDD$APHASIA
7403   AMERIND VERBALIZATION ORAL$VERBAL$APRAXIC
7403   OBJECTIONS$TO$TERM APRAXIA$OF$SP
7403   PICA
7403   PICA$INTERPRETATION
7403   STUDY PROGNOSIS APHASIC
7404   AVERAGE$ENCEPHALIC$R APHASICS LINGUISTIC$NONLINGUISTIC
       $AUD$STIMULI
7404   EFFECTS PROGRAM TOKEN$TEST TEACHING$COMPREHENSION
       $SKILLS APHASICS
7405   COMMUNICATIONS$CLUB COMMUNITY$SOLUTION NEEDS CHRONIC
       $APHASIC
7408   THERAPY DEV$APRAXIA$SP
7412   DIFFERENCES R AUD$VERBAL$MATERIALS APHASIC
7417   AUD$SYNTACTIC$PREFERENCES BRAIN$DAMAGED$ADULTS
```

7417    AUD$SYNTACTIC$PREFERENCES BRAIN$DAMAGED$ADULTS
7417    EFFECTS PROCESSING$TIME VERBAL$RECOGNITION APHASICS
7504    DISIMON1 SHORTENING PICA
7504    DUFFY PANTOMIME$RECOGNITION APHASICS
7522    GARDNER HUMOROUS$MATERIAL, COMP APPRECIATION FOLLOWING
        BRAIN DAMAGE
7522    HOWES REACTION$TIME FOCAL$IMPAIRMENT LESIONS RIGHT
        $HEMISPHERE
7526    KELTER CONCEPT STRUCTURE APHASIC SCHIZOPHRENIC PATIENTS
        SORTING$TASK
7527    BLISS APHASIC NONAPHASIC$CHILDREN SENTENCE$REPETITION
7527    BROOKSHIRE RECOGNITION AUD$SEQUENCES APHASIC$BRAIN-DAMAGED
        $SUBJECTS
7527    HELMICK EFFECTS STIMULUS$REPETITION NAMING$BEHAVIOR
        APHASIC$ADULT
7527    LASS CHILDRENS$PERFORMANCE TOKEN$TEST
7527    LILES PAUSE$TIME AUD$COMPREHENSION APHASIC$SUBJECTS
7529    BROOKSHIRE PROMPTING SPONTANEOUS$NAMING PICTURES APHASIC
        $SUBJECTS
7532    DENNIS COMPREHENSION SYNTAX INFANTILE$HEMIPLEGICS
        HEMIDECORTICATION
7532    GADDES SPREEN-BENTON$APHASIA$TESTS
7532    GLEASON RETRIEVAL SYNTAX BROCA'S$APHASIA
7532    KEITH SINGING$THERAPY APRAXIA APHASIA
7532    KERTESZ INTELLIGENCE APHASIA RAVEN'S$MATRICES(RCPM)
7532    MARTIN APHASIA: PHONOLOGICAL MORPHOLOGICAL$INTERACTIONS
        ERROR$PERF
7532    MOHR THALAMIC$HEMORRAGE APHASIA
7532    NEBES INTERNAL$SP APHEMIA
7532    OSCAR-BERMAN BRAIN$DAMAGE PROCESSING$SP
7532    RIKLAN VERBAL$FUNCTIONS THALAMIC$LESIONS
7532    SASANUMA KANA+KANJI$PROCESSING JAPANESE$APHASICS
7532    WAGENAAR SPONTANEOUS$SPEECH APHASIC
7603    BOONE WRITING APHASIA$REHABILITATION
7603    DUFFY VERBAL$COMPREHENSION SPEECH READING WRITING
        ADULT$APHASIA
7603    HELMICK SPOUSES'$UNDERSTANDING COMMUNICATION$DISABILITIES
        APHASIC
7603    MARSHALL WORD$RETRIEVAL APHASIC$ADULTS
7603    SPARKS MELODIC$INTONATION$THERAPY APHASIA
7604    BLISS ADULT$APHASICS SENTENCE$EVAL+REVISION$TASK
7604    CHAPEY DIVERGENT$SEMANTIC$BEHAVIOR APHASIA
7613    THOMSEN TRAUMATIC$APHASIA FOCAL$LESIONS
7622    HEILMAN APHASIA, MIXED$TRANSCORTICAL INTACT$NAMING
7627    BROOKSHIRE TASK$DIFFICULTY SENTENCE$COMP APHASIC
7627    HANSON RECALL SENTENCE$MEANING APHASIC

7627   HELMICK PERSEVERATION BRAIN-INJURED$ADULTS
7627   OELSCHLAEGER TRAUMATIC$APHASIA CHILDREN
7627   WATAMORI RECOVERY$PROCESS BILINGUAL$APHASIC
7629   GLASS BILINGUAL$CUBAN-AMERICAN$APHASIC BODY$PART$IDEN
7632   ALBERT STM APHASIA
7632   BROWN NEURAL$ORGANIZATION LANG APHASIA LATERALIZATION
7632   BRYDEN VISUAL$HEMIFIELD$DIFFERENCES TYPEFACE
7632   BRYDEN VISUAL$HEMIFIELD$DIFFR
7632   CARAMAZZA RIGHT-HEMISPHERIC$DAMAGE VERBAL$PROBLEM
       $SOLVING
7632   CARAMAZZA ALGORITHMIC + HEURISTIC$PROCESSES LANG$COMP
       APHASIC
7632   CARMON VISUAL$HEMIFIELD$DIFFERENCES PERCEP VERBAL
       $MATERIAL
7632   CERMAK REHEARSAL$STRATEGIES ALCOHOLIC$KORSAKOFF$PATIENTS
7632   CERMAK VERBAL$RETENTION APHASIC+AMNESIC
7632   DENNIS LANG$ACQUISITION HEMIDECORTICATION
7632   DENNIS NAMING+LOCATING$BODY$PARTS TEMPORAL$LOBE$RESECTION
7632   GAINOTTI COMPREHENSION SYMBOLIC$GESTURES APHASIA
7632   GARDNER READING APHASIA
7632   GOODGLASS SEMANTIC$FIELD,NAMING AUD$COMPREHENSION
       APHASIA
7632   GREENBLATT ALEXIA AGRAPHIA HEMIANOPSIA
7632   HECAEN APHASIA CHILDREN HEMISPHERIC$SPECIALIZATION
7632   HEILMAN MEMORY BROCA'S+CONDUCTION$APHASIA
7632   KIM DEFICITS TEMPORAL$SEQUENCING VERBAL$MATERIAL LATERALITY
       LESION
7632   KIMURA IMPAIRMENT NONLINGUISTIC$HAND$MOVEMENTS DEAF
       $APHASIC
7632   LASKY LING$COMPLEX RATE PAUSE AUD-VERBAL$COMPREHENSION
       ADULT$APHASIC
7632   LECOURS SCHIZOPHASIA JARGONAPHASIA
7632   MOHR DYSLEXIA DYSGRAPHIA
7632   SAFFRAN SP$PERCEP WORD$DEAFNESS
7632   SASANUMA APHASIC COMPREHENSION SENTENCES TEMPORAL
       $ORDER
7632   SCHLANGER PERCEP EMOTIONALLY$TONED$SENTENCES RT$HEMIS
       $DAMAGED APHASIC
7632   TALLAL SP$PERCEPTION+PRODUCTION CHILDREN DYSPHASIA
7632   WECHSLER APHASIA ILLITERATE$DEXTRAL
7632   WEIDNER RATE COMPLEXITY STIMULUS PERF ADULT$APHASIC
7703   CHAPEY APHASIA
7703   DARLEY APHASIA
7703   DISIMONI DYSFUNCTION SCHIZOPHRENIC$PATIENS APHASIA
       $BATTERY
7703   LAPOINTE $PROGRAMMED$STIMULATION APHASIA

7703     LOVE CUEING$TECHNIQUES BROCA'S$APHASIA
7703     MARTIN APHASIA$TESTING PICA
7704     COHEN VALIDITY SKLAR$APHASIA$SCALE
7704     GROHER LANG MEMORY$DISORDERS CLOSED$HEAD$TRAUMA
7704     JOHNSON DICHOTIC$EAR PREFERENCE APHASIA
7704     PODRAZA EFFECTS AUD$PRESTIMULATION NAMING APHASIA
7704     WARREN SHORT—TERM$MEMORY APHASIA
7705     PORTER TRANSACTIONAL$ANALYSIS THERAPY WIVES ADULT
         $APHASIC
7722     KERTESZ RECOVERY$PATTERNS PROGNOSIS APHASIA
7722     MCGLONE SEX$DIFFERENCES CEREBRAL$VERBAL$FUNCTIONS
         $BRAIN$LESIONS
7722     WINNER COMP METAPHOR BRAIN—DAMAGED$PATIENTS
7725     AMMON APHASICS PERCEP CONNOTATIVE$MEANING
7725     BASSO PHONEMIC$ID APHASIA
7725     BRUHN REACTION$TIME EPILEPTIC BRAIN—DAMAGED
7725     DERENZI SPACIAL$MEMORY HEMISPHERIC$LOCUS LESION
7725     DUNLOP LINGUISTIC$AU
7725     DUNLOP LINGUISTIC$ARTIC$ASPECTS SINGLE$WORD APRAXIA
7725     FARMER SELF—CORRECTIONAL$STRATIES
7725     FARMER SELF—CORRECTIONAL$STRATEGIES SP APHASICS ADULTS
7725     FARMER SELF—CORRC
7725     GALLAGHER WH—QUES APHASICS
7725     GARDNER MUSICAL$DETONATION$CONNOTATION ORGANIC$PATIENTS
7725     JUST APHASIC NORMAL$ADULTS SENTENCES—VERIFICATION
         $TASK
7725     KUMAR STM NONVERBAL$TACTUAL$TASK CEREBRAL$COMMISSUROTOMY
7725     OCKLEFORD FORM$PERCEP MACAQUES LESIONS
7725     RAUSCH OLFACTORY$MEMORY ANTERIOR$TEMPORAL$LOBECTOMY
7725     REYNOLDS TACTILE$PERCEP MOTOR$COORDINATION AGENESIS
         CORPUS$CALLOSUM
7729     SNYDER SYNTACTICAL$ASPECTS DEV$APRAXIA
7729     STICK CLOZE$PROCEDURE MORPHOLOGICAL SEMANTIC$BASED
         $TREATMENT APHASICS
7732     AXELROD ORAL$REPORT WORDS WORD$APPROXIMATIONS VISUAL
         $FIELD
7732     BENTON GERSTMANN$SYNDROME
7732     BURNS PHONEMIC$BEHAVIOR APHASIC
7732     DAVIS HEMISPHERIC$ASYMMETRIES INFANTS
7732     EFRON PERCEP DICHOTIC$CHORDS HEMISPHERECTOMIZED
7732     FAY TEMPORAL$CAPABILITIES ECHOLALIC$CHILD
7732     FENNELL RELIABILITIES LATERALITY$TESTS
7732     HEFFNER DEV$AUD$AGNOSIA MR$ADOL
7732     HIER ORAL+WRITTEN NAMING WERNICKE'S$APHASIA
7732     JAUHAINEN AUD$PERCEP SP APHASIA
7732     KERTESZ NUMERICAL$TAXONOMY APHASIA

7732    LURIA ASSESSMENT APHASIA
7732    LURIA QUASI-APHASIC$SP LESIONS DEEP$STRUCTURES BRAIN
7732    MALY BRAIN$PERFUSION NEUROPSYCHOLOGICAL$TEST APHASICS
7732    MARTINDALE SYNTACTIC + SEMANTIC$CORRELATES VERBAL
        $TICS GILLES$TOURETTE
7732    MATEER IMPAIRMENT NONVERBAL$ORAL$MOVEMENTS APHASIA
7732    PEUSER UNIVERSALITY LANG$DISSOLUTION TURKISH$APHASIC
7732    SHALLICE AUD-VERBAL$STM CONDUCTION$APHASIA
7732    STACHOWIAK TEXT$COMPREHENSION APHASIA
7732    TILLMAN CLUSTERING APHASICS FREE$RECALL
7732    VOINESCU APHASIA POLYGLOT
7732    WEIGL TRANSCODING$PROCESSES PATIENTS AGRAPHIA$DICTATION
7803    BROOKSHIRE CLINICAL$INTERACTION ANALYSIS$SYSTEM OBSERVATIONAL
        $RECORDIN
7803    COOPER ACQUIRED$AUD$VARBAL$AGNOSIA SEISURES CHILDHOOD
7804    DUMOND PRESENTATION ORDER$OF$DIFFICULTY$TASKS APHASIA
7804    LINEBAUGH DICHOTIC$EAR$PREFERENCE APHASIA
7804    WALLER INFLUENCE CONTEXT AUDITORY$COMPREHENSION PARAGRAPHS
        APHASIC
7809    DUDLEY APHASIC$NAMING$PERFORMANCE
7812    SIMPSON RATE$VARIABILITY AUD$PROCESSING APHASIC$PATIENTS
7813    DUFFY PANTOMIME$SYMBOLISM RECOGITION APHASICS
7813    FARMER ERROR$SELF-CORRECTION APHASICS
7813    HUBER JARGON WERNICKE,S$APHASIA
7813    MATTES TOTAL$APHASIA
7822    BEAUVOIS BILATERAL$TACTILE$APHASIA TACTO-VERBAL$DYSFUNCTION
7822    COUGHLAN WORD-COMPREHENSION WORD-RETRIEVAL PATIENTS
        CEREBRAL$LESIONS
7822    HOREL NEUROANATOMY AMNESIA HIPPOCAMPAL$MEMORY$HYPOTHESIS
7822    LEVINE VISUAL$DEFECT VERBAL$ALEXIA SIMULTANAGNOSIAS
7825    ARCHIBALD TIME HEMISPHERE-DAMAGED PERCEP$MAZE$TEST
7825    BLACK DIGIT$REPETITION BRAIN$DAMAGE
7825    BLACK DIGIT$REPETITION BRAIN$DAMAGE
7825    BOLLER DAF APHASIA
7825    BUCKINGHAM ALLITERATION ASSONANCE JARGON$APHASIA
7825    CERMAK APHASIC$AMNESIC VERBAL$NONVERBAL$RETENTIVE
        $ABILITIES
7825    CERMAK APHASIC AMNESIC RETENTIVE$ABILITIES
7825    DERENZI SHORTENED$VERSION TOKEN$TEST
7825    DERENZI NORMATIVE$DATA SCREENING$POWER SHORTENED$TOKEN
        $TEST
7825    DERENZI TEST EXPRESSIVE$DISTURBANCES APHASICS
7825    GORDON LEFT$HEMISPHERE$DOM RHYTHM DICHOTICALLY-PRESENTED
        $MELODIES
7825    PARADOWSKI UNILATERAL$BRAIN$DAMAGE CLEM$REACTIONS
7825    PEASE CUING PICTURE$NAMING APHASIA

7825    SCHWARTZ SIGN$COMPREHENSION GLOBAL$APHASIA
7825    SCHWARTZ SIGN$COMPREHENSION GLOBAL$APHASIA
7825    SEMENZA ANALYTIC + GLOBAL$STRATEGIES COPYING$DESIGNS
        BRAIN-DAMAGED
7825    STROHNER SEMANTIC + ACOUS$ERRORS APHASIC SCHIZOPHRENIC
        SOUND-PIC$MATCH
7825    WAPNER VISUAL$AGNOSIA ARTIST
7827    LOZANO DAF DYSPRAX1A SP
7827    NOLL ERRORS APHASIC$SUBJECTS TOKEN$TEST
7827    PTACEK AUD$PATTERN$RECOGNITION APHASIC
7827    TOPPIN TOKEN$TEST$PERFORMANCE APHASIC$SUBJECTS
7829    CAMPBELL EXPRESSIVE$SP$PROGRAM CHILD ACQUIRED$APHASIA
7829    HARTMAN WRITING EXPRESSION APHASIA


                    0402

5403    CASE RETARDED$SP
5503    CONSIDERATION ETIOLOGIES SP$RETARDATION
5609    SLOW$TO$TALK
5703    CASE$STUDY DELAYED$LANG
6013    DIAGNOSIS$TREATMENT LATE$SP$LANG$DEV CHIL
6113    DEV$LANG$DISORDERS
6114    CONGENITAL$LANG$DISABILITY STUDY MODEL EVOLUTION$COMM
6403    ORAL$LANG PREMATURE$CHIL
6413    ORAL$LANG IMMATURE$CHIL
6804    ECHOLALIA IQ DEV$DICHOTOMY SP$LANG$SYSTEMS
6903    DELAYED$LANG$DEV
7104    STABILITY VALIDITY MEAS$INTELLIGENCE CHIL DELAYED
        $LANG$DEV
7303    VOICE$THERPY LANG$DELAYED$CHIL
7304    DEV BASE$SYNTAX LINGUISTICALLY$DEVIANT$CHIL
7403    LANG$DELAYED$CHIL ADOL
7403    PARENT-ASSISTED$TREATMENT$PROGRAM PRESCH$LANG$DEL
        $CHIL
7413    LINGUISTIC$APPROACHES DEV$LANG$DIS
7504    ARAM LANG CHILD DEV$LANG$DIS
7512    PANAGOS PHONOLOGY$GRAMMATICAL$REDUCTION DELAYED$SP
7529    ILLERBRUN COMP SPACIAL$ADJECTIVES CHILD NORMAL$DEVIANT
        $LANG$DEV
7603    SCHIFF COMMUNICATION$PROBLEMS HNG$CHILDREN DEAF$PARENTS
7604    FREEDMAN SEMANTIC$RELATIONS LANG-IMPAIRED$CHILDREN
7604    LEONARD SEMANTIC$RELATIONS LANG-DISORDED$CHILDREN
7604    TALLAL RAPID$AUD$PROCESSING DISORDERED$LANG
7703    CRAMBLIT VERBAL$ENVIRONMENT LANG-IMPAIRED$CHILD

7713   FARMER STOP$COGNATE$PROD ADULT ATHETOTIC CEREBRAL-PASIED
7723   KODGON MULTI-FUNCTIONAL$APPROACH SINGLE-WORD$USAGE
7812   MELINE COMP PROD VERBS LANG-DISORDERED$CHILD
7812   PANAGOS PHONOLOGY GRAMMATICAL$REDUCTION DELAYED$SP
       DEV
7826   AFFOLTER SP-SOUND$PRODUCTION LANG-IMPAIRED$CHIL


## 0403


5513   PREDICTION$FUTURE READING$DISABILITIES CHIL ORAL$LANG
       $DISORDERS
5804   ASSESSING LANG$DEV
5904   REL LANG$NONLANG$MEAS SCH$CHIL
6004   LANG$MEAS RELIABILITY SIZE LANG$SAMPLES
6103   EVAL CHIL LANG$DELAY
6204   STUDY TEMPORAL$RELIABILITY LANG$MEAS
6304   TEMPORAL$RELIABILITY LANG$MEAS
6603   DEV$SENTENCE$TYPES METHOD COMPARING NORMAL$DEVIANT
       $SYNTACTIC$DEV
6703   DIFFERENTIAL$DIAGNOSIS APHASIC SCHIZOPHRENIC$LANG
       CHIL
6714   VALIDITY PROBE-LATENCY$TECHNIQUE ASSESSING LANG$STRUCTURE
6715   PURDUE$PEGBOARD SCREENING$TEST BRAIN$DAMAGE MR NONVERBAL
       $CHIL
6904   STANDARDIZED$METHOD OBTAINING SPOKEN$LANG$SAMPLE
7003   SCREENING$TEST SYNTAX$DEV
7004   STANDARDIZED$METHOD OBTAINING SPOKEN$LANG$SAMPLE
7010   CLOZENTROPY PROCEDURE TESTING LANG$PROFICIENCY FOREIGN
       $STUDENTS
7103   DEV$SENTENCE$SCORING CLINICAL$PROCEDURE ESTIMATING
       SYNTACTIC$DEV
7103   DIAGNOSTIC$SIGNIFICANCE SENTENCE$REPETITION LANG-IMPAIRED
       $CHIL
7104   REL SP$DISCRIM LANG$ABILITIES SCH$CHIL
7108   EDUC-DIAGNOSTIC$APPROACH LANG$PROBLEMS
7117   INTELLIGENCE$TESTS CHIL LANG$ANALYSIS
7204   COMPARISON RESULTS REVISED$VERSION BERKOS$TEST$MORPHOLOGY
7204   PROBLEM LANG$DIS LENGTH$VS$STRUCTURE
7204   REL COMPONENTS GRAMMAR LANG$DIS
7208   VARIABILITY$TEST$SCORES FORM$A$B PPVT
7212   ADULT-CHIL$DIALOGUE DIAGNOSTIC$IMPLICATIONS
7212   ADULT-CHIL$DIALOGUE DIAGNOSTIC$IMPLICATIONS
7212   COMPUTERIZED$SCORING ITPA
7214   TRANSFORMATIONAL$GRAMMARS AGRAMMATICAL$PATIENTS

```
7305   LANG$ASSESSMENT
7312   LANG$ASSESSMENT RESTRICTING$STRUCTURE
7313   DIAGNOSIS$DEV$LANG$DIS
7314   VALIDATING PERMUTATIONAL$TEST GRAMMATICALITY
7403   ELICITED$IMITATIONS ASSESSING$GRAMMATICAL$STRUCTURE
       CHIL
7403   OPEN$SYLLABLE SYMPTOM$LANG$DIS
7403   PREDICTING$LANG$LOSS AR$REFLEX
7403   SCREENING$LANG SP$DEV
7412   COMPARATIVE$STUDY CHIL TOKEN$TEST NSST PPVT
7503   PRUTTING EXPRESSIVE$PORTION NSST SPONTANEOUS$LANG
       $SAMPLE
7503   RATUSNIK INTERNAL$CONSISTENCY NSST
7504   CRONKHITE SCORING ITPA MULTIVARIATE$ANALYSIS NORMATIVE
       $DATA
7504   DAVIS PRONOUN$ASSESSMENT FREE$SP$TECHNIQUE
7504   DISIMONI SHORTENING PICA
7504   JOHNSON RELIABILITY DSS SCORING FUNCTION SAMPLE$SIZE
7511   LASS CHILD$PERFORMANCE TESTS RECEPTIVE$LANG$ABILITIES
7511   LASS CHILDREN'S$PERFORMANCE TESTS RECEPTIVE$LANG
7512   MASLAND NEUROLOGICAL CORRELATES LANG$DISABILITIES
7522   HOWES REACTION$TIME FOCAL$IMPAIRMENT LESIONS RIGHT
       $HEMISPHERE
7527   LASS CHILDRENS$PERFORMANCE TOKEN$TEST
7532   GADDES SPREEN-BENTON$APHASIA$TESTS
7603   ARNOLD GRAMMATIC$CLOSURE ITPA BLACK CHILDREN
7603   LARSON RESPONSE$PATTERNS PRE-SCHOOL$CHILDREN NSST
7603   TOLER INTERROGATIVE$MODEL EVALUATE MOTHERS' QUESTION
       $FORMS
7603   TORONTO DEVELOPMENTAL$ASSESSMENT SPANISH$GRAMMAR
7611   ROBB CHIL TOKEN$TEST DEV$TEST$SCH$READINESS GRAMMATICAL
       $CONCEPTS$TEST
7611   TROMBOLI MIDDLE-CLASS + ECONOMICALLY-DEPRIVED$CHIL
       TOKEN$TEST
7627   MARTINO TOKEN$TEST APHASICS
7703   ARNDT PSYCHOMETRIC$EVAL NSST
7703   BYRNE NSST
7703   HUBBELL FACILITATING SPONTANEOUS$TALKING CHIL
7703   LILES JUDGMENTS GRAMMATICALITY LANG-DISORDERED$CHIL
7703   RUEDA COMPARISON SPANISH$TESTS RECEPTIVE$LANG
7704   BLISS STORY$COMPLETION MEAS LANG$DEV CHILD
7704   WILLWIMS VALIDITY PPVT MENTALLY$RETARDED$CHILD
7708   DUCHAN R BLACK$CHILDREN GRAMMATIC$CLOSURE ITPA
7708   LONGHURST DSS HEAD$START$CHILDREN
7708   SILVESTRI DEV$ANALYSIS ACQUISITION COMPOUND$WORDS
7722   LEDOUX COGNITION COMMISSUROTOMY
```

7722    WINNER COMP METAPHOR BRAIN-DAMAGED$PATIENTS
7732    FENNELL RELIABILITIES LATERALITY$TESTS
7732    LURIA ASSESSMENT APHASIA
7732    MALY BRAIN$PERFUSION NEUROPSYCHOLOGICAL$TEST APHASICS
7803    KIRK USES ABUSES ITPA
7803    MILLER EARLY$CHILD$LANG$DISORDERS COMM$INTERACTIONS
7803    OLSWANG ELICITOR$EFFECTS LANG LANG-IMPAIRED CHILD
7803    SCOTT COMPARISON HOME+CLINIC$GATHERED$LANG$SAMPLES
7805    LEONARD NONSTANDARDIZED$APPROACHES ASSESSMENT LANG
        $BEHAVIORS
7812    MELINE COMP PROD VERBS LANG-DISORDERED$CHILD
7825    DERENZI NORMATIVE$DATA SCREENING$POWER SHORTENED$TOKEN
        $TEST
7825    DERENZI SHORTENED$VERSION TOKEN$TEST
7827    CULATTA RELATIONSHIP PERCEPTUAL$DYSFUNCTION LANG$DISORDERS
7827    FRANK PSYCHOLINGUISTIC$FINDINGS GILLES$DE$LA$TOURETTE
        $SYNDROME
7827    MULAC TESTING SYNTACTIC$STRUCTURE
7827    NOLL ERRORS APHASIC$SUBJECTS TOKEN$TEST
7827    SALVATORE TOKEN$TEST$COMMANDS EXPERIENCED INEXPERIENCED
        $EXAMINERS


                            0404


6305    LANG$MODIFICATIONS DISRUPTION CULTURAL$VERBAL$HABITS
6703    LANG$SP$DEFICITS CULTURALLY$DISADVANTAGED$CHIL IMPLICATIONS
6805    LANG ECONOMICALLY$DISADVANTAGED$CHIL
6819    EFFECT CULTURAL$DEPRIVATION LANG$DEV
6904    LANG$DEFICIENCY DISADVANTAGED$CHIL
7004    COMMENT LANG$DEFICIENCY DISADVANTAGED$CHIL
7012    LANG$PEDAGOGY TEACHERS DEPRIVED$CHIL
7105    PLURALISM RELEVANCE LANG$INTERVENTION CULTURALLY$DEPRIVED
        $CHIL
7212    LANG DEPRIVED$CHIL
7508    MUN VERBAL$EXPRESS SOCIOECON$STATUS
7527    GEFFNER COGNITIVE$USE LANG DISADVANTAGED$CHILDREN


                            0405


5403    ENVIRONMENTAL$INFLUENCE VERBAL$OUTPUT MR$CHIL
5413    FINDINGS SP$VOICE$THERAPY MR$CHIL
5703    ANALYSIS SP$DEFECTS INSTITUTIONALIZED$MR

5803   SP$THERAPY MR$CHIL
5810   REL SPEAKING$ABILITY MENTAL$ABILITIES VERBAL$COMPREHENSION
5903   LONGITUDINAL$STUDY SP$LANG$DEV BRAIN$DAMAGED$MR$CHIL
5903   SITUATIONAL$SP$THERAPY MR$CP$CHIL
5907   RESEARCH$NEEDS SP$PATH$AUDIOLOGY MR DELAYED$SP$LANG
       $DEV
5914   EFFECTS WORD$LEARNING IMBECILES
5918   SP$THERAPY MR
6003   LANG MENTATION PHENYLKETONURIC$CHIL
6004   LISTENING$TRNG MR$CHIL
6013   SP$LANG$HNG DISORDERS ENCEPHALOPATHY
6103   MOWRERS$THEORY SP$HABILITATION MR
6203   SP$LANG$PROGRAM EDUCABLE$HANDICAPPED$CHIL
6205   TRNG MR$CHIL ORAL$COMM
6307   ADULT$VERBAL$BEHAVIOR PLAY$THERAPY MR$CHIL
6307   ADULT$VERBAL$BEHAVIOR PLAY$THERAPY MR$CHIL
6307   ASSESSMENT SP$LANG MR$CHIL PARSONS$LANG$SAMPLE
6307   ASSESSMENT SP$LANG MR$CHIL PARSONS$LANG$SAMPLE
6307   RF VOCAL$R CANDY$VOCAL$SMILING$RF MR
6307   VERBAL$BEHAVIOR MR$CHIL
6307   VERBAL$BEHAVIOR ADULTS INSTITUTIONALIZED$MR$CHIL
6307   VERBAL$BEHAVIOR ADULTS INSTITUTIONALIZED$MR$CHIL
6307   VERBAL$BEHAVIOR MR$CHIL
6404   EST MEAN$LENGTH$R CHIL$MR
6405   CONCEPTS SP$RESEARCH MR$CHIL
6604   AUD$DISCRIM MR$CHIL
6604   EFFICACY SP$THERAPY EMR$CHIL
6703   CLIENT-CENTERED$COMM$THERAPY MR$DELINQUENTS
6703   SP$LANG$PROBLEMS MONGOLISM REVIEW$LITERATURE
6704   SP$HNG$CHARACTERISTICS FAMILIAL$DYSAUTONOMIA
6714   VERBAL$LABELLING LEARNING DISCRIMINATION MR$CHIL
6804   ACQUISITION ENG$MORPHOLOGY EMR$CHIL
6813   AUD$PROBLEMS MR$CHIL
6814   STM SYNTACTIC$STRUCTURE MR$CHIL
6913   LANG MR$CHIL
7003   PROGRAMMED$COMM$THERAPY AUTISTIC$MR$CHIL
7003   SP$HNG$LANG DE$LANGE$SYNDROME
7013   SP$MR$CHIL
7014   PERFORMANCE MR$BOYS BERKOS$TEST$MORPHOLOGY
7117   SURVEY SCH$SP$HNG$CLINICIANS CHIL$EMR
7203   SP$LANG$HNG$PROBLEMS LAURENCE-MOON-BIEDL$SYNDROME
7204   ASSESSMENT MODIFICATION VERBAL$IMITATION MR$CHIL
7204   FREE$SP MR$CHIL
7213   VOICE CHIL DOWN$SYNDROME
7314   SYNTACTIC$INDICES LANG$USE MR$CHIL
7403   SP$LANG$DEV CHIL MYELOMENINGOCELE$HYDROCEPHALUS

7404    NONSP$NOUN$USAGE$TRNG MR$CHIL
7504    MONTAGUE COMPUTER$ANALYSIS VERBAL$BEHAVIOR RETARDED
        $CHILD
7504    NAREMORE LANG EMR NORMAL$CHILD
7508    MITCHELL LANG ACADEMICS REATARDED$CHILD
7512    BLOM PSYCHOEDUCATION APPROACHES LEARNING$DISABILITIES
7522    BANICK DOWN,S SYNDROME BIOCHEMICAL$STUDIES
7604    DUCHAN RETARDED$CHILD UNDERSTANDING SEMANTIC$RELATIONS
        VERBAL$CONTEXTS
7613    MEAR-CRINE VERBAL$BEHAVIORS MENTALLY RETARDED CHILDREN
7704    WILLWIMS VALIDITY PPVT MENTALLY$RETARDED$CHILD
7708    LINVILLE SIGNED$ENGLISH MENTALLY$RETARDED
7708    MITCHELL TRAINABLE$CHILDREN ADJECTIVES$POLARS$PREPOSITIONS
7732    HEFFNER DEV$AUD$AGNOSIA MR$ADOL
7804    BEDROSIAN COMMUNICATIVE$PERFORMANCE MR CONVERSATIONAL
        $SETTING
7804    BLISS SENTENCE$STRUCTURES MENTALLY$RETARDED

## 0406

5816    IMPROVING TEACHING LANG
6015    INCREASE$VOCAB
6017    PSYCHOLOGICAL$ASPECTS REHAB CHIL ORGANIC$LANG$DIS
6103    LEARNING$PRINCIPLES TEACHING SP$LANG
6109    AUDIO-LINGUAL$AIDS LANG$TRNG USES LIMITATIONS
6204    SP$THERAPY CHIL$LINGUISTIC$SKILLS
6215    BOOKS TEACHING$READING
6217    GAME$APPROACH LANG$UNIT SP$THERAPY
6303    EFFECTS SP$THERAPY LINGUISTIC$SKILLS SCH$CHIL
6304    COMMENT SP$THERAPY CHIL$LINGUISTIC$SKILLS
6315    LANG$PROBS SP$THER ADOL
6413    R NON-LANG$CHIL$TRNG
6416    PROGRAMMED$INSTRUCTION LANG$DIRECTIONS
6514    PREDICTABILITY$WORDS FUNCTION AUD$CONTEXTUAL$CUES
6803    RADIO$TELEMETRY MONITORING$VERBAL$BEHAVIOR
6815    LANG$PATTERNING
6815    TEACHING NONVERBAL$CHIL
6903    THERAPEUTIC$CONSTRUCT NONVERBAL$BOYS
7003    BEHAVIORAL$STRATEGY LANG$TRNG AUTISTIC$CHIL
7007    RF$PROCEDURES FUNCTIONAL$SP BRAIN-INJURED$CHIL
7007    RF$PROCEDURES ESTABLISHING$MAINTAINING ECHOIC$SP NONVERBAL
        $CHIL
7012    HYPOTHESIS$TESTING TECHNIQUES FACILITATE LANG$LEARNING
7108    LANG$INTERVENTION

| 7203 | BASES DECISION LANG$TRNG |
|------|--------------------------|
| 7303 | LINGUISTICS LANG$THERAPY SENTENCE$CONSTRUCTION$BOARD |
| 7305 | PROBLEM$SOLVING DELAYING$SP STRATEGIES TEACHING$LANG |
| 7306 | RHYTHMIC$UNITS SYNTACTIC$UNITS PROD PERCEP |
| 7315 | LANG MR$DEAF$CHIL PROJECT$LIFE |
| 7315 | LEARNING$LANG COMPUTER |
| 7317 | STUDY EFFECTS PROGRAMMED$INSTRUCTION LINGUISTIC$ABILITY |
| 7403 | ENVIRONMENTAL$LANG$INTERVENTION RULES$CONTEXT$GENERALIZATION |
| 7403 | GENERALIZATION LANG$TRNG |
| 7403 | LANG$COMPREHENSION$PROCEDURES |
| 7403 | LANG$TRNG APPLIED$LINGUSTICS |
| 7403 | PARENT-ASSISTED$TREATMENT$PROGRAM PRESCH$LANG$DEL $CHIL |
| 7403 | SYNTACTIC$SLOT-FILLER SENTENCE$CONSTRUCTION$BOARD |
| 7404 | NONSP$NOUN$USAGE$TRNG MR$CHIL |
| 7407 | SYSTEMATIC$PROCEDURES TRNG$CHIL$LANG |
| 7408 | PLANNING CHIL$CHANGE LANG DEV$REMEDIATION$PROGRAMS TEACHERS$PARENT |
| 7408 | REACTION$PARENT COORDINATING$LANG$REMEDIATION TEACHERS $PARENTS |
| 7408 | TREATMENT DEVELOPMENTAL$APRAXIA SPEECH |
| 7413 | STRUCTURAL$LINGUISTICS LOGOPEDICS$SP$THERAPY |
| 7414 | TEACHING CONSTRUCTED$R LANG$THERAPY |
| 7503 | APPLEMAN CONDITIONING LANG NONVERBAL$CHILD SPECIAL $EDUCATION |
| 7503 | LONGHURST APPLIED$COMMUNICATION$GAME COMMENT MUMA |
| 7503 | MUMA COMMUNICATION$GAME DUMP$PLAY |
| 7508 | BROOKNER TOTAL$COMM NONDEAF$CHILD |
| 7508 | LEONARD MODELING LANG$TRAINING |
| 7508 | SIMON TALK$TIME LANG$DEV READINESS$CLASSES |
| 7512 | KLEFFNER TEACHING CHILDREN AUD$PROCESSING LEARNING $DISABILITIES |
| 7516 | ESL$APPROACH TEACHING ENGLISH |
| 7527 | MCDEARMON REPRESENTATIONAL$PROMPTS APHASIA$THERAPY |
| 7532 | KEITH SINGING$THERAPY APRAXIA APHASIA |
| 7604 | COURTRIGHT IMITATIVE$MODELING INSTRUCTING LANG$DIS $CHILDREN |
| 7605 | MAYBERRY CHIMP SIGN$LANG NONVERBAL$CLIENT |
| 7613 | SEGRE AUTOBIOGRAPHICAL APHASIC$REHAB |
| 7627 | FRIEDMAN CLINICIAN$FEEDBACK CHILD$INITIATED$VERBALIZATION LANG$TRNG |
| 7627 | SHEWMAN FACILITATING$SENTENCE$FORMULATION |
| 7703 | CONNELL CRITERIA EVALUATION LANGUAGE$PROGRAMS |
| 7703 | HUBBELL FACILITATING SPONTANEOUS$TALKING CHIL |
| 7703 | LAHEY PLANNING FIRST$LEXICON |
| 7703 | SEYMOUR THERAPEUTIC$MODEL COMMUNICATIVE$DISORDERS CHIL BLACK$ENGLISH |

7708   ANDREWS LANG-IMPAIRED$CHILD MATHEMATICS SP$PATHOLOGIST
7708   CHAPPELL COGNITIVE-LINGUISTICS$INTERVENTION CONCEPT
       $FORMATION
7708   MOORE SEMANTIC$CONTEXTUAL$COMPONENTS LANG
7708   MUMA LANG$INTERVENTION$STRATEGIES
7713   EISENSON REHAB APHASIC$ADULTS
7713   JORDAL TREATMENT LANG$DIS CHILDREN
7729   WITZEL TRAINING$PROCEDURES MOTHER CHILD$STATEMENTS
7803   SHELTON ASSESS PARENT-ADMINISTERED$LISTENING$TRAINING
       PRESCHOOL$CHILD
7803   WEAVER EFFECT GESTURAL$PROMPT SYNTAX$TRAINING
7804   WILCOX WH$QUESTIONS LANG-DISORDERED$CHIL
7812   DIXON RECEPTIVE$LABEL$TRAINING
7827   LOZANO DAF DYSPRAXIA SP
7827   SCHWARTZ ELICITED$IMITATION LANG$ASSESSMENT
7829   CAMPBELL EXPRESSIVE$SP$PROGRAM CHILD ACQUIRED$APHASIA
7829   WARYAS LANG$INTERVENTION$PROGRAMMING


                              0407


5409   AUD$DIS CHIL MANUAL DIFFERENTIAL$DIAGNOSIS
5915   MEAS LEARNING$ABILITIES
6205   DIS$NEUROLOGICAL$INTEGRATIVE$MECHANISMS
6703   VERBAL$SEQUENCE$DISCRIMS$TRNG LANG$IMPAIRED$CHIL
6804   DISTURBANCE PERCEP AUD$SEQUENCE CHIL MINIMAL$CEREBRAL
       $DYSFUNCTION
7011   AUD$FIGURE-GROUND$PERCEP NI$CHIL
7012   DISABILITIES LEARNING$SYMBOLS
7014   CONCEPT$LEARNING STM CONTRIBUTION THEORY
7212   AUD$PERCEP$TRNG
7212   READING$DISABILITY LANG$DIS
7215   WRITING CHIL LANG READING$DEFICIENCIES
7303   AUD$INTEGRATIONAL$PROBLEM LANG$DISABILITY ADULT$MENTAL
       $PATIENT
7303   AUD$PROCESSING LANG$DIS
7304   LEARNING$DISABLED$CHIL
7312   DYSLEXIA
7408   LAC ADD TEACHERS SP$SPECIALISTS
7417   SP$THERAPY LEARNING$DISABILITY$SCH
7505   STARK READING$FAILURE LANG
7522   YAMADORI ALEXIA, IDEOGRAM$READING
7527   PANTALOS SENTENCE$LENGTH-DURATION$RELATIONSHIPS AUD
       $ASSEMBLY$TASK
7532   GOLDSTEIN AUD$AGNOSIA CORTICAL$DEAFNESS

7532   OSCAR-BERMAN BRAIN$DAMAGE PROCESSING$SP
7532   SAFFRAN MEM WORD$LISTS+SENTENCES DEFICIENT$AUD$STM
7604   TALLAL RAPID$AUD$PROCESSING DISORDERED$LANG
7632   DENCKLA NAMES OBJECT-DRAWINGS DYSLEXIA+LEARNING DISABLED
       $CHILDREN
7632   ELLIOTT HYPERLEXIA
7632   KIM DEFICITS TEMPORAL$SEQUENCING VERBAL$MATERIAL LATERALITY
       LESION
7632   MOHR DYSLEXIA DYSGRAPHIA
7632   SAFFRAN SEMANTIC$MECHANISMS PARALEXIA
7632   SAFFRAN SP$PERCEP WORD$DEAFNESS
7632   STACHOWIAK FUCTIONAL$DISCONNECTION ALEXIA COLOR$NAMING
7703   MANNING CHIL AUDITORY$PERCEPTUAL$DISORDERS TIME-COMPRESSED
       $SP$DISCRIM
7703   OELSCHLAEGER TIME-COMPRESSED$SP$DISCRIM CENTRAL$AUD
       $DIS PEDIATRIC
7704   MORAN MASTERY VERB$TENSE$MARKERS LD$CHILD
7708   WITKIN AUD$PROCESSING CHILDREN
7716    COGNITION+COMM$PATTERNS CLASSROOMS
7722   LEDOUX COGNITION COMMISSUROTOMY
7804   FREEMAN DISCRIM TIME-ALTERED$APPROX CHIL READING$PROBS
7812   SCHUBERT RELIABILITY GOLDMAN-FRISTOE-WOODCOCK$TEST
       LD CHILD
7812   SIMPSON RATE$VARIABILITY AUD$PROCESSING APHASIC$PATIENTS
7825   KAPUR RECOGNITION$READING PARALEXIA
7825   LINDGREN FINGER$LOCAALIZATION READING$ABILITY
7825   SPELLACY DYSCALCULIA GERSTMANN$SYNDROME CHIL
7827   LILES PAUSE$TIME AUDITORY$COMPREHENSION LANG$DISORDERED
       $CHIL
7827   ROGOW COMPREHENSION QUESTIONS NONSPEAKING$CHIL


                              0408


5403   LANG$DIS PARENT-CHILD$REL
5603   LANG$INVEST CHIL FAMILIAL$DYSAUTONOMIA
5713   LANG$SYMPTOMS FAMILIAL$DYSAUTONOMIA
5803   ORIENTING$REFLEX$DISTURBANCES CENTRAL$AUD LANG$HANDICAPPED
       $CHIL
6005   PROGRESS RESEARCH NEUROLOGICAL$SENSORY$DIS
6103   SOCIAL$PARTICIPATION NONLANG$CHIL
6215   AUDIOMETRIC$FINDINGS CHIL PROGRAM LANG$DIS
6314   REL INDUCED$DYSNOMIA PHONEME$FREQ
6503   LANG$DIS CHIL REORGANIZATION$THINKING
6704   MITIGATED$ECHOLALIA CHIL

6903    LANG$DEV$PROGRAM BLIND$LANG-DIS$PRESCH$GIRL
6904    COGNITIVE$FUNCTIONING LANG$DEFICIENT$CHIL
7114    RACIAL$DIFFERENCES ASSOCIATIVE$STYLE
7117    RACE$IDENTIFICATION BASIS BIASED$SP$SAMPLES
7203    DEVIANT$LANG
7303    CHIL LANG$DISORDERS
7303    DIFFERENTIAL$LANG NEUROLOGIC$CHARACTERISTICS CEREBRAL
        $INVOLVEMENT
7303    NONVERBAL$CHIL
7303    REGULARITIES$ABNORMAL$CHIL$PHONOLOGY
7314    MOTHERS NON-MOTHERS SEMANTIC$ADAPTATION DEVIANT$SP
7405    PEDIATRIC$PSYCHOPHARMACOLOGY LANG-LEARNING$IMPAIRED
        $CHIL
7410    LANG$ATTITUDE ANALYSIS TEACHER$DIFFERENCES
7503    SHEWAN LANG-DISORDERED$CHILD COMMUNICATION$GAME DUMP
        $PLAY
7527    SCHUSTER LANG$INTERVENTION$LEXICON
7532    DARLEY LANG NEUROSURGERY PARKINSONISM
7532    DENNIS COMPREHENSION SYNTAX INFANTILE$HEMIPLEGICS
        HEMIDECORTICATION
7604    LEONARD SEMANTIC$RELATIONS LANG-DISORDED$CHILDREN
7627    KASTEIN EMOTIONAL$STRESS LANG$DEV VISUALLY$IMPAIRED
        $CHILDREN
7632    CARAMAZZA RIGHT-HEMISPHERIC$DAMAGE VERBAL$PROBLEM
        $SOLVING
7632    CARMON VISUAL$HEMIFIELD$DIFFERENCES PERCEP VERBAL
        $MATERIAL
7632    CERMAK REHEARSAL$STRATEGIES ALCOHOLIC$KORSAKOFF$PATIENTS
7632    CERMAK VERBAL$RETENTION APHASIC+AMNESIC
7632    DENNIS LANG$ACQUISITION HEMIDECORTICATION
7632    DENNIS NAMING+LOCATING$BODY$PARTS TEMPORAL$LOBE$RESECTION
7632    LAKE HANDEDNESS SEX HEMISPHERIC$ASYMMETRY
7632    SCHLANGER PERCEP EMOTIONALLY$TONES$SENTENCES RT$HEMIS
        $DAMAGED APHASIC
7703    ARCHER BLISSYMBOLICS NONVERBAL$COMM
7703    HALL DISFLUENCIES LANG-DISORDERED$CHIL
7703    MADISON COMMUNICATIVE COGNITIVE$DETERIORATION DIALYSIS
        $DEMENTIA
7703    STARKWEATHER DISORDERS NONVERBAL$COMMUNICATIONS
7703    WERTZ RIGHT-HEMISPHERE$LANG$DOMINANCE LEFT-HEMISPHERE
        $MALFORMATION
7704    GROHER LANG MEMORY$DISORDERS CLOSED$HEAD$TRAUMA
7708    ANDREWS LANG-IMPAIRED$CHILD MATHEMATICS SP$PATHOLOGIST
7732    BENTON GERSTMANN$SYNDROME
7732    DAVIS HEMISPHERIC$ASYMMETRIES INFANTS
7732    FAY TEMPORAL$CAPABILITIES ECHOLALIC$CHILD

7732    FERGUSON AGRAPHIA SYNTACTIC$WRITING MOTOR$SP + MOVEMENTS
        $DIS
7732    WEIGL TRANSCODING$PROCESSES PATIENTS AGRAPHIA$DICTATION
7803    HALL FOLLOWUP$STUDY CHILD ARTIC+LANG$DISORDERS
7804    GALLAGHER CONVERSATIONAL$ASPECTS SP LANG-DISORDERED
        $CHIL
7822    BEAUVOIS BILATERAL$TACTILE$APHASIA TACTO-VERBAL$DYSFUNCTION
7822    COUGHLAN WORD-COMPREHENSION WORD-RETRIEVAL PATIENTS
        CEREBRAL$LESIONS
7822    SHIBASAKI ELECTROENCEPHALOGRAPHIC$STUDIES MYOCLONUS
7827    SCHMAUCH CONSONANT$PRODUCTION LANG-DISORDERED$CHIL


                          0409

7522    YAMADORI ALEXIA, IDEOGRAM$READING
7727    MALAC PROGRAM SYNTAX LANG$DELAYED$CHILDREN


                          0410

5403    EMOTIONAL$INVOLVEMENTS MUTISM
5814    VERBAL$DYSFUNCTION MENTAL$ILLNESS COMPARATIVE$STUDY
5914    EXAMINATION GIBBERISH MULTILINGUAL$SCHIZOPHRENIC$PATIENT
6003    OPERANT$CONDITIONING VERBAL$BEHAVIOR PSYCHOTICS
6204    VOCAB$DIVERSITY SCHIZOPHRENICS
6303    REINSTATEMENT VERBAL$BEHAVIOR PSYCHOTIC RF$METHODS
6303    REINSTATEMENT VERBAL$BEHAVIOR PSYCHOTIC RF$METHODS
6703    DEV$LANG AUTISTIC$CHIL
6703    EVAL COMM AUTISTIC$CHIL
6703    EXPERIMENTAL$SP$LANG$PROGRAM PSYCHOTIC$CHIL
6703    REINSTATING$SP EMOTIONALLY$DISTURBED$MR$WOMAN
6703    SP THOUGHT COMM$DIS CHILDHOOD$PSYCHOSES THEORETICAL
        $IMPLICATIONS
6703    SP THOUGHT COMM$DIS CHILDHOOD$PSYCHOSES THEORETICAL
        $IMPLICATIONS
6706    COMM$THERAPY AUTISTIC$CHIL
6803    EMOTIONALLY$DISTURBED$CHIL SP$CLINIC CONSIDERATIONS
6803    INCREASING VERBAL$BEHAVIOR AUTISTIC$CHIL
6803    INCREASING VERBAL$BEHAVIOR AUTISTIC$CHIL
6914    EMPHASIS MEANING RECALL AUTISTIC$CHIL
6914    PSYCHOLINGUISTIC$STUDY SCHIZOPHRENIC$SP
7003    AUTISTIC$CHIL
7003    BEHAVIORAL$STRATEGY LANG$TRNG AUTISTIC$CHIL

```
7103   AUTISTIC$PRONOUNS
7103   PARENT-CLINICIANS LANG$TRNG AUTISTIC$CHIL
7203   USE WRITTEN$LANG COMM$SYSTEM AUTISTIC$CHIL
7303   ECHOLALIA BLIND AUTISTIC$CHIL
7303   LANG$TERAPY CHIL$SCHIZOPHRENIA MONITORING$FEEDBACK
         $APPROACH
7403   LANG$TRNG$PROGRAM NONVERBAL$AUTISTIC$CHIL
7414   LANG AUTISTIC$ECHOLALIA
7503   BALTAXE LANG CHILDHOOD$PSYCHOSIS
7513   SEDLACKOVA DEVELOPMENT AUTISTIC$CHILDREN VERBAL$EXPRESSION
7513   SURIA ACOUSTIC$IMPEDANCE AUTISTIC$CHILDREN
7522   HAUSER INFANTILE$AUTISM$PNEUMOGRAPHIC$FINDINGS
7532   FROMKIN SCHIZOPHRENIC$LANG
7603   BONVILLIAN SIGN$LANGUAGE$ACQUISITION MUTE$AUTISTIC
7603   RATUSNIK THERAPEUTIC$MILIEU COMMUNICATION PSYCHOTIC
         $CHIL
7606   BURNS NONSPECTRAL$PITCH
7632   LECOURS SCHIZOPHASIA JARGONAPHASIA
7703   DISIMONI DYSFUNCTION SCHIZOPHRENIC$PATIENTS APHASIA
         $BATTERY
7727   KONSTANTAREAS SIMULTANEOUS$COMM AUTISTIC$DYSFUNCTIONAL
         $CHILDREN
7732   DURBIN SP MANIA SYNTACTIC$ASPECTS
7732   ROCHESTER THOUGHT-PROCESS$DISORDER SCHIZOPHRENIA
7826   SHAPIRO NEGATION AUTISTIC$CHIL
```

## 0501

```
5409   STUDY LANG
5409   SURVEY VERB$FORMS EASTERN$USA
5509   LINGUISTICS BLOOMFIELD
5609   LANG MEANING REALITY STUDY SYMBOLISM
5615   ACTION$VERBS MEANINGS
5709   AREA SEMANTICS
5709   READINGS LINGUISTICS DEV$DESCRIPTIVE$LINGUISTICS AMERICA
5804   APPLICATION DESCRIPTIVE$LINGUISTICS CHIL$LANG
5809   COURSE MODERN$LINGUISTICS
5814   PSYCHOLINGUISTICS
5906   RELATIVE$OCCURRENCE PHONEMES AMERICAN$ENG
5909   READINGS ENG$LINGUISTICS
5914   BEHAVIORISM LINGUISTICS
5914   LINGUISTICS
5914   QUANTITATIVE$STUDY SYNTAX SP$AUSTRALIAN$CHIL
5914   QUANTITATIVE$TYPOLOGY LANG
```

| | |
|---|---|
| 6014 | LINGUISTIC$PHILOSOPHY MODERN$LINGUISTICS |
| 6014 | THEORY DISTRIBUTIONAL$SYNTAX |
| 6114 | CHARACTERISTICS WORD$CLASSIFICATION |
| 6114 | INDEX MEAS CONTINGENCY ENG$SENTENCES |
| 6114 | MEAS GRAMMATICAL$CONSTRAINTS |
| 6114 | RESULTS RESOLUTION AMBIGUITY SYNTACTIC$FUNCTION LINEAR $CONTEXT |
| 6114 | SYNTACTIC$PROCEDURES ZELLIG$HARRIS |
| 6204 | PSYCHOLOGY LANG$STRUCTURE |
| 6209 | LINGUISTIC$ANALYSIS ORAL$WRITTEN$STYLE |
| 6214 | LINGUISTIC$CODES HESITATION$PHENOMENA INTELLIGENCE |
| 6309 | SEMANTIC$ANALYSIS LANG |
| 6404 | GRAMMATICAL$CLASS VARIABLE VERBAL$SATIATION |
| 6409 | LINGUISTIC$STUDY |
| 6414 | APPROACH SEMANTIC$GENERALIZATION |
| 6414 | LINGUISTIC$STUDY WRITTEN$COMPOSITIONS CHIL |
| 6414 | STUDY GRAMMATICAL$CLASS VARIABLE VERBAL$SATIATION |
| 6415 | HYPHENATED$SUBJECT |
| 6509 | LINGUISTICS SCIENCE |
| 6514 | COGNITIVE$NEUROCHEMICAL$DETERMINATION SENTENCE$STRUCTURE |
| 6515 | DESCRIPTIVE$GRAMMAR |
| 6614 | COGNITION LANG PROBLEM$SOLVING KNOWLEDGE$ENG$NAVAHO |
| 6617 | APPLICATION GENERAL$SEMANTICS NON-VERBAL$COMM |
| 6714 | EXPERIMENTAL$MANIPULATION PROD ACTIVE$PASSIVE$VOICE CHIL |
| 6714 | JUNCTURE$PHENOMENA SEGMENTATION LINGUISTIC$CORPUS |
| 6714 | PROBLEM DESCRIPTION GRAMMAR NATURAL$LANG |
| 6814 | COMPARISON SYNTACTIC$STRUCTURES SP PRESCH$CHIL |
| 6814 | DISTINCTIVE$FEATURES PLURALIZATION$RULES ENG$SPEAKERS |
| 6814 | EYE-VOICE$SPAN ACTIVE$PASSIVE$SENTENCES |
| 6814 | PROMPTED$WORD$REPLACEMENT ACTIVE$PASSIVE$SENTENCES |
| 6817 | APPROACHES STUDY LANG |
| 6817 | IMPLICATIONS TRANSFORMATIONAL$GRAMMAR LANG$THERAPY |
| 6903 | SURFACE$STRUCTURE DEEP$STRUCTURE TRANSFORMATIONS MODEL SYNTACTIC$D |
| 6904 | SOCIAL$CLASS$DIFFERENCES CHIL$SYNTACTIC$PERFORMANCE |
| 6909 | PSYCHOLINGUISTIC$ASPECTS ACTIVE$PASSIVE$SENTENCES |
| 6914 | REL SEMANTIC$SYNTACTIC$FACTORS LANG$STRUCTURE |
| 6914 | TRANSFORMATIONS UNDERSTANDING SENTENCES |
| 7007 | SP$ARTIC ORAL$MORPHOLOGY |
| 7008 | APPROACHES STUDY LANG |
| 7014 | PSYCHOLINGUISTIC$MODEL SYNTACTIC$COMPLEXITY |
| 7014 | PSYCHOLOGICAL$SCALING LINGUISTIC$PROPERTIES |
| 7103 | PIVOT$GRAMMAR |
| 7104 | COMPREHENSION SYNTACTIC$STRUCTURES ADULTS |
| 7104 | SYNTAX PRESCH$FLUENT$DISFLUENT$SP TRANSFORMATIONAL $ANALYSIS |

7114 CHIL$IMITATION COMPREHENSION SENTENTIAL$SINGULARITY
     PLURALITY
7114 COMPREHENSION RECODING-TIME TRANSFORMED$SENTENCES
7114 INCIDENCE FILLED$PAUSES REL PART$OF$SP
7114 INTERACTION SENTENCE$CHARACTERISTICS MODE$PRESENTATION
     RECALL
7114 SEMANTICS SENTENCE$SUBJECTS
7114 SYMMETRY CLAUSES PSYCHOLOGICAL$SIGNIFICANCE LEFT-BRANCHING
7114 SYNTHESIS RULE RETROFLEX$SP
7114 TEST INDEPENDENCE LINGUISTIC$DIMENSIONS
7206 WORD-FINAL$CONSONANTS AMERICAN$ENG
7214 COMPARISON SENSITIVITY SURFACE$DEEP$STRUCTURE SENTENCES
     CHIL
7214 EXPERIMENTAL$TECHNIQUE INVEST LINGUISTIC$PHENOMENA
7214 GRAMMAR WORKING$MIDDLE$CLASS$CHIL ELICITED$IMITATIONS
7214 PAUSES CLAUSES SENTENCES
7214 SOCIOLINGUISTIC$STUDY ADJECTIVE ADVERB
7214 STRESS$RULES PERFORMANCE
7214 VERBAL$PRODUCTIVITY ADJECTIVE$USAGE
7303 LINGUISTIC$ANALYSIS$SP$SAMPLES
7303 LINGUISTIC$ANALYSIS CHIL$SP COMPARISON$PROCEDURES
7304 COMPREHENSION LINGUISTIC$CONCEPTS LOGICAL$OPERATIONS
7304 DEV PHRASE$STRUCTURE$RULES TAG$QUESTIONS CHIL
7310 ANALYSIS SPOONERISMS PSYCHOLINGUISTIC$PHENOMENA
7312 CROSS$LANG$STUDY SP$PROD CHIL AUDIO$AUDIO-VISUAL$MODALITIES
7314 ALL-PURPOSE$R VERBAL$BEHAVIOR
7314 COMPARISON FACTORIAL$STRUCTURE WRITTEN$CODING$PATTERNS
     MIDDLE$CLAS
7404 INDIVIDUAL$DIFFERENCE SPOKEN$SYNTAX SCH$CHIL
7406 RULE-SYNTHESIS SP WORD$CONCATENATION
7409 RESOLUTION GENERATIVE$SEMANTICS PSYCHOLINGUISTIC$ANALYSIS
7414 ACCEPTABILITY LINGUISTIC$CONNECTIVES FUNCTION REL
     REFERENT$EVENTS
7414 COMPARISON FACTORIAL$STRUCTURE ORAL$CODING$PATTERNS
     MIDDLE-CLASS
7414 INVEST WORD$ORDER PARENT-CHILD$INTERACTION FREE$ORDER
     $LANG
7504 DAVIS PERCEP$STRATEGIES NORMAL-HEARING+HEARING-IMPAIRED
     $CHILD COMPREHE
7504 DAVIS STRATEGIES NORMAL-HNG + HI$CHIL COMPREHENSION
     RELATIVE$CLAUSES
7506 BARRETT LEXICAL$DEVELOPMENT OVEREXTENSION CHILD$LANG
7521 GALLAGHER RELATIONSHIP LEXICAL$BOUNDARIES SP$PROD
     CHILD
7521 LEWIS APICAL$COARTIC JUNCTURE$BOUNDARIES
7523 ANDERSEN CUPS GLASSES LEARNING BOUNDERIES VAGUE

7523    CARTER TRANSFORMATION SENSORIMOTOR$MORPHEMES DEVELOPMENT
        'MORE' 'MINE'
7523    DORE HOLOPHRASES SP LANG$UNIVERSALS
7523    GARDNER CHILDREN'S$METAPHORIC$PRODUCTIONS PREFERENCES
7523    GARVERY REQUESTS RESPONSES CHILDREN'S$SP
7523    MACWHINNEY MORPHOLOGICAL$FORMATIONS HUNGARIAN$CHIL
7523    MURRY PERCEPTUAL$RESPONSE INFANT$CRYING MATERNAL$RECOGNITION
        SEX$JUDGE
7523    THIEMAN IMITATION RECALL OPTIONALLY$DELETABLE$SENTENCES
7523    TOWNSEND CHIL$STRATEGIES INTERPRETING COMPLEX$COMPARATIVE
        $QUESTIONS
7526    KEMPER SURFACE STRUCTURE INFINITIVE-COMPLEMENT$SENTENCES
7526    KORIAT SYMBOLIC IMPLICATIONS VOWELS ORTHOGRAPHIC REPRESENTATION
7526    MALGADY EFFECTS PHRASE$SIMILARITY INTERPRETATION FIGURATIVE
        $SENTENCES
7526    SAUSE SEX$DIFFERENCES LANG CHILD
7526    TAYLOR SIMILARITY FRANCH ENGLISH WORDS
7533    MALECOT FRENCH$LIAISON GRAMMATICAL$PHONETIC PARALINGUISTIC
        $VARIABLES
7603    TORONTO DEVELOPMENTAL$ASSESSMENT SPANISH$GRAMMAR
7606    KLATT LINGUISTIC$USES SEGMENTAL$DURATION ENGLISH ACOUS+PERCEP
        $EVIDENCE
7606    LEHISTE ROLE DURATION DISAMBIGUATING SYNTACTICALLY
        $AMBIGUOUS$SENTENCES
7606    STREETER EFFECTS LEARNING$ENG SECOND$LANG ACQUI PHONEMIC
        $CONTRAST
7621    BRASINGTON INHIBITIONS UNIVERSAL$RULES
7621    COOPER SYNTACTIC$CONTROL TIMING SP$PROD COMPLEMENT
        $CLAUSES
7621    ROCA WHO IS AFRAID UNIVERSAL$STATEMENTS
7623    ANTINUCCI CHIL$TALK WHAT$HAPPENED
7623    BALDIE ACQUISITION PASSIVE$VOICE
7623    EHRI COMPREHENSION PRODUCTION ADJECTIVES SERIATION
7623    LIMBER COMPETENCE PERFORMANCE PRAGMATICS SP YOUNG
        $CHIL
7623    MACRAE MOVEMENT LOCATION ACQUISITION DEICTIC$VERBS
7623    MACWHINNEY HUNGARIAN$RESEARCH ACQUISITION MORPHOLOGY
        SYNTAX
7623    OLNEY ADULT$JUDGEMENTS AGE LINGUISTIC$DIFFERENCES
        INFANT$VOCALIZATIONS
7623    RAMER SYNTACTIC$STYLES EMERGING$LANG
7623    RICHARDSON LINGS$MATURITY COMPOSITIONS CHIL NATL$CHIL
        $DEV$STUDY
7623    SACHS CHILDREN'S$USE AGE-APPROPRIATE$SP SOCIAL$INTERACTION
        ROLE-PLAY
7623    TOWNSEND CHIL INTERPRET COMPARATIVE$ADJECTIVES OPPOSITES

7623    WEBB STAGES EGOCENTRISM CHILDREN'S$USE 'THIS' 'THAT'
7632    SCHACHTER SEMANTIC$PREREQUISITES MODEL$LANG
7633    RICHMAN /E/-/E/ FRENCH$VERB$ENDINGS
7706    COOPER FUNDAMENTAL$FREQUENCY$CONTOURS SYNTACTIC$BOUNDARIES
7706    COOPER SYNTACTIC$BLOCKING PHONOLOGICAL$RULES SP$PRODUCTION
7706    HOUSE IDENTIFICATION LANG UTTERANCE
7706    OLLER EFFECT FINAL-SYLLABLE$POSITION VOWEL$DURATION
        INFANT$BABBLING
7716     FOOTNOTE ANTHROPOLOGICAL$LINGUISTICS
7721    FOX DENTAL$FLAPS VOWEL$DURATION RULE$ORDERING AMERICAN
        $ENGLISH
7721    LEHISTE ISOCHRONY RECONSIDERED.
7723    BLOUNT FEATURES PARENT-CHILD$SP ENGLISH SPANISH
7723    KARMILOFF-SMITH CHILDREN'S$UNDERSTANDING POST-ARTICLES
7723    LUST CONJUNCTIONS$REDUCTION CHILD$LANG
7723    SCHLESINGER COGNITIVE$DEVELOPMENT LINGUISTIC$INPUT
        LANG$ACQUISITION
7733    HO INTONATION MANDARIN INTERROGATIVE$EXCLAMATORY$DECLARATIVE
7733    MCCASLAND ENGLISH STOPS AFTER /S/ MEDIAL$WORD-BOUNDARY
7804    CARROLL FUNCTIONAL$CLAUSES SENTENCE$SEGMENTATION
7821    CUTLER PHONEME-MONITORING CONTEXT PHONETIC$SEQUENCES
7821    ELUGBE WIDER$APPLICATION "TAP"
7821    HIGGS PHONOLOGICAL$PERCEPTION OBSTRUENT$COGNATES
7821    MACARI PSYCHOPHYSICAL$EVIDENCE NATURAL$PHOLOGICAL
        $PROCESSESS
7821    ROBINSON GENERATIVE$PHONOLOGY PHONOLGICAL$IDENTIFICATION
7823    CLARK STRATEGIES ACQUISITION DEIXIS
7823    COKER SYNTACTIC$SEMANTIC$FACTORS ACQUISITION 'BEFORE'
        $'AFTER'
7823    FOLGER PRAGMATIC$ANALYSIS SPONTANEOUS$IMITATIONS
7823    GILBERT TEMPORAL$SEQUENTIAL$CONSTRAINTS PHONOLOGICAL
        $PRODUCTIONS
7823    HOPMANN DEVELOPMENTAL$STUDY FACTIVITY NEGATION COMPLEX
        $SYNTAX
7823    HORGAN DEVELOPMENT FULL$PASSIVE
7823    KAIL DEVELOPMENTAL$PRODUCTION UTTERANCES LEXEMES
7823    LEONARD ASPECTS CHILD$PHONOLOGY IMITATIVE SPONTANEOUS
        $SP
7823    MARTLEW LANGUAGE$USE ROLE CONTEXT FIVE-YEAR-OLD
7823    PARK PLURALS CHILD$SP
7823    SHIBAMOTO LEXICAL SYLLABIC$PATTERNS PHONOLOGICAL$ACQUISITION
7826    GREENFIELD PSYCHOLOGICAL$RELATIONS ACTION LANG$STRUCTURE


0502


5410    FREQ OCCURRENCE CONSONANTS WORDS SP$CHIL$SCH

5603    SIBLING$INFLUENCE CHIL$SP
5703    BABBLING ECHOLALIA LANG$THEORY
5709    LANG$SKILLS CHIL DEV INTERREL
5710    COMPARISON CHAIN$ASSOC PRESCH$SCH$CHIL ACTION-PICTURE
        $STIMULI
5803    HNG SPEAKING LANG$LEARNING
5814    EFFECTS EARLY$DEPRIVATION SP$DEV
5815    DEV CONNECTED$LANG$SKILLS
5815    READING$EVAL CONTINUING$STUDY
5815    REL SP$LANG$DEV INTELLIGENCE SOCIO-ECONOMIC$STATUS
5904    LANG$SKILLS MALE$FEMALE SCH$CHIL
6004    INF$SP EFFECT SYSTEMATIC$READING$STORIES
6103    AGE$FIRST$WORD REVIEW$RESEARCH
6103    CONCEPTS SP$DEV
6103    ORGANISMIC$DEV ORAL$LANG
6104    EDUC$A CHIL LANG$DEV
6115    LANG$DEV
6203    METHODS PRESENTING$INFO SP$LANG$DEV
6314    SOCIAL$CLASS$DIFFERENCES LANG$DEV STUDY WRITTEN$WORK
6413    EVOLUTIONARY$SOURCES HUMAN$LANG
6414    ACQUISITION$WORD
6415    BUILDING$LANG$FOUNDATION PRESCH$LEVEL
6504    INFLUENCE HOME$BACKGROUND DEV$COMM$SKILLS CHIL
6515    DEV$LANG VERTICAL$LEARNING HORIZONTAL$ASSOCIATION
6515    INF$SP$LANG$DEV
6615    CAPACITY LANG$ACQUISITION
6704    ERRORS ECHOIC$BEHAVIOR PRESCH$CHIL
6713    CHIL$ECHOLALIA
6803    DEV AUD$COMPREHENSION LANG$STRUCTURE CHIL
6804    ECHOLALIA IQ DEV$DICHOTOMY SP$LANG$SYSTEMS
6813    PREREQUISITES LANG$DEV
6815    BEGINNING FUNCTIONAL$LANG
6820    VERBAL$OUTPUT SCH$CHIL
6903    REVIEW MEAN$LENGTH$R MEAS EXPRESSIVE$LANG$DEVL CHIL
6903    REVIEW MEAN$LENGTH$R MEAS EXPRESSIVE$LANG$DEVL CHIL
6905    STUDIES LANG$ACQUISITION
7004    LATENCY ECHOIC$R PRESCH$CHIL
7004    STRESS WORD$POSITION DETERMINANTS IMITATION LANG$LEARNERS
7005    DEV COMM$SKILLS URBAN$MINORITY$POPULATIONS
7008    STUDIES LANG$ACQUISITION
7013    TWINS GRAMMATICAL$DEVELOPMENT
7014    DEV$ANALYSIS SUBJECT$PREDICATE$SENTENCE
7104    REL SP$DISCRIM LANG$ABILITIES SCH$CHIL
7107    DEV$ASPECTS SP$LANG
7112    CHIL ACQUISITION PHONETIC$BEHAVIOR
7112    LANG$LEARNING SWITCH$MECHANISM

7112    LINGUISTIC$THEORY CHIL
7114    ELLIPSIS DISCOURSE LINGUISTIC$ANALYSIS COMPUTER CHIL
        $ACQUISITION$L
7114    VOCAB PRONUNCIATION$ACQUISITION BILINGUALS$MONOLINGUALS
7203    REL MEAS EARLY$LANG$DEV
7204    EVAL INTRAVERBAL$R CHIL
7212    CHIL EVOLVING$SP CODING$PROCESS
7212    FEEDBACK LANG$ACQUISITION
7214    DEV CONNOTATIVE$DENOTATIVE$MEANING MIDDLE$LOWER-CLASS
        $CHIL
7303    IMITATION EARLY$STAGES SP$ACQUISITION
7304    DEV$ENGLISH$MORPHOLOGY BLACK$AMERICAN CHIL LOW$SOCIOECONOMIC
        $BACKG
7314    ASPECTS SEMANTIC$PHONOLOGICAL$DEV CHIL$FIRST$WORDS
7314    LANG$ACQUISITION CLASSICAL$CONDITIONING
7315    PRELINGUISTIC$IMAGERY$COGNITION
7404    CHIL DISCRIM RHYME
7404    COMM$DEV FIRST$THREE$YEARS$LIFE
7414    DESIGN MULTIVARIATE$ANALYSIS LANG$BEHAVIOR LANG$DEV
7414    INFORMATION$UNITS ACQUISITION$LANG
7414    LANG$DEV CHIL$PRESCH
7415    CHIL DEV$LANG
7503    GIATTINO FATHER'S$SP LANG-LEARNING$CHILD
7503    HOLLAND LANG$THEORY CHIL
7503    REES LANG$DEVELOPMENT
7504    CHAPMAN WORD$ORDER EARLY UTTERANCES PRODUCTION COMPPREHENSICN
7504    DAVIS STRATEGIES NORMAL-HNG + HI$CHIL COMPREHENSION
        RELATIVE$CLAUSES
7504    EILERS FRICATIVE$DISCRIMINATION INFANCY
7504    EISELE INFANT$SUCKING$R CHANGES SPL AUDITORY$STIMULI
7504    FAY CHILD ECHOIC$R INTERLOCUTORY$QUESTIONS$TYPES
7504    LODGE ACQUISITION IDIOMS ENGLISH
7521    GALLAGHER RELATIONSHIP LEXICAL$BOUNDARIES SP$PROD
        CHILD
7521    MOSKOWITZ ACQUISITION FRICATIVES PHONETICS PHONOLOGY
7523    ANDERSEN CUPS GLASSES LEARNING BOUNDERIES VAGUE
7523    BRUNER ONTOGENESIS SP
7523    CARTER TRANSFORMATION SENSORIMOTOR$MORPHEMES DEVELOPMENT
        'MORE' 'MINE'
7523    GARDNER CHILDREN'S$METAPHORIC$PRODUCTIONS PREFERENCES
7523    HARRIS INFERENCES SEMANTIC$DEVELOPMENT
7523    SAVIC ADULT-CHILD$COMMUNICATION QUESTION$ACQUISITION
7523    TOWNSEND CHIL$STRATEGIES INTERPRETING COMPLEX$COMPARATIVE
        $QUESTIONS
7526    BRANIGAN SYLLABIC$STRUCTURE ACQUISITION CONSONANTS
7526    BUIUM INTERROGATIVE$TYPES PARENTAL$SP LANG$LEARNING
        $CHILD

7526   EILERS TELEGRAPHIC$SP CHILD
7526   FOX SPOKEN$LANG WORDS$SYLLABLES$PHONEMES
7526   FROMBERG SYNTAX MODEL GAMES LANG EARLY EDUC
7526   HARNER CHILD$UNDERATANDING LINGUISTIC PAST FUTURE
7526   KEENAN COHERENCY CHILD$DISCOURSE
7526   LESSER DOUBLE$FUNCTION$TERMS
7526   MOERK PROCESSES PRODUCTS IMITATION
7526   OYAMA SENSITIVE$PERIOD ACQUISITION NONNATIVE$PHONOLOGICAL
       $SYSTEM
7526   RAMER DEVELOPMENT SYNTACTIC$COMPLEXITY
7526   WHITEHURST LANG$ACQUIRED IMITATION
7529   HOLDGRAFER COMP PROD CHILD$ACQUISITION MORPHOLOGICAL
       $RULES
7529   ILLERBRUN COMP SPACIAL$ADJECTIVES CHILD NORMAL$DEVIANT
       $LANG$DEV
7603   BEASLEY CHILDREN'S$PERCEP TIME-COMPRESSED$SP SP$DISCRIM
7603   HOLDSTEIN KIBBUTZ CITY$CHILDREN SYNTACTIC ARTICULATORY
7603   LARSON RESPONSE$PATTERNS PRE-SCHOOL$CHILDREN NSST
7603   PRUTTING IMITATION
7603   TOLER INTERROGATIVE$MODEL EVALUATE MOTHERS' QUESTION
       $FORMS
7603   TORONTO DEVELOPMENTAL$ASSESSMENT SPANISH$GRAMMAR
7604   BECKWITH RECOGNITION LABELS PICTURED$OBJECTS$EVENTS
       INFANTS
7604   DUCHAN RETARDED$CHILD UNDERSTANDING SEMANTIC$RELATIONS
       VERBAL$CONTEXTS
7604   FREEDMAN SEMANTIC$RELATIONS LANG-IMPAIRED$CHILDREN
7604   MILLER CATEGORICAL$SP$DISCRIM INFANTS
7604   RAMER IMITATION CHILD$LANG
7611   ROBB CHIL TOKEN$TEST DEV$TEST$SCH$READINESS GRAMMATICAL
       $CONCEPTS$TEST
7621   COOPER SYNTACTIC$CONTROL TIMING SP$PROD COMPLEMENT
       $CLAUSES
7623   ANTINUCCI CHIL$TALK WHAT$HAPPENED
7623   BALDIE ACQUISITION PASSIVE$VOICE
7623   BARTLETT ACQUISITION MEANING DIMENSIONAL$ADJECTIVES
7623   DORE TRANITION$PHENOMENA EARLY$LANG$ACQUISITION
7623   EDWARDS SP$CODES SP$VARIANTS CHILDREN'S$SP
7623   KIMBROUGH INFANT$BABBLING SP
7623   LIMBER COMPETENCE PERFORMANCE PRAGMATICS SP YOUNG
       $CHIL
7623   MACRAE MOVEMENT LOCATION ACQUISITION DEICTIC$VERBS
7623   MACWHINNEY HUNGARIAN$RESEARCH ACQUISITION MORPHOLOGY
       SYNTAX
7623   RAMER SYNTACTIC$STYLES EMERGING$LANG
7623   RICHARDSON LING$MATURITY COMPOSITIONS CHIL NATL$CHIL
       $DEV$STUDY

7623    RUKE-DRAVINA 'MAMA' 'PAPA' CHILD$LANG
7623    SACHS CHILDREN'S$USE AGE-APPROPRIATE$SP SOCIAL$INTERACTION
        ROLE-PLAY
7623    SCHACHTER EVERYDAY$CARETAKER$TALK
7623    TOWNSEND CHIL INTERPRET COMPARATIVE$ADJECTIVES OPPOSITES
7623    WEBB STAGES EGOCENTRISM CHILDREN'S$USE 'THIS' 'THAT'
7627    KASTEIN EMOTIONAL$STRESS LANG$DEV VISUALLY$IMPAIRED
        $CHILDREN
7704    EILERS DEV$CHANGES SP$DISCRIM INFANTS
7704    GALLAGHER REVISION$BEHAVIORS SP NORMAL$CHILD
7704    LINARES-ORAMA EVALUATION SYNTAX PUERTO$RICAN$CHILD
7704    SPRING DISCRIM LINGUISTIC$STRESS INFANCY
7706    EILERS CONTEXT-SENSITIVE$PERCEPTION CONSONANTS INFANTS
7706    OLLER EFFECT FINAL-SYLLABLE$POSITION VOWEL$DURATION
        INFANT$BABBLING
7708    SILVESTRI DEV$ANALYSIS ACQUISITION COMPOUND$WORDS
7723    CLARK WHAT'S IMITATION?
7723    EDELSKY SPANISH$LANG$ACQUI AGE SCHOOL CONTEXT R 'DILE'
        $'PREGUNTALE'
7723    KARMILOFF-SMITH CHILDREN'S$UNDERSTANDING POST-ARTICLES
7723    KUCZAJ INFLUENCES CHILDREN'S$COMPREHENSION 'YOUNGER'
        'OLDER'
7723    LI ACQUISITION TONE MANDARIN-SPEAKING$CHIL
7723    LITOWITZ LEARNING DEFINITIONS
7723    LUST CONJUNCTION$REDUCTION CHILD$LANG
7723    MURRY ACOUSTICAL$CHARACTERISTICS INFANT$CRIES FUNDEMENTAL
        $FREQUENCY
7723    PETRETIC COMPREHENSION PROD DEV CHIL$R TELEGRAPHIC
        $SENTENCES
7723    SCHLESINGER COGNITIVE$DEVELOPMENT LINGUISTIC$INPUT
        LANG$ACQUISITION
7723    TYACK CHILDREN'S$PRODUCTION COMPREHENSION QUESTIONS
7723    WODE STAGES DEVELOPMENT LI$NEGATION
7732    DUYNE DEV EAR$ASYMMETRY CODING$PROCESSES MEMORY CHILDREN
7803    SNYDER-MCLEAN VERBAL$INFO$GATHERING CHILD$USE LANG
        ACQUIRE$LANG
7804    BAUMGARDNER ACQUISITION COMPREHENSION VERB$PHRASE
        $ANAPHORA
7804    CHAPMAN COMPREHENSION$STRATEGIES ANIMATE$AGENTS PROBABLE
        $EVENTS
7804    FOLGER LANG SENSORIMOTOR$DEVELOPMENT REFERENTIAL$SP
7804    GALLAGHER STRUCTURAL$CHARACTERISTICS MONOLOGUES CHIL
7806    WILLIAMS DISCRIM YOUNG$INFANTS VOICED$STOP
7823     RATNER GAMES,SOCIAL$EXCHANGE ACQUISITION LANG
7823    BARRETT LEXICAL$DEVELOPMENT OVEREXTENSION CHILD$LANG
7823    BERNDT DEVELOPMENT VAGUE$MODIFIERS LANG PRE-SCHOOL
        $CHILDREN

7823    CAIRNS WHO,WHY,WHEN HOW DEV$STUDY
7823    CLARK STRATEGIES ACQUISITION DEIXIS
7823    COKER SYNTACTIC$SEMANTIC$FACTORS ACQUISITION 'BEFORE'
        $'AFTER'
7823    CORRIGAN LANG$DEVELOPMENT OBJECT$PERMANENCE$DEVELOPMENT
7823    COTTON NOUN-PRONOUN$PLEONASMS ROLE AGE SITUATION
7823    HOPMANN DEVELOPMENTAL$STUDY FACTIVITY NEGATION COMPLEX
        $SYNTAX
7823    KAIL DEVELOPMENTAL$PRODUCTION UTTERANCES LEXEMES
7823    LEONARD ASPECTS CHILD$PHONOLOGY IMITATIVE SPONTANEOUS
        $SP
7823    LINDHOLM LANG$MIXING BILINGUAL$CHILDREN
7823    MARTLEW LANGUAGE$USE ROLE CONTEXT FIVE-YEAR-OLD
7823    NINIO ACHIEVEMENT ANTECEDENTS LABELLING
7823    PARK PLURALS CHILD$SP
7823    SACHS COMPREHENSION TWO-WORD$INSTRUCTIONS CHIL ONE-WORD
        $STAGE
7823    SEGALOWITZ AGENT-PATIENT$WORD-ORDER$PREFERENCE ACQUISITION
        TAGLOG
7823    SHATZ CHILDREN'S$COMPREHENSION MOTHER'S$QUESTION-DIRECTIVES
7823    SHIBAMOTO LEXICAL SYLLABIC$PATTERNS PHONOLOGICAL$ACQUISITION
7823    STARK FEATURES INFANT$SOUNDS EMERGENCE COOING
7823    TSE TONE$ACQUISITION CANTONESE
7823    TYLER DEVELOPMENTAL$ASPECTS SENTENCE$PROCESSING MEMORY
7823    VOLTERRA DEVELOPMENT LANG BILINGUAL$CHILDREN
7826    DEPAULO LANG$DEVELOPMENT SPEECH CHIL
7826    JAMES LISTENER$AGE SITUATION POLITENESS CHILDREN'S
        $DIRECTIVES
7826    LYONS AGE-AT-ACQUISITION WORD$RECOGNITION
7826    MONTGOMERY SENTENCE$REPETITION EFFECTS LENGTH COMPLEXITY
        FAMILIARITY
7826    NICOLICH IMITATIVE$LANG SINGLE-WORD$PERIOD
7834    BOYNTON CONVERSATIONAL$EXPANSION YOUNG$CHIL


                         0503


5709    VOCAB COLLEGE$STUDENTS CLASSROOM$SPEECHES
5814    PLURAL$NUMBER NOUNS
5815    BASIC$VOCAB
5910    WORD-COMPOUNDING AMERICAN$SP
6314    INVEST DENOTATIVE$ASPECTS WORD-MEANING
6414    PROBABILISTIC$PAIRS GRPS$WORDS TEXT
6514    PROBABILISTIC$PROCEDURE GROUPING$WORDS$INTO$PHRASES
6703    SEMANTICS VOICE

6717    FREEDOM WORD$USAGE
7314    VOCABS ORAL$LANG GRAPHIC$LANG
7404    EFFECTS AGE WORD$FREQUENCY OBJECT$RECOGNITION NAMING
        CHIL
7523    CARTER TRANSFORMATION SENSORIMOTOR$MORPHEMES DEVELOPMENT
        'MORE' 'MINE'
7523    HARRIS INFERENCES SEMANTIC$DEVELOPMENT
7526    HIGGINS PRESUPPOSITIONAL$NATURE COMPARATIVES
7526    LAZERSON ANATONMY TEN COLOR-NAMES
7526    RICHARDSON LEXICAL DERIVATION
7623    CHAMBERS CHILDREN'S$UNDERSTANDING AMERICAN$KIN$TERMS
7623    RUKE-DRAVINA 'MAMA' 'PAPA' CHILD$LANG
7623    SCHACHTER EVERYDAY$CARETAKER$TALK
7632    SCHACHTER SEMANTIC$PREREQUISITES MODEL$LANG
7723    FRENCH COMPREHENSION BEFORE AFTER LOGICAL ARBITRARY
        $SEQUENCES
7723    KUCZAJ INFLUENCES CHILDREN'S$COMPREHENSION 'YOUNGER'
        'OLDER'
7723    LITOWITZ LEARNING DEFINITIONS
7823    CAIRNS WHO,WHY,WHEN HOW DEV$STUDY
7823    NINIO ACHIEVEMENT ANTECEDENTS LABELLING


                        0504


5506    PHONEMIC$CONFUSION$VECTORS
5706    REL INTELLIGIBILITY FREQ$OCCURRENCE ENG$WORDS
5810    REL SPEAKING$ABILITY MENTAL$ABILITIES VERBAL$COMPREHENSION
6114    PHONEMIC$SIGNIFICANCE
6310    REL SENTENCE$ORDER COMPREHENSION
6404    SEMANTIC$COMPONENTS QUALITY PROCESSED$SP
6413    AUD$MEM LANG
6506    DISTINCTIVE$FEATURES ERROR SHORT-TERM$MEM ENGLISH
        $VOWELS
6510    EFFECTS ASPECTS SENTENCE$STRUCTURE IMMEDIATE$RECALL
6515    LANG PERCEP
6606    DISTINCTIVE$FEATURES ERRORS STM ENG$CONSONANTS
6614    IMMEDIATE$VERBAL$MEM LINGUISTIC$SOPHISTICATION CHIL
6614    ROLE RELATIVE$INDETERMINACY WORD$INITIALS$FINALS STUDY
6706    PHONEME$GROUPING SP$RECOGNITION
6714    COMPARATIVE$SKILLS MONOLINGUALS$BILINGUALS PERCEP
        PHONEMIC$SEQUENC
6804    AUD$SEQUENCE$LEARNING CHIL
6811    DEV AUD$PERCEPTUAL$SKILLS MATURATION PILOT$STUDY
6814    RECALL ANSWERS CONDUCIVE$QUESTIONS

6814    TRANSFORMATIONAL$COMPLEXITY SHORT$TERM$RECALL
6904    STM ORAL$PERCEP EXPERIMENTAL$SOUND$LEARNING
6906    SEQUENTIAL$AUD$INFORMATION$PROCESSING
7004    REL READING AUD$ABILITIES CHIL
7006    DEPTH SEQUENTIAL$AUD$INFORMATION$PROCESSING
7014    PHONEME$REPETITION STRUCTURE$LANG
7014    STRUCTURAL$APPERCEP ABSENCE SYNTACTIC$CONSTRAINTS
7017    SHORT-TERM$MEM PHONOTACTIC$RULES
7103    PHONETIC$CONTEXTS SP-SOUND$RECOGNITION PROD$PRACTICE
7106    AUD$MEM TONES
7106    DEPTH SEQUENTIAL$AUD$INFO$PROCESSING
7106    SIGNAL$PROCESSING COCKTAIL$PARTY$EFFECT
7108    AUD$PERCEP LANG$DEV
7114    PROCESSING RECALL COMPATIBLE$INCOMPATIBLE$QUESTION
        $ANSWER$PAIRS
7114    ROLE UNDERDETERMINACY REFERENCE SENTENCE$RECALL CHIL
7114    SENTENCE$PROCESSING FUNCTION SYNTAX STM AGE MEANINGFULNESS
        $STIMULU
7204    ARTIC$EFFECTIVENESS STIMULABILITY CHIL$PERFORMANCE
        PERCEP$MEM$TASK
7204    AUD$COMPREHENSION ENG MONOLINGUAL$BILINGUAL$PRESCH
        $CHIL
7204    AUD$COMPREHENSION ENG MONOLINGUAL$BILINGUAL$PRESCH
        $CHIL
7304    AUD$ASSEMBLY SEGMENTED$SENTENCES CHIL
7304    AUD$PERCEPS RHYMING CHIL
7304    AUD$REASSEMBLY$ABILITIES BLACK$WHITE$CHIL
7304    CHIL RECALL APPROXIMATIONS$ENG
7304    SENTENCE$COMPREHENSION CHIL PAUSE$POSITION ABSENCE
        $PAUSES
7312    AUD$PROCESSING
7312    INTERCONSONANTAL$DISTANCES REL IMMEDIATE$RECALL
7314    CHIL CODING STM
7314    COARTIC$EFFECTS POST-CONSONANTAL$VOWELS SHORT-TERM
        $RECALL
7314    ROLE INTONATION RECALL LINGUISTIC$STIMULI
7314    SENTENCE$IMITATION PRESCH$CHIL
7404    USE PROSODY SYNTACTIC CHIL COMPREHENSION$SPOKEN$SENTENCES
7412    AUD$CLOSURE AUD$DISCRIM CHIL
7412    AUD$MEM AUD$SEQUENCING
7414    REMEMBERING TRIVIA
7504    LOCKE MEMORY SP
7511    HICKS INTERFERENCE NONSYMBOLIC$AUDITORY$INFORMATION
7511    MASTERSON PSYCHOACOUSTIC$PROCESSING DICHOTIC$SENTENCES
        PRE-SCHOOL
7511    MASTERSON PSYCHOACOUS$PROCESSING DICHOTIC$SENTENCES
        PRE-SCH$CHILD

7512 PISONI MECHANISMS AUD$DISCRIM CODING LINGUISTIC$INFO
7512 WOOD ASSESSMENT AUD$PROCESSING
7526 FISHER OBJECT IMAGE OBJECT
7526 SHELDEN STRADEGIES PROCESSING$RELATIVE$CLAUSES CHILD
     ADULTS
7532 MOLFESE BRAIN$LATERALIZATION SP+NONSPEECH
7532 SANIDES NEUROLOGY TEMPORAL$LOBE PRIMATES SP
7606 LEHISTE ROLE DURATION DISAMBIGUATING SYNTACTICALLY
     $AMBIGUOUS$SENTENCES
7632 BOND INPUT$UNITS SP$PERCEP
7632 WARREN EEG$ALPHA WORD$PROCESSING RECALL
7632 YUND DICHOTIC$COMPETITION TONE$BURSTS SP
7704 MARSHALL STM ORAL$RETENTION
7706 REMINGTON PROCESSING PHONEMES SP SPEED-ACCURACY STUDY
7706 SAWUSCH PERIPHERAL$CENTRAL$PROCESSES ADAPT PLACE$ARTIC
     STOP$CONSONANTS
7708 WITKIN AUD$PROCESSING CHILDREN
7723 FOWLES COMPETENCE TALENT VERBAL$RIDDLE$COMPREHENSION
7725 HEESCHEN PRAGMATIC-SEMANTIC$SYNTACTIC$FACTORS EAR
     $DIFFERENCES DICHOTIC
7725 MCKEEVER VISUAL$AUD$LANG$PROCESSING$ASYMMETRIES
7732 NATALE PERCEP NONLINGUISTIC$AUD$RHYTHMS SP$HEMISPHERE
7803 BURROWS READING$SKILLS AUD$COMP ACADEMIC$ACHIEVEMENT
7803 REES UNDERSTAND MEAN COMP
7823 OLNEY ADULT$PERCEPTION ONE-WORD$UTTERENCES
7823 TYLER DEVELOPMENTAL$ASPECTS SENTENCE$PROCESSING MEMORY
7825 GEFFEN R$EAR$ADVANTAGE DICHOTIC$LISTENING
7825 SPELLACY DIRECTED$ATTENTION PERCEPTUAL$ASYMMETRY MONAURAL
     $TONES
7825 ZOCCOLOTTI LATERALIZATION VERBAL + CONFIGURATIONAL
     $PROCESSING
7826 DALE INFLUENCE QUESTION$FORM TESTIMONY PRESCHOOL$CHIL
7826 DEPAULO LANG$DEVELOPMENT SPEECH CHIL
7826 GOURLEY CHILD$COMP GRAMMATICAL$STRUCTURES
7826 HARDYCK RECOGNITION$MEMORY LANG$DOMINANCE BILINGUALISM
7826 HOMZIE CHILDREN'S$REPRODUCTIONS
7826 INHELDER LANG THOUGHT CHOMSKY PIAGET
7826 MEHLER SENTENCE$PERCEPTION
7826 MONTGOMERY SENTENCE$REPETITION EFFECTS LENGTH COMPLEXITY
     FAMILIARITY

0505

5509 ASPECTS LANG

```
5606   LINGUISTIC$PREREQUISITES SP$WRITER
5703   LINGUISTIC$FUNCTIONING BILINGUAL$MONOLINGUAL$CHIL
5703   PREDICTION MISSING$WORDS SENTENCES
5709   ORIGINS PREHISTORY LANG
5814   NOTE INFORMATIVENESS PARTS$WORDS
5814   PREDICTABILITY$WORDS$IN$CONTEXT LENGTH$PAUSES
5814   REL FUNCTIONAL$BURDENING$PHONEMES FREQ$OCCURRENCE
5904   SCALING ABSTRACTION$LEVEL SINGLE$WORDS
5914   FRIES WORD$CLASSES
5914   LINEAR$CONTEXT LEXICAL$AMBIGUITY
5914   SOCIAL INDIVIDUAL LANG
5915   CONVERSATIONAL$LANG
6009   LINGUISTIC$INTERPRETATION SP PROBLEMS FOREIGN$STUDENTS
6009   ORIGINS$SP COMM$FUNCTION
6014   COMM VERBAL$MODES$EXPRESSION
6014   CONTROL$TOWER$LANG
6014   ORGANIZATION RUSSIAN-ENG$STEM$DICTIONARY MAGNETIC
       $TAPE
6106   LINGUISTIC$CONSIDERATIONS PORPOISE
6114   ANALOGIES LANG LIFE
6114   CHARACTERISTICS WORD$CLASSIFICATION
6114   SOCIAL$CLASS LINGUISTIC$CODES GRAMMATICAL$ELEMENTS
6214   EXPERIMENT SLIPS$OF$THE$TONGUE WORD$ASSOCIATION
6215   LANG READING
6310   REL SENTENCE$ORDER COMPREHENSION
6314   MULTIVARIATE$ANALYSIS LATIN$ELEGIAC$VERSE
6314   PRELIMINARY$STUDIES MACHINE$GENERATED$INDEX$VOCABS
6410   VERBAL$BEHAVIOR SPEAKER FUNCTION RF$CONDITIONS
6414   CONSCIOUSNESS LINGUISTIC$CONTACT EMPIRICAL$FINDINGS
       CRITIQUE
6414   FACTOR$ANALYSIS SEMANTIC$DIFFERENTIAL$RATINGS SCALES
6414   MODEL CONTINUOUS$LANG$BEHAVIOR
6414   SOCIAL$CLASS$LANG$DIFFERENCES GRP$DISCUSSIONS
6414   TYPING$ERRORS CLUES SERIAL$ORDERING$MECHANISMS LANG
       $BEHAVIOR
6504   SP AURAL$COMPREHENSION FOREIGN$STUDENTS
6514   BILINGUALISM BICODALISM
6514   COGNITIVE$NEUROCHEMICAL$DETERMINATION SENTENCE$STRUCTURE
6514   VISUAL$ANALOGIES VERBAL$OPERATIONS
6614   COGNITION LANG PROBLEM$SOLVING KNOWLEDGE$ENG$NAVAHO
6614   SOUND-MEANING$CORRELATIONS ENG$WORDS
6615   IMPLICATIONS LANG COGNITION
6615   LANG$RESEARCH FOREIGN$COUNTRIES
6714   ANALYSIS WORD$FREQ SPOKEN$LANG CHIL
6714   SOCIAL$PSYCHOLOGICAL$FACTORS REL VARIABILITY ANSWERING
       $BEHAVIOR CH
```

```
6806   PRIMATE$VOCALIZATIONS HUMAN$LINGUISTIC$ABILITY
6807   BRAINS$DOMINANT$HEMISPHERE
6807   BRAINS$DOMINANT$HEMISPHERE
6814   PROBLEM$SOLVING FUNCTION LANG
6814   SEMANTIC$DIFFERENTIAL$PROFILES REL MONOLINGUAL$BILINGUAL
       $TYPES
6814   SENTENCE$CONSTRUCTION GERMAN-ENGLISH$BILINGUALS
6914   EXPERIMENTS QUEER$SENTENCES
6914   SOCIAL$CLASS NOMINAL$GRP REFERENCE
7011   PREDICTABILITY$WORDS SENTENCES
7012   CYBERNETIC$ASPECTS SYMBOL$MANAGEMENT
7014   VERBAL$BEHAVIOR SOCIAL$DISTANCE
7112   CONCEPTS CEREBRAL$DOMINANCE HANDEDNESS LANG
7114   SEMANTIC$THEORY
7114   SOCIAL$CLASS$DIFFERENCES EXPRESSION UNCERTAINTY CHIL
7207   VERBAL$ENVIRONMENT LANG-LEARNING$CHIL
7209   CONCEPTS LANG MEANING COMPARATIVE$STUDY
7214   ORAL$WRITTEN$LANG COGNITIVE$DEV AFRICA USA
7303   NONCOMM$FUNCTION LANG CHIL
7305   NONVERBAL$COMM
7305   SOCIAL$CLASS$BASES LANG
7408   COMPARISON LANG$SAMPLES SITUATIONS
7414   EFFECT DEFINITE$ARTICLE SALIENCE NOUN
7414   REL PERCEIVED$GENERALITY AMBIGUITY SET$WORDS
7414   SOCIAL$CLASS REFERENCE$CONTEXT
7414   STATUS$PERCEP SYNTAX
7505   CUTTING REL SP LANG AUGUST
7523   DEVILLIERS FACTS
7523   MACWHINNEY MORPHOLOGICAL$FORMATIONS HUNGARIAN$CHIL
7523   MURRY PERCEPTUAL$RESPONSE INFANT$CRYING MATERNAL$RECOGNITION
       SEX$JUDGE
7523   SAVIC ADULT-CHILD$COMMUNICATION QUESTION$ACQUISITION
7523   SODERBERGH LANG EAR EYE
7526   WINKLEMAN SEMANTIC$REPRESENTATION$OF$KINSHIP$SYSTEMS
7532   BROWN NEURAL$ORGANIZATION LANG THALAMIC$CORTICAL$REL
7532   FEDIO MEMORY$PERCEP$DEFICITS ELECTRICAL$STIM THALAMUS
       $PARIETAL$SUBCORT
7532   GARDNER UNIMODAL$DEFICIT OPERATIONAL$THINKING
7532   OJEMANN OBJECT$NAMING RECALL THALAMIC$STIMULATION
7603   HOLDSTEIN KIBBUTZ CITY$CHILDREN SYNTACTIC ARTICULATORY
7611   ROBB CHIL TOKEN$TEST DEV$TEST$SCH$READINESS GRAMMATICAL
       $CONCEPTS$TEST
7623   EDWARDS SP$CODES SP$VARIANTS CHILDREN'S$SP
7623   OLNEY ADULT$JUDGEMENTS AGE LINGUISTIC$DIFFERENCES
       INFANT$VOCALIZATION
7623   SCHACHTER EVERYDAY$CARETAKER$TALK
```

7632    LEIBER LEXICAL$DECISIONS CEREBRAL HEMISPHERES
7632    MOORE BILATERAL$TACHISTOSCOPIC$WORD$PERCEP STUTTERERS
        NORMAL
7632    MOSCOVITCH LANG RIGHT$HEMISPHERE
7632    SCHACHTER SEMANTIC$PREREQUISITES MODEL$LANG
7703    WERTZ RIGHT-HEMISPHERE$DOMINANCE LEFT-HEMISPHERE$MALFORMATION
7721    FOX DENTAL$FLAPS VOWEL$DURATION RULE$ORDERING AMERICAN
        $ENGLISH
7723    HOMZIE CHIL$REPROD EVENT$ORDER IMPLIED$VS$DIRECTLY
        $STATED$CAUSATION
7723    PETRETIC COMPREHENSION PROD DEV CHIL$R TELEGRAPHIC
        $SENTENCES
7732    AXELROD ORAL$REPORT WORDS WORD$APPROXIMATIONS VISUAL
        $FIELD
7732    DUYNE DEV EAR$ASYMMETRY CODING$PROCESSES MEMORY CHILDREN
7732    GILBERT CROSS-MODAL$MATCHING+ASSOCIATION SODIUM$AMYTAL
7732    NATALE PERCEP NONLINGUISTIC$AUD$RHYTHMS SP$HEMISPHERE
7732    PIROZZOLO HEMISPHERIC$SPECIALIZATION READING WORD
        $RECOGNITION
7733    FANT LARYNX LANG
7821    BUCKINGHAM NEURAL$MODEL LANG SP
7823    AEGALOWITZ AGENT-PATIENT$WORD-ORDER$PREFERENCE ACQUISITION
        TAGLOG
7823    LINDHOLM LANGUAGE$MIXING BILINGUAL$CHILDREN
7823    STEFFENSEN METHODS ANSWERING$YES/NO$QUESTIONS
7825    ARNDT COGNITIVE$MODE ASYMMETRY CEREBRAL$FUNCTIONING
7825    ARNDT COGNITIVE$MODE ASYMMETRY CEREBRAL$FUNCTION
7825    BIRKETT HEMIS$DIFFERENCES RECOGNITION NONSENSE$SHAPES
7825    MARTIN VERBAL + SPATIAL$ENCODING VISUAL$STIMULI
7825    MCGLONE SEX$DIFFERENCES FUNCTIONAL$BRAIN$ASYMMETRY
7825    REYNOLDS HEMIS$SPECIALIZATION ALPHABETICAL$STIMULI
7825    ROY HANDEDNESS KINESTHETIC$SPATIAL$LOCATION
7825    SHALLICE FRONTAL$LOBES COGNITIVE$ESTIMATION
7825    ZOCCOLOTTI LATERALIZATION VERBAL + CONDIGURATIONAL
        $PROCESSING


                            0506


6404    COMPARISON GRAMMAR$CHIL FUNCTIONALLY$DEVIANT$SP
6514    PREDICTABILITY$WORDS FUNCTION AUD$CONTEXTUAL$CUES
6814    SEMANTIC$DIFFERENTIAL$PROFILES REL MONOLINGUAL$BILINGUAL
        $TYPES
7012    SYMBOLIC$FOUNDATIONS APTITUDE
7312    CROSS$LANG$STUDY SP$PROD CHIL AUDIO$AUDIO-VISUAL$MODALITIES

7504    DAVIS PRONOUN$ASSESSMENT FREE$SP$TECHNIQUE
7523    HART ADULT$CUES LANG$COMPETENCE CHIL
7523    THIEMAN IMITATION RECALL OPTIONALLY$DELETABLE$SENTENCES
7526    JAMES MEMORY ACTIVE PASSIVE$SENTENCES
7526    LEFEVER FIELD INDEPENDENCE SENTENCE$DISAMBIGUATION
7526    LEONARD SYNTACTIC SEMANTIC$FEATURES EMERGING$GRAMMARS
7526    TWENEY SEMANTIC$ORGANIZATION DEAF HRING SS
7606    KLATT LINGUISTIC$USES SEGMENTAL$DURATION ENGLISH ACOUS+PERCEP
        $EVIDENCE
7623    LLOYD ELICITING$TRUE/FALSE$JUDGEMENTS CHIL
7629    BARTHOLOMEUS EVALUATION LANG$CONVERSATIONNEL
7723    HOMZIE CHIL$REPROD EVENT$ORDER IMPLIED$VS$DIRECTLY
        $STATED$CAUSATION
7804    HUDGINS SENTENCE$STRUCTURE ELICITED$IMITATION
7823    FOLGER PRAGMATIC$ANALYSIS SPONTANEOUS$IMITATIONS

## 0601

5403    BIBLIOGRAPHY ESO$SP
5503    ARTIFICIAL$LARYNX ESO$SP
5506    IMITATION DUTCH$VOWELS$WORDS HEMILARYNGECTOMIZED$SUBJECT
5506    THROAT$LOUDSPEAKER PSEUDOLARYNX
5609    LARYNGECTOMEES ORGANIZE
5609    SP LARYNGECTOMY
5907    RESEARCH$NEEDS SP$PATH$A VOICE$SP$PROBLEMS LARYNGECTOMY
6113    X-RAY$STUDY LARYNGECTOMIZED$SPEAKERS
6203    ESO$SP ADOL$BOY CASE$REPORT
6203    WHISTLE$TECHNIQUE ESO$SP
6205    TRNG ESO$SP
6303    CLINICAL$MEAS ESO$SP
6303    CLINICAL$MEAS ESO$SP METHODOLOGY CURVES$SKILL$ACQUISITION
6303    FACTORS REL SP$PROFICIENCY LARYNGECTOMIZED
6303    RELATIVE$INTELLIGIBILITY ESO$SP ARTIFICIAL$LARYNX
        $SP
6313    X-RAY$PICTURE HYPOPHARYNX PSEUDOGLOTTIS$ESO VOCAL
        REHAB LARYNGECTO
6403    CASE$REPORT ENDENTULOUS$APHASIC$LARYNGECTOMEE
6503    AIR$VOLUME AIR$FLOW REL MALE$ESO$SPEAKERS
6503    AIR$VOLUME AIR$FLOW REL MALE$ESO$SPEAKERS
6503    ROLE LARYNGECTOMEE POST-LARYNGECTOMY$VOICE$INSTRUCTION
6513    COMPARISON INTELLIGIBILITY ESO$SP
6513    VOCAL$AIR$CHARACTERISTICS SUPERIOR$MALE$ESO$SPEAKER
6713    CINE$OBSERVATION TONGUE$ESO$APEAKERS
6713    REL FREQ$PITCH ESO$VOICE

6803    LARYNGECTOMEE ARTIFICIAL$LARYNX
6806    COMPARISON SUBGLOTTAL$ESO$PRESSURE SP
6903    LARYNGECTOMEES$VIEWPOINT INTELLIGIBILITY ESO$SP
7003    CLINICAL$EXPECTATIONS ESO$SP
7003    ESO$SP
7003    LARYNGECTOMEE ARTIFICIAL$LARYNX
7003    SIMILARITIES GLOSSOPHARYNGEAL$BREATHING INJECTION
        $METHODS AIR$INTA
7103    TECHQNIUE TEACHING LARYNGECTOMIZED TRAP$AIR PROD ESO
        $SP
7104    STUDY BUCCAL$SP
7104    STUDY TALKER$SEX$RECOGNITION ESO$VOICES
7203    CONVERSION ASAI ESO$SP
7203    USE CRISIS-INTERVENTION REHAB LARYNGECTOMEES
7204    ACOUS$CHARACTERISTICS ESO$SP FEMALE$LARYNGECTOMEES
7204    COMPARISON FUND$FREQ ESO$SP MEAS WAVE-BY-WAVE AVERAGING
        $BASIS
7204    FORMANT$FREQ$CHARACTERISTICS ESO$SP
7213    ACOUS$AERODYNAMIC SUPERIOR$ELECTROLARYNX$SPEAKER
7217    ACQUISITION ESO$SP VARIABLES
7303    ELECTROLARYNX TEMPORARY$TRACHEOSTOMIES
7303    PHONATION TRACHEO-ESOPHAGEAL$SHUNT TOTAL$LARYNGECTOMY
7303    SP LARYNGOESOPHAGECTOMY$COLONY$TRANSPLANT
7303    SP TOKYO$ARTIFICIAL$LARYNX
7303    SP$LANG$TRNG LARYNGECTOMIZED$CHIL
7303    STUDY PHARYNGEAL$SP
7304    ACCEPTABILITY$RATINGS ESOPHAGEAL ARTIFICIAL$LARYNX
        SP
7404    REL ESO$SP$PROFICIENCY AUD$FUNCTION
7404    SOCIAL VOCATIONAL$ACCEPTABILITY ESO$SPEAKERS
7417    TRIADIC$INTERVENTION LARYNGECTOMEE$REHAB
7417    TRIADIC$INTERVENTION LARYNGECTOMEE$REHAB
7503    ZWITMAN WESTERN$ELECTRIC$ELECTROLARYNX MOUTH-TYPE
        $INSTRUMENT
7504    HORII INTELLIGIBILITY ESOPHAGEAL$SP MASKING
7513    MURRY INTRAORAL$AIR$PRESSURE ESOPHAGEAL$SPEAKERS
7603    TORGERSON ACQUISITION ESOPHAGEAL$SP PHARYNGEAL$SP
7604    CHRISTENSEN VOWEL$DURATION ESP
7604    CHRISTENSEN VOWEL$DURATION ESOPHAGEAL$SP
7627    NICHOLS CONFUSIONS$PHONEMES$SPOKEN ESOPH$SPEAKERS
        VOWELS$DIPHTHONGS
7627    NICHOLS CONFUSIONS$PHONEMES$SPOKEN ESOPHAGEAL$SPEAKERS
        INITIAL
7727    NICHOLS CONFUSIONS$PHONEMES ESOPHAGEAL$SPEAKERS TERMINAL
7803    WEINBERG REED-FISTULA$SP PHARYNGOLARYNGECTOMY
7803    ZWITMAN DEV TESTING INTRAORAL$ELECTROLARYNX

7804   CHRISTENSEN VOT ESOPHAGEAL$SP
7827   LIGHT SP$AID ESOPHAGEAL$SPEAKER HEMIPARESIS$TONGUE

## 0602

5403   PITCH$LEVEL NASALITY
5506   COMPARISON HYPONASALITY HYPERNASALITY VOICE$QUALITY
       INTELLIGIBILIT
5804   HARSHNESS GLOTTAL$ATTACK
5903   ANALYSIS VOLUNTARY$MUTISM
6104   PHONETIC$ELEMENTS PERCEP NASALITY
6203   HARSHNESS OR$TIME
6204   ACOUS$STUDY NASALITY
6217   METHODS IMPROVING DYSPHONIC$VOICE
6303   BREATHINESS PHONATION$LENGTH
6313   VOCAL$FRY
6313   VOCAL$FRY
6403   VOICE$SYMPTOMATOLOGY FUNCTIONAL$DYSPHONIA$APHONIA
6410   FUND$FREQ$ANALYSIS HARSH$VOCAL$QUALITY
6503   FUNCTIONAL$APHONIA ADOL$BOY CASE$REPORT
6513   NEURO-PSYCHIATRIC$ASPECTS SPASTIC$DYSPHONIA
6603   INCIDENCE$STUDY CHRONIC$HOARSENESS CHIL
6603   PSYCHIATRIC$SYMPTOMATOLOGY FUNCTIONAL$DYSPHONIA$APHONIA
6603   TREATMENT FUNCTIONAL$APHONIA CHIL ADULT
6803   PSYCHOGENIC$DYSPHONIAS
6804   ADOL$VOICE$QUALITY$ABERRATIONS PERSONALITY SOCIAL
       $STATUS
6804   FUND$FREQ$INVEST VOCAL$FRY HARSHNESS
6804   PERCEP$DIFFERENTIATION VOCAL$FRY HARSHNESS
6804   VOCAL$FRY PHONATIONAL$REGISTER
6903   PSYCHOGENIC$APHONIA
6913   DIAGNOSIS$HOARSENESS
6913   HYPERNASALITIES
6913   PITCH$PERTURBATION FUNCTION SUBJECTIVE$VOCAL$CONSTRICTION
6913   VOCAL$FOLD$LENGTH VOCAL$FRY
7011   PITCH$PERTURBATIONS NORMAL$PATHOLOGIC$VOICES
7013   FALSETTO$VOICE$QUALITY
7017   EVAL VELO$MECHANISM HYPERNASAL$SPEAKERS
7103   CASE$STUDY PSYCHOGENIC$HOARSENESS
7103   CASE$STUDY PSYCHOGENIC$HOARSENESS
7103   EARLY$MOTOR$UNIT$DISEASE PSYCHOGENIC$BREATHY$DYSPHONIA
7104   PHYSIOLOGIC$CORRELATES VOCAL$FRY
7104   SEVERITY NASALITY SP$TASKS
7104   SEVERITY NASALITY SP$TASKS

7106   LOCATION SLOPE$DISCONTINUITIES GLOTTAL$PULSE$SHAPES
       VOCAL$FRY
7108   EVAL VELO$MECHANISM HYPERNASAL$SPEAKERS
7203   DIAGNOSIS TREATMENT VOICE$DIS SCH$CHIL
7313   ACOUS$PARAMETERS PERCEP MODAL$FALSETTO$VOICE
7403   INSTRUMENTAL$MODIFIACTION HYPERNASAL$VOICE MR$CHIL
7403   VELO$INSUFFICIENCY NEURAL$EMOTIONAL$MENTAL$DISORDERS
7503   SILVERMAN CHRONIC$HOARSENESS SCHOOL-AGE$CHIL
7603   WOLFE SPECTROGRAPHIC$COMPARISON SPASTIC$DYSPHONIA
7627   FLETCHER NASALANCE HI
7704   LINDBLOM QUANTITATIVE$EVALUATION HYPERNASALITY
7706   MURRY MULTIDIMENSIONAL $CLASSIFICATION ABNORMAL$VOICE
       $QUALITIES
7713   HIROSE EUNUCHOIDISM VOICE PITCH
7813   GALL PHOTOKYMOGRAPHIC$STATEMENTS FUNCTIONAL$DISORDERS
       PARALYSIS TUMORS


                          0603


5513   VOCAL$REHAB BENIGN$LESIONS VOCAL$CORDS
5713   LARYNGEAL$WHISTLE
5803   VOCAL$REHAB BENIGN$LESIONS VOCAL$CORDS
5813   LARYNGEAL$ASYMMETRY SURGICAL$MEDIOPOSITION VOCAL$CORD
6103   CHIL VOCAL$NODULES
6203   APHONIA$RELIEF BONE$PASTE$INJECTIONS
6203   APHONIA$RELIEF BONE$PASTE$INJECTIONS
6203   DYSPHONIA UNILATERAL$VOCAL$CORD$PARALYSIS CASE$STUDY
6203   LARYNGEAL$TISSUE$REACTION HABITUAL$HYPERKINETIC$DYSPHONIA
6203   PATHOGENESIS TREATMENT VOCAL$NODULES
6306   ACOUS$MEAS FUNDAMENTAL$PERIODICITY NORMAL$PATHOLOGIC
       $LARYNGES
6503   ACOUS$PERCEP$FACTORS ACUTE-LARYNGITIC$HOARSENESS
6503   ACOUS$PERCEP$FACTORS ACUTE-LARYNGITIC$HOARSENESS
6613   APPROACH DIAGNOSIS$HOARSENESS
6613   EARLY$DIAGNOSIS ABNORMAL$PALATAL$MOBILITY CINE
6803   SPASTIC$DYSPHONIA VOICE NEUROLOGIC PSYCHIATRIC$ASPECTS
6803   SPASTIC$DYSPHONIA COMPARISON VOICE$TREMOR NEUROLOGIC
6803   VOCAL$ULCERS GER$MALE
6804   PERCEP$DIFFERENTIATION VOCAL$FRY HARSHNESS
6806   PERCEP$STUDY VOCAL$FRY
6903   SPASTIC$DYSPHONIA CASE$PRESENTATION
6906   VOWEL$AMPLITUDE$MODULATIONS PATIENTS LARYNGEAL$DISEASES
6917   EMG LARYNGEAL$DYSPHONIA
7003   OBJECTIVE$EVAL THERAPY VOCAL$NODULES CASE$REPORT

7003  PROGRESSIVE$HOARSENESS APHONIA BLASTOMYCOSIS
7007  RESTORATIVE$TREATMENT DENTOFACIAL$COMPLEX
7013  PHONATION$QUOTIENT PATIENTS$LARYNGEAL$DISEASES
7103  DYSPHONIAS SPINAL$BRACING SCOLIOSIS
7103  DYSPHONIAS SPINAL$BRACING SCOLIOSIS
7103  PAPILLOMATA VOCAL$FOLDS
7103  PATIENTS SPASMODIC$DYSPHONIA
7106  DESCRIPTIONS SP PATIENTS CANCER VOCAL$FOLDS
7106  DESCRIPTIONS SP PATIENTS CANCER VOCAL$FOLDS JUDGMENTS
      AGE VOICE$QU
7113  HYPERFUNCTIONING$ALARYNGEAL$VOICE CHEWING$APPROACH
7303  IMPED SPASINODIC$DYSPHONIA
7313  PARALYTIC$DYSPHONIA
7403  ALARYNGEAL$SP
7403  SUDDEN$ONSET HIGH-PITCHED$VOICE UNILATERAL$VOCAL$CORD
      $PARALYSIS
7412  COMPARISON PERSONALITY$CHARACTERISTICS CHIL NODULES
      RORSCHACH
7503  SHPRINTZEN THERAPEUTIC$TECHNIQUE VELOPHARYNGEAL$INCOMPETENCE
7513  HARMA VOCAL$POLYPS NODULES
7603  DEAL CHILDREN VOCAL$NODULES
7603  WOLFE SPECTROGRAPHIC$COMPARISON SPASTIC$DYSPHONIA
7606  ISHIZAKA COMPUTER$SIMULATION PATHOLOGICAL$VOCAL-CORD
      $VIBRATION
7627  LEEPER VOICE$INITIATION NORMAL$CHILDREN CHILDREN$VOCAL
      $NODULES
7729  CURRY APERIODIC$VOCAL$FOLD$FREQ INTERMITTENT$APHONIA
7729  HARTMAN SEX$IDENTIFICATION ALARYNGEAL$SP
7803  BOWMAN VELO$RELATIONSHIPS CEPHALOMETRICALLY PERSONS
      SUSPECTED$INCOMP
7813  BOENNINGHAUSEN SOUND-ANALYTICAL$STUDIES FORMATION
      SUBSTITUTE$VOICE
7813  ISSHIKI TURBULENT$NOISE DYSPHONIA

## 0604

5403  VOICE$PROBLEMS ACTOR SINGER
5409  KEEP HEALTHY$VOICE
5803  INVEST ABILITY VOICE$DEFECTIVES DISCRIM DIFFERENCES
      PITCH LOUDNESS
5803  VOICE$QUALITY ADENOTONSILLECTOMY
5809  MEDICAL PSYCHOLOGICAL$ASPECTS SP$DIS VOICE$DISTURBANCES
5809  VOICE$DIS
5903  BIBLIOGRAPHY VOICE$DIS

5904   VOICE$QUALITY ANXIETY
6013   LARYNGEAL$SYMPTOMS$GOITRE
6414   VOICE$QUALITY DEPRESSION
6704   PITCH$DISCRIM TONAL$MEM ADULT$VOICE$PATIENTS
6704   SIGNIFICANCE HARMONIC$CHANGES NOISE$COMPONENTS HOARSENESS
6713   SYNDROME$SHORTENED$VELUM INNERVATION$SOFT$PALATE
7103   HYPONASALITY PATULOUS$EUS$TUBES CASE$REPORT
7108   VOICE-DIS$CHIL DESCRIPTIVE$APPROACH
7117   AVOIDANCE LABELS EVAL VOICE$DIS
7203   EFFECTS ADENOIDECTOMY SP CHIL POTENTIAL$VELO$DYSFUNCTION
7503   BRODNITZ AGE CASTRATO$VOICE
7606   ISHIZAKA COMPUTER$SIMULATION PATHOLOGICAL$VOCAL-CORD
       $VIBRATION
7703   MOORE VOICE$DISORDERS RESEARCH SP$SCIENCE
7724   SHPRINTZEN INCONGRUOUS$MOVEMENTS VELUM LATERAL$PHARYNGEAL
       $WALLS
7727   COMSTOCK STAMMERING$SYSTEM$ELOCUTION
7803   MURRY SPEAKING$FF$CHAR VOICE$PATHOLOGIES
7813   BRUNNER INFLUENCE VOCAL STRESS VIENNA$BOYS$CHOIR
7813   MONTAGUE PITCH FUNDEMENTAL$FREQUENCY DOWN'S$SYNDROME
       $CHIL

## 0605

5503   METHOD THERAPY PARALYTIC$CONDITIONS
5613   TREATMENT$VOCAL$DISORDERS SPONTANEOUS$IMAGERY
5803   THERAPY NASAL$RESONANCE
5903   CYBERNETICS TREATMENT VOICE$DIS
5903   SP$REHAB LARYNGOPLASTY
6017   PROBLEMS VOICE$THERAPY
6313   TACTILE$APPROACH VOICE$PLACEMENT
6313   X-RAY$PICTURE HYPOPHARYNX PSEUDOGLOTTIS$ESO VOCAL
       REHAB LARYNGECTO
6506   METHOD TRNG SPEAKER PHONATE FUND$FREQ
6605   TRNG$STUDENTS MANAGEMENT VOICE$DIS
6713   VOCAL$REHAB RECONSTRUCTIVE$SURGERY LARYNGEAL$CANCER
7003   VELO$CLOSURE MODIFIED$TONGUE-ANCHOR$TECHNIQUE
7103   SP$REHAB ASAI$METHOD LARYNGOPLASTY
7104   PHYSIOLOGIC$CORRELATES VOCAL$FRY
7203   CONTINGENCIES BIOELECTRIC$MODIFICATION NASALITY
7303   MODIFICATION VELAR$MOVEMENT
7303   SILENT$COUGH$METHOD
7303   SILENT$COUGH$METHOD VOCAL$HYPERFUNCTION
7303   VOICE$THERPY LANG$DELAYED$CHIL

7313   PERCEP$SKILLS CLINICAL$MANAGEMENT NASALITY
7313   VOCAL$CHANGE ATYPICAL$PITCH$INTENSITY LEVELS
7403   DISMISSAL$CRITERIA VOICE$THERAPY
7403   TREATMENT$VOCAL$ABUSE VOCAL$INTENSITY$CONTROLLER
7403   VOICE$PROD RADIOTHERAPY LARYNGEAL$CANCER
7403   VOICE$THERAPY SURGERY$CONTACT$GRANULOMA
7404   SPECTROGRAPHIC$ANALYSIS FUND$FREQ HOARSENESS VOCAL
       $REHAB
7408   PROPRIOCEPTIVE$TACTILE$KINESTHETIC$FEEDBACK VOICE
       $THERAPY
7503   BRODY VISUAL$FEEDBACK NORMAL$VOCAL$INTENSITY RETARDED
       $ADULTS
7503   ZWITMAN TEFLON$INJECTION LOWER$VOCAL$PITCH
7508   ANDREWS COMM$PROB VOICE$THERAPY CHILD
7603   DRUDGE SHAPING$BEHAVIOR VOICE$THERAPY
7613   BERGENDAL MUSICAL$TALENT PROGNOSTIC$INSTRUMENT VOICE
       $TREATMENT
7613   SMITH CHANGES SP (THE ACCENT$METHOD)
7629   KASTON TREATMENT SPASTIC$DYSPHONIA
7803   PROSEK EMG$BIOFEEDBACK TREATMENT HYPERFUNCTIONAL$VOICE
7803   REICH TEFLON$LARYNGOPLASTY


                          0606


7727   COMBE FELIX VOISIN'S CAUSES CURES STAMMERING


                          0607


5403   MERITS BACKWARD$PLAYING$SP SCALING VOICE$QUALITY$DIS
6003   TECHNIQUES TESTING HYPERNASAL$VOICE
6113   PHONIATRIC$CONTRIBUTIONS LANG$RESEARCH
6313   LARYNGEAL$ANALOG SYNTHESIS$HARSH$VOICE$QUALITY
6613   EARLY$DIAGNOSIS ABNORMAL$PALATAL$MOBILITY CINE
6613   LARYNGEAL$ANALOG SYNTHESIS$JITTER$SHIMMER AUD$PARAMETERS
       $HARSHNESS
6704   AIR$FLOW VOCAL$FRY
6713   STUDY VELO$FUNCTION PERCEIVED$NASALITY VOWELS CINE
       $TV$MONITOR
6917   ROLE PHONETIC$CONTEXTS ARTIC$MOVEMENTS FACILITATION
       ESO$TONE
7003   SIMILARITIES GLOSSOPHARYNGEAL$BREATHING INJECTION
       $METHODS AIR$INTA

7104   SUBGLOTTAL$PRESSURE AIR$FLOW$MEAS VOCAL$FRY
7203   ADULT$VOICE$SCREENING
7313   LAMINAGRAPHIC$STUDY VOCAL$FRY
7512   KIM CLINICAL$SUPRASEGMENTAL$FEATURE$SYSTEM
7603   HESS ASSESSMENT VELOPHARYNGEAL$ADEQUACY MANOMETRIC
7603   WOLFE SPECTROGRAPHIC$COMPARISON SPASTIC$DYSPHONIA
7603   ZWITMAN ASSESS ORAL$TELESCOPE RADIOGRAPHIC$EXAM VELO
       $INADEQUACY
7606   ISHIZAKA COMPUTER$SIMULATION PATHOLOGICAL$VOCAL-CORD
       $VIBRATION
7613   BERGENDAL MUSICAL$TALENT PROGNOSTIC$INSTRUMENT VOICE
       $TREATMENT
7624   FLETCHER "NASALANCE" VS LISTENER$JUDGEMENTS NASALITY
7624   KRISCHER MATHEMATICS TREATMENT$EVALUATION
7624   SHELTON EVALUATION VELO$CLOSURE
7624   WATSON PPVT INTELLIGENCE CHIL PALATAL$PROBLEMS
7629   STARK RELIABILITY VOICE$PROFILING$SYSTEM
7703   DALY BIOELECTRONIC$MEASUREMENT NASALITY TMR CHIL
7710   MONTGOMERY INTERACTIVE EFFECTS SEX ANDROGYNY
7724   VANDEMARK PREDICTIVE$VALUE IPAT
7729   HARTMAN SEX$IDENTIFICATION ALARYNGEAL$SP
7803   NETSELL NONINVASIVE$METHOD ESTIMATING$SUBGLOTTAL$AIR
       $PRESSURE
7813   BOENNINGHAUSEN SOUND-ANALYTICAL$STUDIES FORMATION
       SUBSTITUTE$VOICE
7813   GORDON AIR$FLOW MECHANICAL$DYSPHONIA
7813   KLINGHOLZ EVALUATION HOARSENESS
7813   PFAU PERSONALITY PHONIATRIC DIAGNOSIS
7829   HARTMAN MANAGEMENT HYPERFUNCTIONAL$VOICE$DIS CHILD
7829   PENNER OCCUPATIONAL$ACCEPTABILITY NASALITY


## 0701

7605   PICKERING BILINGUAL+BICULTURAL$EDUCATION SP$PATHOLOGIST
7833   ADAMS CORRELATES STRESS NATIVE NON-NATIVE SPEAKERS
       ENGLISH


## 0702

5503   REHAB ADULTS DYSARTHRIC$SP
5603   ARTIC$PROBLEMS PLACEMENT ORTHODONTIC$APPLIANCES
5618   STUDY DEFECTIVE$SP OPEN-BITE$MALOCCLUSION

5813   DYSARTHRIA FROM AMYOTROPHIC$MYOTONIA
6103   ARTIC REL DENTAL$ABNORMALITIES
6303   DYSARTHRIA OROPHARYNGEAL$REFLEXOLOGY
6403   COMPARATIVE$STUDY NORMAL$DEFECTIVE$ARTIC REL MALOCCLUSION
       DEGLUTIT
6403   LONGITUDINAL$STUDY ARTIC DEGLUTITION MALOCCLUSION
6403   SEVERE$ARTIC$DIS MOTOR$ABILITY
6507   EFFECTS OROFACIAL$ANOMALIES SP
6603   LISPING THUMB-SUCKING CHIL OPEN-BITE$MALOCCLUSIONS
6603   TONGUE-PALATE$CONTACT PALATE$DEFECTS
6613   LISTENER$CONFUSIONS R DYSARTHRIC$SP
6804   CEPHALOMETRIC$STUDY DEFECTIVE$S$ARTIC VARIATIONS INCISOR
       $DENTITION
6903   EVAL VELO$FUNCTION DYSARTHRIA
6903   HYPOPLASIA TONGUE
6903   VOICE$ARTIC$DEFECTS PARALYSIS$GLOMUS
6904   CHANGES OROPHARYNGEAL$CAVITY$SIZE DYSARTHRIC$CHIL
6904   CLUSTERS DEVIANT$SP$DIMENSIONS DYSARTHRIAS
7003   ANALYSIS ARTIC PARTIAL$TOTAL$GLOSSECTOMY
7004   LIST EST DYSARTHRIC$SINGLE$WORD$INTELLIGIBILITY
7004   PHONEMIC$VARIABILITY APRAXIA$SP
7007   MODIFICATION ORAL-FACIAL$FUNCTION SP
7007   RESTORATIVE$TREATMENT DENTOFACIAL$COMPLEX
7103   COMPENSATORY$PHYSIOLOGIC$PHONETICS GLOSSECTOMEE
7103   COMPENSATORY$PHYSIOLOGIC$PHONETICS GLOSSECTOMEE
7103   LIP$TAPING BUCCAL-LABIAL$INSUFFICIENCY
7104   EFFECTS MOTOR$SENSORY$DISRUPTION SP DESCRIPTION ARTIC
7203   CHANGES PHONATORY$ASPECTS GLOSSECTOMEE$INTELLIGIBILITY
7203   CHANGES PHONATORY$ASPECTS GLOSSECTOMEE$INTELLIGIBILITY
7204   DYSARTHRIA MS
7303   MODIFICATION$LIP$HYPRRTONIA DYSARTHRIA EMG$FEEDBACK
7314   GLOSSOLALIA REGRESSIVE$SP
7404   DEVELOPMENTAL$APRAXIA$SP CHIL DEFECTIVE$ARTIC
7404   DYSARTHRIA WILSON'S$DISEASE
7503   KENT CINERADIOGRAPHIC$ASSESSMENT ARTICULATORY$MOBILITY
       DYSARTHRIAS
7513   MOORE PHONETIC$CONTEXTS INTELLIGIBILITY CLEFT-PALATE
       $SPEAKERS
7527   LA POINTE PHONEMIC CHARACTERISTICS APRAXIA
7532   KEITH SINGING$THERAPY APRAXIA APHASIA
7603   DABUL THERAPEUTIC$APPROACHES APRAXIA
7603   NETSELL PAROXYSMAL$ATAXIC$DYSARTHRIA
7629   SLOTIUK DYSARTHRIA PARKINSONISM
7632   LECOURS PHONETIC$DISINTEGRATION$SYNDROME ANARTHRIA
7703   BEUKELMAN COMMUNICATION DYSARTHRIC
7703   DISIMONI PHONEME$DURATION$CONTROL UTTERANCE-LENGTH
       APRACTIC

7704    HARDISON EFFECTS LINGUISTIC$VARIABLES APRAXIA
7713    DORDAIN VOICE SP WILSON'S$DISEASE
7729    SLOTUIK OCCLUSION$RELATIONSHIPS ARTIC$BEHAVIOR SCHOOL-AGE
        $CHILD
7729    TUOMI DIADOCHOKINESIS ARTIC IMPAIRMENT
7732    FERGUSON AGRAPHIA SYNTACTIC$WRITING MOTOR$SP + MOVEMENTS
        $DIS
7732    MARTINDALE SYNTACTIC + SEMANTIC$CORRELATES VERBAL
        $TICS GILLES$TOURETTE
7732    MATEER IMPAIRMENT NONVERBAL$ORAL$MOVEMENTS APHASIA
7803    DEAL MODIFICATION EIGHT-STEP$CONTINUUM TREATMENT APRAXIA
        ADULTS
7803    HIROSE ANALYSIS ABNORMAL$ARTIC$DYNAMICS DYSARTHRIC
7804    LARSON EFFECTS CEREBELLAR$LESIONS MONKEY$JAW$FORCE
        $CONTROL
7825    SHANE RHYTHMIC$STIM ARTIC$ACCURACY APRAXIA

## 0703

5403    RATING DEFECTIVE$SP TRAINED$UNTRAINED$OBSERVERS
5403    REL AUD$DISCRIM ARTIC$DEFECTS CHIL NON-ORGANIC$IMPAIRMENT
5407    EFFECT LATENCY STIMULATION R REPROD$SOUNDS
5407    INFLUENCE ORAL$VS$PICTORIAL$PRESENTATION ARTIC$TESTING
5407    RELIABILITY EVAL ARTIC STIMULATION$TESTING
5407    SPONTANEOUS$IMPROVEMENT ARTIC R ORAL PICTURE$ARTIC
        $TESTS
5503    MEAS SEVERITY ARTIC$DEFECTIVENESS
5503    RELIABILITY INDIV$RATINGS SEVERITY DEFECTIVE$ARTIC
5503    STUDY REL ARTIC$ABILITY LANG$ABILITY
5506    ARTIC$TESTING STANDARDS ARTIC$TESTS
5703    SCALING$METHODS ARTIC$DEFECTIVENESS
5710    PREDICTIVE$EFFICIENCY BATTERY$ARTIC$DIAGNOSITC$TESTS
5803    PROGNOSTIC$TESTING FUNCTIONAL$ARTIC$DIS CHIL
5810    OBSERVED$PREDICTED$ESTIMATES RELIABILITY SP$ARTIC
        $RATING$SCALE
5814    ARTIC$TESTS INTELLIGIBILITY
5903    SP$ERROR$RECOGNITION$ABILITY
5904    PHONETIC$STUDY MISARTIC$R
6003    FUNCTIONAL$ARTIC$DEFECT PERFORMANCE NONVERBAL$TASK
6003    NUMERICAL$MEAS ARTIC
6003    PREDICTION ARTIC$ABILITY KINDERGARTEN$TESTS
6004    ARTIC$TEST$MEAS LISTENER$RATINGS ARTIC$DEFECTIVENESS
6004    PROCEDURES SCALING ARTIC
6004    REL AUD$PERCEP$FACTORS ARTIC$ABILITY

| | |
|---|---|
| 6004 | SCALING DEFECTIVE$ARTIC DIRECT$MAGNITUDE$ESTIMATION |
| 6104 | ARTIC$TEST VELO$CLOSURE |
| 6104 | PITCH$DISCRIM ARTIC |
| 6203 | EXPERIENCE ARTIC$EXAMINERS |
| 6203 | EXPERIENCE ARTIC$EXAMINERS |
| 6203 | NUMERICAL$MEAS ARTIC |
| 6203 | PASSAGE SP$SCREENING SCH |
| 6203 | PICTURE$ARTIC$TEST |
| 6204 | ANALYSIS CORRELATIONS ARTIC$DEVIATIONS |
| 6204 | MOTOR$AUD$ABILITIES CHIL ARTIC$DEVIATIONS |
| 6204 | PREDICTIVE$SCREENING$TEST ARTIC$MATURATION |
| 6303 | ARTIC$DEVIATIONS R CLINICAL$MEAS SOUND$DISCRIM |
| 6303 | INFLUENCE TESTING$INSTRUMENT ARTIC$R CHIL |
| 6303 | INFLUENCE TESTING$INSTRUMENT ARTIC$R CHIL |
| 6303 | PHONOLOGICAL$ANALYSIS DYSLALIA |
| 6303 | REL SP$DISCRIM ARTIC$DEFECTS |
| 6303 | SP$DEFECTS ORAL$FUNCTIONS |
| 6303 | TEMPORAL$RELIABILITY ARTIC$TESTING |
| 6304 | ANALYSIS ARTIC$R SCH$CHIL |
| 6304 | EFFECTS GRP$PRESSURE JUDGMENTS SP$SOUNDS |
| 6306 | INVESTIGATION PRECISION ARTIC$TESTING$PROGRAM |
| 6403 | AUD$DISCRIM CONSISTENCY ARTIC$R$PHONEME |
| 6404 | COMPARISON GRAMMAR$CHIL FUNCTIONALLY$DEVIANT$SP |
| 6404 | INTELLIGIBILITY$MEAS DYSARTHRIC$SP |
| 6406 | ARTIC*TEST CONTROL CIRCUITS |
| 6410 | COMPARATIVE$STUDY SOUND$SUBSTITUTIONS |
| 6504 | ORAL$LANG$SKILLS CHIL DEFECTIVE$ARTIC |
| 6506 | ARTIC-TESTING$METHODS CONSONANTAL$DIFFERENTIATION CLOSED-R$SET |
| 6603 | PERSISTENCE OPEN$SYLLABLE DEFECTIVE$ARTIC |
| 6604 | MEAS ARTIC$MERIT |
| 6605 | CASE$SELECTION SCH ARTIC$DIS |
| 6703 | AUD$DISCRIM ARTIC |
| 6703 | DEV FILMSTRIP$ARTIC$TEST |
| 6703 | USE TV STUDY ARTIC$PROBLEMS |
| 6704 | ARTIC$PROBLEMS ABILITY STORE$PROCESS$STIMULI |
| 6704 | NOMOGRAM ARTIC$PROD |
| 6704 | TASK EVAL ARTIC$CHANGE COMPARISON TASK$SCORES BASELINE |
| 6704 | TASK EVAL ARTIC$CHANGE DEV$METHODOLOGY |
| 6706 | RHYMING$MINIMAL$CONTRASTS DIAG$ARTIC$TEST |
| 6711 | EFFECT BACKGROUND$SP PHONEME$DISCRIM CHIL DEFECTIVE $ARTIC |
| 6804 | COMPARISON TRADITIONAL$CONDENSED$ARTIC$TESTS NUMBER $SOUNDS |
| 6804 | PHONETIC$DISTORTIONS SERIAL$TRANSMISSION SHORT$SP $SAMPLES |

| | |
|---|---|
| 6817 | DISTINCTIVE$FEATURE$ANALYSIS ARTIC$ERRORS SIBLINGS |
| 6820 | ARTIC$RATE ARTIC$DIS CHIL |
| 6903 | PREDICTIVE$SCREENING$TEST$ARTIC |
| 6904 | DIFFERENTIAL$DIAGNOSTIC$PATTERNS DYSARTHRIA |
| 6904 | PROCEDURE TESTING$POSITION$GENERALIZATION ARTIC$TRNG |
| 6904 | REL ARTIC AUD$ABILITIES VARIABLES |
| 6904 | RELIABILITY$JUDGMENTS ARTIC$PROFICIENCY |
| 6904 | TASK EVAL ARTIC$CHANGE IMITATIVE$TASK$SCORES SPONTANEOUS $TASK$SCOR |
| 6906 | COMMENTS LEARNING ARTIC$TESTING MISTUNED$SINGLE-SIDEBAND $LINKS |
| 6910 | CORRELATIONS TIMBRE$DISCRIM ARTIC$SCORING |
| 6911 | PITCH$DISCRIM SP$DISCRIM ARTIC$DEFECTIVE$CHIL |
| 6913 | LINGUAL$PRESSURE CHIL$ARTIC$DIS |
| 6913 | R$CHIL REDUCED$PHONEMIC$SYSTEMS SEASHORE$MEAS$MUSICAL $TALENTS |
| 6914 | EXPERIMENTALLY$ELICITED ARTIC$BEHAVIOR |
| 6917 | ARTIC$TESTING INSTRUCTIONAL$MOTIVATION |
| 7003 | ANALYSIS ARTIC$BEHAVIOR SP-DEFECTIVE$CHIL CONNECTED $SP ISOLATED$WO |
| 7003 | GENERATIVE$STUDIES CHIL$PHONOLOGICAL$DIS |
| 7004 | COMMENT REL ARTIC$DEFICITS SYNTAX SPEECH$DEFECTIVE $CHIL |
| 7004 | CONSISTENCY JUDGMENTS ARTIC$PROD |
| 7006 | REPLY PITFALLS ADAPTIVE$TESTING |
| 7007 | ARTIC$ASSESSMENT |
| 7008 | CASE$SELECTION SCH ARTIC$DIS |
| 7014 | ARTIC$TEST LINGUISTIC$TECHNIQUE |
| 7014 | GENERAL$LANG$DEFICITS CHIL$ARTIC$DIS |
| 7103 | DISTINCTIVE$FEATURE$ANALYSIS CHIL$MISARTIC |
| 7103 | PRELIMINARY$VIEW INFORMATION$THEORY ARTIC$OMISSIONS |
| 7104 | CONSONANT$INTELLIGIBILITY RELIABILITY VALIDITY SP $ASSESSMENT |
| 7203 | ARTIC$DIS CLINICAL$APPLICATIONS DISTINCTIVE$FEATURE $THEORY |
| 7204 | ANALYSIS SUBSTITUTION$ERRORS STANDARD$ENG$SPEAKING $CHIL |
| 7204 | ANALYSIS SUBSTITUTION$ERRORS STANDARD$ENG$SPEAKING $CHIL |
| 7204 | EFFECTS SIMILARITY SOUND$SUBSTITUTIONS RETENTION |
| 7204 | IMITATIVE$SPONTANEOUS$ARTIC$ASSESSMENT PRESCH$CHIL |
| 7204 | ITEM$CONTEXT S$PHONE$ARTIC$TEST$RESULTS |
| 7204 | LANG$COMPREHENSION AUD$DISCRIM ARTIC$DEFICIENT$CHIL |
| 7212 | SP$DISCRIM ARTIC$DEFECTIVE$CHIL |
| 7214 | DISTINCTIVE$FEATURE$ANALYSIS CONSONANTAL$SUBSTITUTION $PATTERN |

7303   DENVER$ARTICULATION$SCREENING$EXAM
7304   SHORT-TERM$MEMORY LANG$SKILLS ARTIC-DEFICIENT$CHIL
7312   STUDY SPONTANEOUS$REMISSION ARTIC$DEFECTS SCH$CHIL
7314   CHIL ATTENTION ARTIC
7317   ORAL$VIBROTACTILE$THR ORAL$FACIAL$ANOMALIES ARTIC
       $DEFECTS
7403   COUNTING$TO$TWENTY MEAS DIADOCHOKINETIC$SYLLABLE$RATE
7403   MARKEDNESS$THEORY ARTIC$ERRORS
7403   REVIEW DENVER$ARTICULATION$SCREENING$EXAM
7404   NEUROPSYCHOLOGICAL$INVEST FUNCTIONAL$DIS$ARTIC
7404   REL ARTIC$DEFECTS SOUND$IDENTIFICATION
7408   RELATIONSHIP SELF$CONCEPT REMISSION ARTICULATORY$ERRORS
7503   MCREYNOLDS ARTICULATORY-DEFECTIVE$CHIL$DISCRIM PRODUCTION
       $ERRORS
7503   PETERSON NASAL$EMISSION MISARTICULATION$SIBILANTS
       $AFFRICATES
7503   SHRIBERG RESPONSE$EVOCATION$PROGRAM
7504   WILLIAMS REL DISCRIM ARTICULATION$TRAINING CHILD MISARTICULATIONS
7508   BARRETT PREDICTIVE$ARTIC SCREENING
7513   LARIVIERE INTELLIGIBILITY GLOSSECTOMEE PERCEP ACOUS
7513   MOORE PHONETIC$CONTEXTS INTELLIGIBILITY CLEFT-PALATE
       $SPEAKERS
7527   ALLISON RELATIONSHIP ARTIC$DIS SELF-MONITORING$AUD
       $DISCRIM
7527   WILSON INFLUENCE PRE-INFORMATION RATING$ARTICULATION
7603   MANNING AUDITORY$MASKING AUTOMATIZATION ARTICULATORY
       $PRODUCTION
7604   MOORE STIMULABILITY ARTIC$/S/ CLUSTER FREQ$OCCURRENCE
7627   LASS TIME-EXPANDED$SP DIAGNOSIS ARTIC
7703   KUEHN CINE$INVESTIGATION CHILDREN'S$SUBSTITUTIONS
7703   MULLEN STIMULUS$PICTURE$IDENTIFICATION ARTICULATION
       $TESTING
7703   PAYNTER IMITATIVE SPONTANEOUS ARTICULATORY$ASSESSMENT
       CHIL
7704   ARNDT IDEN DESCRIPTION HOMOGENEOUS$SUBGROUPS MISARTIC
       $CHIL
7704   HOFFMAN CONTEXTUAL-COARTICULATORY$INCONSISTENCY R
       $MISARTICULATION
7704   MCNUTT ORAL$SENSORY MOTOR$BEHAVIORS CHILD MISARTICULATIONS
7704   PARNELL SUBJECTIVE$EVAL ARTIC$EFFORT
7704   SHELTON DELAYED$JUDGEMENT$DISCRIM ARTIC$STATUS
7708   MASON OROFACIAL$EXAM$CHECKLIST
7713   ANDREWS INTELLIGIBILITY CEREBRAL PALSIED SP
7727   KELLY VIBROTACTILE$SENSATION CHILDREN NORMAL$DEFECTIVE
       $ARTIC
7727   STEPHENS FACTORS AFFECTING JUDGEMENT

7729   TUOMI DIADOCHOKINESIS ARTIC IMPAIRMENT
7733   CHRISTE LINGUISTIC$INTRODUCTION ARTIC SP
7803   DUBIOS COMPARISON METHODS OBTAINING$ARTIC$R
7804   ELBERT MISARTICULATING$CHILDREN'S$GENERALIZATION
7804   JORDAN PERFORMANCE CHIL GOOD + POOR$ARTICULATION TONGUE
       $PLACEMENT
7812   KIM CLINICAL$SUPRASEGMENTAL$FEATURE$SYSTEM
7827   YORKSTON MEAS INTELLIGIBILITY DYSARTHRIC$SP

## 0704

5403   DEV ·EVAL SP$IMPROVEMENT$PROGRAM SCH$CHIL
5403   STUDY RECORDED$ARTIC$EXERCISES
5407   EFFECTIVENESS COMBINED$VISUAL-AUD$STIMULATION IMPROVING
       ARTIC
5407   INFLUENCE INCREASED$STIMULATION PROD UNFAMILIAR$SOUND
       FUNCTION TIM
5420   SP$THERAPY CONSIDERATIONS CHIL FUNCTIONAL$ARTIC$DIS
5703   COMPARISON AURAL$STIMULATION$METHODS TEACHING$SP$SOUNDS
5703   EVAL SPECIAL$SCH SP$DEFECTIVE$CHIL
5703   USE NONSENSE$SYLLABLE ARTIC$THERAPY
5709   TEACHING$SP
5715   TECHNIQUE DEV POST-PLOSIVE$ASPIRATION
5810   EFFECT CREATIVE$ACTIVITIES ARTIC$CHIL SP$DIS
5904   TRNG$PARENTS CHIL FUNCTIONAL$MISARTIC
6003   TV-CLASSROOM ARTIC$PROGRAM
6103   EFFECTS SP$THERAPY SP$IMPROVEMENT ARTIC READING
6103   THERAPEUTIC$ORAL$DEVICE LATERAL$EMISSION
6104   MATERNAL$ENVIRONMENTAL$FACTORS REL SUCCESS SP$IMPROVEMENT
       $TRNG
6116   SP$IMPROVEMENT ARTIC$TRNG
6117   SP$IMPROVEMENT MATERIALS METHODS
6203   EFFECTS DURATIONS SP$IMPROVEMENTS ARTIC READING
6203   EFFECTS DURATIONS SP$IMPROVEMENTS ARTIC READING
6304   PHONEME-SOUND$GENERALIZATION FUNCTION PHONEME$SIMILARITY
       VERBAL$UN
6403   EFFECTS MATERNAL$ATTITUDES IMPROVEMENT ARTIC MOTHERS
       TRAINED
6403   EFFECTS MATERNAL$ATTITUDES IMPROVEMENT ARTIC MOTHERS
       TRAINED
6405   TIME$ALLOCATION ARTIC$PROGRAM
6510   MODIFICATION FUNCTIONAL$ARTIC$ERRORS INSTRUMENTAL
       $CONDITIONING
6517   INTERFERENCE$THEORY ARTIC$CORRECTION

| | |
|---|---|
| 6703 | APPROACH CORRECTION DEFECTIVE$PHONEME$R |
| 6703 | APPROACH CORRECTION DEFECTIVE$PHONEME$R |
| 6704 | EFFECTIVENESS ARTIC$THERAPY SCH$CHIL |
| 6704 | EFFECTS TYPES$STIMULATION ARTIC$R SP$DEFECTIVE$CHIL |
| 6807 | REGULATING$ROLE SP FORMATION VOLUNTARY$MOVEMENTS |
| 6903 | EVAL SP$THERAPY PRECISION$RECORDING |
| 7003 | EFFECTS R$CONTINGENT$PUNISHMENT DEFECTIVE$ARTIC$R |
| 7003 | PATTERNING DEVIANT$ARTIC |
| 7003 | PROGRAM ARTIC$THERAPY ADMINISTERED$BY$MOTHERS |
| 7004 | FACTORS EFFECTIVENESS ARTIC$THERAPY EMR$CHIL |
| 7007 | STIMULUS$CONTROL PHONEME$ARTIC OPERANT$TECHNIQUES |
| 7015 | ARTIC$TRNG VISUAL$SP |
| 7103 | STUDY EFFECTIVENESS S-PACK$PROGRAM ELIMINATION FRONTAL $LISPING CHI |
| 7103 | TRANSFER$TRNG ARTIC$THERAPY |
| 7104 | AUTOMATED$PROGRAM$THERAPY ARTIC$CORRECTION |
| 7104 | PREDICTION ARTIC$IMPROVEMENT THERAPY EARLY$LESSON $SOUND$PROD |
| 7108 | EFFECT FREQ SP$THERAPY MEAS ARTIC$PROFICIENCY |
| 7108 | PROCEDURES COUNTING CHARTING TARGET$PHONEME |
| 7108 | STRUCTURED$PROGRAM MODIFYING$R$MISARTIC |
| 7203 | DISTINCTIVE$FEATURE$GENERALIZATION ARTIC$TRNG |
| 7203 | GENERALIZATION OPERANT$SP$THERAPY MISARTIC |
| 7203 | STRUCTURING$SP$THERAPY$CONTINGENCIES ORAL$APRAXIC $CHIL |
| 7204 | EFFECTS TIMED$CORRECT$SOUND$PROD CARRYOVER |
| 7204 | TEACH$UNFAMILIAR$SOUNDS$ISOLATION |
| 7208 | SELF-DIRECTING$APPROACH ARTIC$THERAPY |
| 7208 | USE BEEP$TAPE SPEED$UP$ARTIC$R |
| 7211 | SP$TRNG MUSICAL$EAR-TRNG PITCH-DEFICIENT$CHIL ARTIC $DEFECTS |
| 7212 | DISTINCTIVE$FEATURE$MODEL DIAGNOSIS PROGNOSIS THERAPY |
| 7214 | ARTIC$GENERALIZATION ARTIC$TRNG |
| 7303 | LEXICAL$APPROACH REMEDIATION FINAL$SOUND$OMISSIONS |
| 7317 | EFFECTS SCHEDULING ARTIC$THERAPY |
| 7408 | EFFECTIVENESS S-PACK CHIL |
| 7408 | FIELD$STUDY PROGRAMMED$ARTICULATION$THERAPY |
| 7408 | SHORT-TERM$LISP$CORRECTION DISTRIBUTION$CLINICIANS $TIME |
| 7503 | ELBERT TRANSFER /R/ CONTEXTS |
| 7503 | SHRIBERG RESPONSE$EVOCATION$PROGRAM |
| 7508 | BOWN TECHNIQUES CORRECTING$R$MISARTIC |
| 7508 | COSTELLO ARTIC$INSTRUC DISTINCTIVE$FEATURE$TREORY |
| 7508 | GALLOWAY PARAPROFESSIONAL$PERSONNEL ARTIC THERAPY |
| 7508 | HALL THERAPY NASAL$LISP |
| 7508 | RUSCELLO WORD$POSITION ARTIC THERAPY |

```
7512    IRWIN PAIRED$STIMULI$MONOGRAPH
7512    KIM SEGMENTAL$FEATURE ENGLISH NUCLEI$SEMIVOWELS CONSONANTS
7512    MCCABE MULTIPLE$PHONEMIC$APPROACH ARTIC$THERAPY
7603    COSTELLO MODIFICATION ARTICULATION DISTINCTIVE$FEATURE
        $THEORY
7603    COSTELLO GENERALIZATION ARTICULATION$INSTRUCTION
7603    DABUL THERAPEUTIC$APPROACHES APRAXIA
7603    MANNING AUDITORY$MASKING AUTOMATIZATION ARTICULATORY
        $PRODUCTION
7627    COSTELLO PUNISHMENT$CONTINGENCIES ARTIC$INSTRUCTION
7627    COSTELLO MODIFICATION INCORRECT$R OFF-TASK$BEHAVIORS
        ARTIC$INSTRUCTION
7627    RITTERMAN THERAPIST$HABITUATION CLIENT$PROGRESS ARTIC
        $THERAPY
7629    CAMPBELL COMPETING$SP DISMISSAL$DECISIONS ARTIC$THERAPY
7629    FAHEY PARENT$CONDUCTED ARTIC$MODIFICATION
7629    HOLDGRAFER TRANSFER ARTIC$TRAINING MORPHOLOGICAL$CONTEXTS
7703    GERBER PROGRAMMING ARTICULATION$MODIFICATION
7703    MANNING CORRECT$PRODUCTION ARTICULATORY$ACQUISITION
7708    WATERS PRECISION$THERAPY
7727    CHAPEY ADULT$ARTIC$ERRORS BASED DISTINCTIVE$FEATURE
        $THERAPY
7727    PAYNTER EFFECTS EXAMINER RACE ARTIC BLACK$CHILDREN
7727    RIEBER HISTORICAL THEORY THERAPY STUTTERING
7803    HALL FOLLOWUP$STUDY CHILD ARTIC+LANG$DISORDERS
7803    SHELTON ASSESS PARENT-ADMINISTERED$LISTENING$TRAINING
        PRESCHOOL$CHILD
7812    KIM KIM,S$SEGMENTAL$FEATURE SYSTEM DEVIANT$ARTIC$MOTOR
        $BEHAVIOR
7829    GUESS BEHAVIORAL$APPROACH SP$DEFICIENT$CHILD
```

## 0705

```
5603    PARENTAL$ATTITUDES DEV$SP$PROBLEMS
5713    DYSLALIA TWIN$GIRLS
6003    LITERATURE$SURVEY ARTIC$MATURATION
6204    DIFFERENCES CHIL SPONTANEOUSLY$OUTGROW CHIL RETAIN
        $FUNCTIONAL$ARTI
6403    SEVERE$ARTIC$DIS MOTOR$ABILITY
6603    PERSISTENCE OPEN$SYLLABLE DEFECTIVE$ARTIC
7208    REVIEW DEV$APRAXIA$SP
7417    PSYCHOLOGICAL$DIMENSION SP$THERAPY FUNCTIONAL$ARTIC
7512    PANAGOS PHONOLOGY$GRAMMATICAL$REDUCTION DELAYED$SP
```

## 0706

```
5603    ARTIC$DIS PERSONALITY
```

5610    PARENTAL$OCCUPATIONAL$CLASSIFICATION ARTIC$MATURATION
5713    TONGUEDNESS
5803    REL MISSPELLING MISARTIC
5913    DEFECTS$ARTIC
6003    ATTITUDES MOTHERS ARTIC-IMPAIRED$SP-RETARDED$CHIL
6003    OVERPROTECTIVE$TENDENCIES SP-IMPAIRED$CHIL
6003    PARENTAL$OCCUPATIONAL$CLASS ARTIC$DEFECTIVE$CHIL
6013    TACHYLALIA
6103    VISCERAL$SWALLOWING MALOCCLUSION
6113    PHONIATRIC$CONTRIBUTIONS LANG$RESEARCH
6203    REL MISSING$TEETH CONSONANT$SOUNDS
6305    DYSLALIAS
6503    INCIDENCE VISCERAL$SWALLOW LISPERS
6718    LISP ADULTS
6814    DISTINCTIVENESS DEFECTIVE$FRICATIVE$SOUNDS
7013    TACHYPHEMIA
7303    DEVIANT$ARTIC
7304    PATTERNS$TONGUE$CONTACT LISPING$SPEAKERS
7408    ARTICULATION$ISSUES$NEEDS RESEARCH
7412    LONGITUDINAL$STUDY SPONTANEOUS$REMISSION ARTIC$DEFECTS
        SCH$CHIL
7413    COMPARISON LINGUAL$PRESSURE LISPING
7414    THEORETICAL$CONSIDERATIONS ARTIC$SUBSTITUTIONS
7503    MCREYNOLDS ARTICULATORY-DEFECTIVE$CHIL$DISCRIM PRODUCTION
        $ERRORS
7503    PETERSON NASAL$EMISSION MISARTICULATIONS$SIBILANTS
        $AFFRICATES
7504    PANAGOS SP$COMPREHENSION DEVIENT+NORMAL$SPEAKING$CHILD
7504    WINITZ SELF-RETRIEVAL ARTIC$RETENTION
7513    ONDRACKOVA COMPENSATORY$PRONUNCIATION VELAR$CONSONANTS
7527    ROSEN MORPHOLOGICAL$INFLECTIONS CHILDREN NORMAL IMPAIRED
        ARTIC
7603    SILVERMAN LISTENERS'$IMPRESSIONS LATERAL$LISPS
7703    KUEHN CINE$INVESTIGATION CHILDREN'S$SUBSTITUTIONS
7704    ARNDT IDEN DESCRIPTION HOMOGENEOUS$SUBGROUPS MISARTIC
        $CHIL
7704    MCNUTT ORAL$SENSORY MOTOR$BEHAVIORS CHILD MISARTICULATIONS


                              0801


5403    INTEGRATION PSYCHOTHERAPY SP$THERAPY CONFLICT$THEORY
        STUTTERING
5603    STUTTERING REL GOAL$GRADIENT$HYPOTHESIS
5709    STUTTERING THEORIES THERAPIES

5803   STUTTERING PSYCHIATRIC$VIEWPOINT
5814   DEV$CRISIS$THEORY STUTTERING
5819   PUBLIC$OPINION CAUSES STUTTERING
5918   THEORETICAL$FORMULATION STUTTERING
6003   CONCEPTS$STUTTERING
6004   ANXIETY HOSTILITY STUTTERING
6103   DEV$STUTTERING THEORETICAL$CLINICAL$IMPLICATIONS
6103   MATERNAL$REJECTION STUTTERING
6103   STUTTERING SPINAL$MENINGITIS
6203   GUILT SHAME TENSION GRAPHIC$PROJECTIONS STUTTERING
6303   STUTTERING ENDOCRINE$MALFUNCTION
6309   BLUEMEL$INFLUENCE STUTTERING$THEORY
6413   PGSR$STUTTERERS
6603   ADEQUACY LEARNING$PRINCIPLES INTERPRETATION STUTTERING
6603   STUTTERING LEARNED$BEHAVIOR
6613   STUTTERING AUTOMATIC$CONTROL$VIEW
6704   GRAMMATICAL$FUNCTION REL STUTTERING CHIL
6709   PYKNOLEPSY STUTTERING
6813   LEARNING$PRINCIPLE STUTTERING
6813   STAMMERING CEREBRAL$LESIONS CHIL
6903   STUTTERING PHONETIC$TRANSITION$DEFECT
6913   DISTURBANCES HISTIDINE$METABOLISM HEREDITARY$STAMMERING
6920   STUTTERING$THEORIES
7003   SIGNAL$DETECTION$HYPOTHESIS PERCEP$DEFECT$THEORY STUTTERING
7012   STUTTERING BEHAVIORAL$MODEL
7203   ANTICIPATORY$STRUGGLE$HYPOTHESIS IMPLICATIONS VARIABILITY
       STUTTERI
7304   GRAMMATICAL$FACTOR CHIL$DISFLUENCY CONTINUITY$HYPOTHESIS
7503   LEITH CULTURAL$INFLUENCES TREATMENT BLACK$STUTTERER
7505   LANDER STUTTERING THEORY
7703   SHEEHAN HEREDITY STUTTERING
7727   QUARRINGTON THEORIES STUTTERING THERAPEUTIC APPROACH
7727   SNYDER PSYCHODYNAMIC THEORY THERAPY STUTTERING
7727   WARREN STUTTERING
7727   WEBSTER THEORY STUTTERING EMPIRICISM
7727   WINGATE THEORY THERAPY STUTTERING
7727   WINGATE SOURCE STUTTERING
7728   DALE DYSFLUENT BILINGUAL$CUBAN$AMERICAN
7728   KIDD GENETIC STUTTERING
7728   RECORDS HANDEDNESS STUTTERING
7803   TRAVIS CEREBRAL$DOMINANCE$THEORY STUTTERING
7827   WOODS STIGMA STUTTERER


                        0802


5513   ROLE$REASSURANCE STUTTERING$THERAPY

5603 STUTTERING ANXIETY FUNCTION EXPERIMENTAL$TRNG
5609 STUTTERING PSYCHODYNAMIC$APPROACH UNDERSTANDING TREATMENT
5703 EFFECTS AUD$MASKING SP$STUTTERERS
5703 PSYCHOTHERAPY SP$THERAPY CONFLICT$TECHNIQUES APPROACH
     $AVOIDANCE
5709 STUTTERING THEORIES THERAPIES
5713 SHADOWING TREATMENT$STAMMERING
5803 STUTTERING$THERAPY JAPAN
5804 SPEAKING$TIME$BEHAVIOR STUTTERER SP$THERAPY
5903 COUNSELING PARENTS STUTTERING$CHIL
5903 USE MEBROBAMATE STUTTERING$THERAPY
6003 NEGATIVE$PRACTICE CLINICAL$OBSERVATIONS
6003 SUGAR$PLACEBOS STUTTERING
6003 TRANQUILIZERS STUTTERING
6004 CLIENT-CENTERED$COUNSELING ADULT$STUTTERERS
6004 GENERALIZATION STUTTERING$BEHAVIOR ASSOCIATIVE$LEARNING
6103 CARBON$DIOXIDE$THERAPY MEDICAL$TREATMENT STUTTERING
6103 RETRNG$PROGRAM ADULT$STUTTERER
6105 STUTTERING$THERAPY
6117 ATTITUDES SCH$THERAPISTS TRNG PRACTICES STUTTERING
     $THERAPY
6120 EVAL STUTTERING$THERAPY
6217 PARENTS TEACHERS UNDERSTAND STUTTERING
6303 DISCUSSION NONFLUENCY STUTTERING OPERANT$BEHAVIOR
6303 EXPERIMENTAL$PROGRAMS STUTTERING$THERAPY
6303 USE TRANQUILIZERS TREATMENT STUTTERING
6319 STUTTERING$HABILITATION
6405 SURVEY COMTEMPORARY$AMERICAN$LITERATURE STUTTERING
     $SP$REHAB
6503 MOTOKINESTHETIC$APPROACH PREVENTION SP$DEFECTS STUTTERING
6503 PROCEDURE GRP$CONSENSUS ADULT$STUTTERING$THERAPY
6503 STRUCTURING$THERAPY THERAPIST STUTTERING$CHIL
6504 REL ADAPTATION CONSISTENCY IMPROVEMENT STUTTERING
     $THERAPY
6513 METHOD TREATMENT$STUTTERING KINETIC$DISCHARGE$THERAPY
6603 MMPI PROGNOSIS STUTTERING$THERAPY
6603 UTILIZATION SEMANTIC$SATIATION STUTTERING THEORETICAL
     $ANALYSIS
6604 CLIENT-CLINICIAN$REL FACTORS STUTTERING$THERAPY
6604 CLIENT-CLINICIAN$REL FACTORS STUTTERING$THERAPY
6604 EFFECTS R$CONTINGENT$SHOCK STUTTERING
6604 EFFECTS SIMULTANEOUSLY$PUNISHING$STUTTERING REWARDING
     $FLUENCY
6617 BLENDING PHRASING TECHNIQUES STUTTERING
6617 EARLY$TREATMENT STUTTERING
6703 PERSONAL$EXPERIENCES STUTTER-AID

6704    EFFECT R$CONTINGENT$VERBAL$PUNISHMENT
6704    METHODOLOGY STUDIES RECOVERY STUTTERING
6714    VERBAL$PUNISHMENT DISFLUENCIES SPONTANEOUS$SP
6803    CHIL$PSYCHIATRIST THERAPY STUTTERING
6803    DAF STUTTERING
6803    DAF STUTTERING
6803    STUTTERING$WORKSHOPS GRP$THERAPY RURAL$SCH
6803    THERAPY ADULT$STUTTERER
6804    EFFECT PUNISHMENT EXPECTANCY$STUTTER FREQ SUBSEQUENT
        $EXPECTANCIES
6804    EFFECTS PHYSICAL$TRNG STUTTERING
6804    MASKING AUD$FEEDBACK STUTTERERS$SP
6804    THERAPY$ADAPTATION STUTTERING REL SP$MEAS THERAPY
        $PROGRESS
6804    TIME-OUT$PUNISHMENT STUTTERING
6807    EVAL TREATMENT$STUTTERING CHIL CATAMNESIS
6807    TREATMENT STUTTERING$NEUROSIS PHYSIOLOGICAL$INTERPRETATION
6903    BEHAVIOR$CHANGE STUTTERING SYSTEMATIC$DESENSITIZATION
6903    CONVERSATIONAL$RATE$CONTROL$THERAPY STUTTERING
6903    DAF SP STUTTERERS
6903    DAF SP STUTTERERS
6903    USES SHEEHAN$SENTENCE$COMPLETION$TEST SP$THERAPY STUTTERING
6904    AVERSIVE$STIMULI
6904    AVERSIVE$STIMULI
6904    EFFECTS NEUTRAL$STIMULUS BUZZER MOTOR$R DISFLUENCIES
6904    VERBAL$PUNISHMENT DISFLUENCY AUGMENTATION DISFLUENCY
        RANDOM$DELIVE
6904    VERBAL$PUNISHMENT DISFLUENCY AUGMENTATION DISFLUENCY
        RANDOM$DELIVE
6911    STUTTERING$INHIBITION HIGH$FREQ$NARROW-BAND$MASKING
7003    CLINICAL$REPORT MEAS EFFECTIVENESS DESENSITIZATION
        $TECHNIQUES
7003    IMPROVEMENT REGRESSION STUTTERERS SHORT-TERM$INTENSIVE
        $THERAPY
7003    TAPE-RECORDED$THERAPY$METHOD STUTTERERS CASE$STUDY
7004    COMMENTS TIME-OUT PUNISHMENT STUTTERING
7004    DECREASE$STUTTERING FUNCTION CONTINUOUS$CONTINGENT
        $AUD$MASKING
7004    EFFECTS DAF SPEECH-RELATED$TASK STUTTERERS
7011    STUTTERING$INHIBITION LIVE$VOICE$INTERVENTION MASKING
        $NOISE
7017    COURSE PROGRESS SYSTEMATIC$DESENSITIZATION STUTTERING
        CASE$REPORT
7020    STUTTERING$GUIDELINES BEGINNING$CLINICIAN
7103    APPLICATION FILIAL$THERAPY CHIL STUTTERING
7103    OPERANT$PROCEDURES STUTTERING$THERAPY CHIL

7103    REFLECTIONS CONCEPTUALIZATION STUTTERING$THERAPY THEORETICAL
        $FRAME
7103    USE PORTABLE$VOICE$MASKER STUTTERING$THERAPY
7104    EFFECTS STUTTERING$FREQ PAIRING$PUNISHMENT$R$COST
        $RF
7104    PUNISHMENT EXPECTANCY$R STUTTERERS
7104    THERAPY STUTTERERS
7104    TIME-OUT$PUNISHMENT STUTTERING
7114    EFFECTS REWARD$SCHEDULE$CHANGES CHIL$SP$FLUENCY
7203    AUD$FEEDBACK STUTTERING
7203    BEHAVIOR$THERAPY PSYCHOANALYSIS TREATMENT SEVERE$CHRONIC
        $STUTTERER
7203    EFFECTS R-CONTINGENT$REWARD CONNECTED$SP CHIL$STUTTER
7203    PERSONAL$REACTIONS STUTTERING$ADULT DAF
7204    APPROACH EVAL STUTTERING$THERAPY
7204    EFFECT REHEARSAL FREQ STUTTERING
7204    EFFECTS ANXIETY$DECONDITIONING STUTTERING$FREQ
7204    EFFECTS AUD$MASKING ANXIETY$LEVEL FREQ$DYSFLUENCY
7204    EQUALITY$INTERVALS LEWIS-SHERMAN$SCALE STUTTERING
        $SEVERITY
7204    EVAL TAPE-RECORDED$METHOD STUTTERING$THERAPY IMPROVEMENT
7204    EXPERIMENTAL$TREATMENT PRESCH$STUTTERING$CHIL
7208    TAPE$RECORDER$THERAPY REHAB$STUTTERING
7213    BEHAVIOR$THERAPY$STUTTERING
7214    EFFECTS R$CONTINGENT$NO DISFLUENCIES
7303    BEHAVIOR$THERAPY STUTTERING REVIEW
7303    DESENSITIZATION STUTTERING
7303    MANAGEMENT DISFLUENT$SP SELF-RECORDING$PROCEDURES
7303    REPLACEMENT$STUTTERING NORMAL$SP
7303    REPLACEMENT$STUTTERING NORMAL$SP
7303    TREATMENT$STUTTERING PRECISION$PUNISHMENT COGNITIVE
        $AROUSAL
7304    EFFECT INTERPOSED$CONDITIONS CONSISTENCY$STUTTERING
7304    PROGRAM INITIAL$STAGES FLUENCY$THERAPY
7313    CONDITIONING NONFLUENCIES AVERSIVE$STIMULUS
7313    STUTTER$THERAPY
7317    THERAPY ADULT$STUTTERERS
7403    FLUENT$SP STUTTERS DAF OPERANT$PROCEDURES
7403    STUTTERING$THERAPY SYMPTOM$LEVEL ATTITUDES
7404    EFFECTS LEVEL$AUD$MASKING VOCAL$CHARACTERISTICS FREQ
        $DISFLUENCY
7404    EFFECTS FOUR-WEEK$INTERVAL CONSISTENCY$STUTTERING
7404    IMMEDIATE$VERSUS$DELAYED$CONSEQUENCES STUTTERING$RESPONSES
7404    MODIFICATION CONTROL RATE$ SPEAKING STUTTERERS
7404    STUTTERERS EXPECTANCIES$IMPROVEMENT R TIME-OUT
7417    CONSIDERATION STUTTERING$THERAPY

7503    COSTELLO ESTABLISHMENT$FLUENCY TIME-OUT$PROCEDURES
7503    HANNA BIOFEEDBACK$TREATMENT STUTTERING
7503    LEITH CULTURAL$INFLUENCES TREATMENT BLACK$STUTTERER
7504    CONTURE INFLUENCE NOISE STUTTERS'$DISFLUENCY
7504    GUITAR REDUCTION STUTTERING ANALOG$EMG$FEEDBACK
7504    INGHAM COVERT+OVERT$ASSESSMENT STUTTERU
7504    INGHAM COVERT+OVERT$ASSESSMENT STUTTERING$THERAPY
        $EVALUATION
7504    MARTIN PUNISHMENT NEGATIVE$RF STUTTERING ELECTRIC
        $SHOCK
7513    ADAMCZYK INFLUENCE REVERBERATING STUTTERING
7603    MANNING VERBAL$VS$TANGIBLE$REWARD CHILDREN STUTTER
7603    PRINS STUTTERERS'$PERCEP THERAPY$IMPROVEMENT POSTTHERAPY
        $REGRESSION
7604    CROSS PRESUMED$FLUENCY$RF$STIMULI
7604    GUITAR PRETREATMENT$FACTORS OUTCOME STUTTERING$THERAPY
7604    HEALEY REDUCTION STUTTERING SINGING
7604    JAMES DURATION EFFECTS TIME-OUT SPEAKING
7613    RANTALA TREATMENT STUTTERING
7627    BERECZ COGNITIVE$CONDITIONING$THERAPY TREATMENT STUTTERING
7628    ADAMS VOICE$ONSET ARTIC$CONSTRICTION SP$SEGMENT STUTTERING
        $ADAPT
7628    AINSWORTH TREATMENT STUTTERING
7628    COHEN ASSERTIVE$TRAINING FLUENCY$SHAPING
7629    BOBERG GROUP$THERAPY STUTTERERS
7703    GENDELMAN TREATMENT STUTTERING
7703    HANNA TRANSFER MAINTENANCE FLUENCY STUTTERING$THERAPY
7703    INGHAM TREATMENT GENERALIZATION STUTTERER CONTINGENCY
        SP$RATE$CONTROL
7708    COOPER CASE-SELECTION$PROCEDURES DISFLUENT$CHILDREN
7708    PETERS EFFECT POSITIVE$REINFORCEMENT FLUENCY
7727    AINSWORTH THEORY CLINICIAN$CHARACTERISTICS$THERAPY
        STUTTERS
7727    ALTROWS MASKING$NOISE FLUENCY$STUTTERERS
7727    KATZ PATENTED$ANTI-STUTTERING$DEVICES
7727    MURPHY CREATIVITY STUTTERING$THEORY THERAPY
7727    QUARRINGTON THEORIES STUTTERING THERAPEUTIC APPROACH
7727    SNYDER PSYCHODYNAMIC THEORY THERAPY STUTTERING
7727    WEBSTER MANIPULATION SP STUTTERERS
7727    WINGATE THEORY THERAPY STUTTERING
7728    ADAMS DIFFERENTIATING NORMALLY$NONFLUENT$CHILD INCIPIENT
        $STUTTERER
7728    ANDREWS HALOPERIDOL STUTTERING
7728    BRANDT TECHNIQUE CONTROLLING DISFLUENCIES DAF
7728    COOPER CONTROVERSIES STUTTERING$THERAPY
7728    HAYDEN DAF OVERT$BEHAVIORS STUTTERERS

7728    HEGDE REINFORCING$FLUENCY STUTTERERS
7728    HUTCHINSON METRONOME$PACING AERODYNAMIC$PATTERNS STUTTERED
        $SP
7728    KLEVANS GROUP$TRAINING COMMUNICATION$SKILLS ADULTS
        STUTTER
7728    MANNING IN$PURSUIT$FLUENCY
7728    POPPEN EFFECTS THERAPIES STUTTERING
7728    REED VERBAL$PUNISHMENT PRESCHOOL$STUTTERERS
7728    SCHWARTZ HOLLINS$PRECISION$FLUENCY$SHAPING$PROGRAM
7728    SCHWARTZ EFFICACY PROTRACTED PRECISION$FLUENCY$SHAPING
7728    WEBSTER PSYCHOTHERAPY STUTTERING
7728    YONOVITZ HIERARCHICAL$SIMULATION STUTTERING$MODIFICATION
        DESENSITIZE
7729    BOBERG MAINTENANCE FLUENCY THERAPY
7803    GUITAR STUTTERING$THERAPY ATTITUDE$CHANGE LONG-TERM
        $OUTCOME
7804    INGHAM PERCEPTUAL$ASSESSMENT NORMALCY$SP STUTTERING
        $THERAPY
7813    NOVAK INFLUENCE DAF STUTTERERS
7827    HANSON CONTINGENT$LIGHT-FLASH STUTTEREING ATTENTION
7827    KAPLAN GESTALT$APPROACH STUTTERING
7827    MANNING TIME-EXPANDED$SP IDENTIFICATION REPETITIONS
        STUTTERERS
7829    INGHAM BEHAVIOR$THERAPY STUTTERING
7829    ST LOUIS MOTOR$SP$AWARENESS STUTTERING

## 0803

5403    ADAPTATION$EFFECT STUTTERING REL THORACIC$ABDOMINAL
        $BREATHING
5403    EVAL STUTTERING
5403    MOTOR$PROFICIENCY STUTTERERS
5403    PERSONALITY$INVENTORY ITEM$ANALYSIS INDIV STUTTER
        OTHER$HANDICAPS
5403    REL STUTTERING SPONTANEOUS$SP SP$CONTENT ADAPTATION
5403    STORE$CLERKS$REACTION STUTTERING
5403    STUDY ADAPTATION RECOVERY STUTTERING SELF-FORMULATED
        $SP
5403    STUDY DIAGNOSIS$STUTTERING SEX$RATIO
5413    IMITATION$STUTTERING
5503    INTERPRETATIONS FACIAL$REACTIONS STUTTERING
5503    LISTENER$ADAPTATION SEVERITY$STUTTERING
5503    MASSETER$MUSCLE$ACTION$POTENTIALS STUTTERED$SP
5503    QUESTIONS ELICIT$STUTTERING$ADAPTATION

```
5503    RELIABILITY UTILITY INDIV$RATINGS SEVERITY STUTTERING
5513    PSYCHOSIS$STUTTERING
5603    CORRELATION MEAS SEVERITY STUTTERING
5603    INCIDENCE STUTTERING OLDER$AGE$GRPS
5603    MMPI$PROFILES STUTTERERS$PARENTS FOLLOW-UP$STUDY
5603    PARENTAL$ENVIRONMENT STUTTERING$CHIL
5603    REL SEVERITY$STUTTERING WORD$CONSPICUOUSNESS
5603    SOCIO-ECONOMIC$FACTORS STUTTERING
5613    PERCEP EVAL$FACTORS$STUTTERING
5703    ADAPTATION RECOVERY OR STUTTERERS
5703    COMPARISON STUTTERERS NON-STUTTERERS
5703    OBSESSIVE-COMPULSIVE$REACTIONS STUTTERERS
5703    PARENTAL$DIAGNOSIS STUTTERING CHIL
5703    POINT$OF$VIEW STUTTERING
5703    STUTTERERS$REACTIONS SP$SITUATION
5709    STUTTERING
5713    GLYCEMIC$CURVE$STUTTERERS
5803    PROJECTIVE$STUDIES STUTTERING
5804    BEHAVIORAL$RIGIDITY ADULT$STUTTERERS
5804    LISTENER$R NONFLUENCIES
5804    RATINGS SEVERITY$STUTTERING
5804    STUTTERING$SEVERITY PROLONGED$SPONTANEOUS$SP
5903    DIAGNOSES$STUTTERING ADOL
5904    CALLING$ATTENTION STUTTERING
5904    EFFECTS HYPERVENTILATION TETANY SP$FLUENCY STUTTERERS
5904    FREQ$ANALYSIS EEG STUTTERERS
5904    MEAS STUTTERING$ADAPTATION
5907    STUTTERING RATE FLUENCY
5909    COMPENDIUM RESEARCH THEORY STUTTERING
5909    UNDERSTANDING STUTTERING ONSET FINDINGS IMPLICATIONS
5910    STUDY BLOOD$CHEMISTRY STUTTERERS HYPNOTIC$CONDITIONS
5919    SEVERITY STUTTERING$RATINGS VISUAL$AUD$PRESENTATIONS
6003    AUDIBILITY$AVOIDANCE NONVOCALIZED$STUTTERERS
6003    DEV$STUTTERING DEV$PHASES
6003    DEV$STUTTERING FEATURES
6003    SERVO-MODEL STUTTERING
6003    SOCIAL$DISTANCE$SCALE STUTTERERS
6003    STUTTERER
6004    EXTENSIONAL$DEFINITION ATTITUDE STUTTERING
6004    PARENTS$DIAGNOSES STUTTERING
6007    STUTTERING NORTH$AMERICAN$INDIANS$SOCIETIES
6020    SP YOUNG$STUTTERERS PRESENCE$MOTHERS
6103    PRIMARY$STUTTERING ADULT
6103    STUDENT STUTTERING STUTTERER
6103    STUTTERER LOW$IQ
6103    STUTTERING FAMILIES ADOPTED$STUTTERERS
```

| | |
|---|---|
| 6104 | ADAPTATION$EFFECT SPONTANEOUS$RECOVERY STUTTERING $EXPECTANCY |
| 6104 | CONSISTENCY$EFFECT STUTTERING$EXPECTANCY |
| 6104 | IDENTIFICATION STUTTERING FLUENT$SP |
| 6104 | MEAS ADAPTATION STUTTERING |
| 6104 | PERSEVERATION STUTTERERS |
| 6104 | WHITE$NOISE STUTTERING |
| 6107 | PREDICTING$RATINGS$SEVERITY STUTTERING |
| 6107 | STUDY SP$BEHAVIOR STUTTERERS DAF |
| 6113 | VIEWPOINTS$ON$STUTTERING |
| 6203 | AVERAGE STUTTERING |
| 6203 | AVERAGE STUTTERING |
| 6203 | EVAL STUTTERING ENVIRONMENTAL$STRESS CRITICAL$APPRAISAL SP |
| 6203 | EVAL STUTTERING IDENTIFICATION STUTTERING USE LABEL |
| 6203 | EVAL STUTTERING SP$CHARACTERISTICS CHIL |
| 6203 | NATURE INCIDENCE STUTTERING BANTU$GRP SCH$CHIL |
| 6203 | STUTTERING SOCIAL$STRUCTURE PACIFIC$SOCIETIES |
| 6204 | EXPERIMENTAL$STUDY PROPERTIES STUTTERED$WORDS |
| 6204 | MEAS CONSISTENCY STUTTERING |
| 6204 | MEAS SEVERITY$STUTTERING SHORT$SEGMENTS$SP |
| 6204 | PHONETIC$INFLUENCES STUTTERING |
| 6204 | STUTTERING PERSEVERATION CHIL |
| 6209 | R$EYE-CONTACT |
| 6209 | STUTTERING NON-WESTERNS |
| 6213 | DYSPHATIC$STUTTERING |
| 6213 | ELECTROPHYSIOLOGICAL$FINDINGS STUTTERERS CLUTTERERS |
| 6303 | CLINICAL$OBSERVATION FINAL$STUTTERING |
| 6303 | FREQ SYLLABLE$REPETITION STUTTERER$JUDGMENT |
| 6304 | ADAPTATION$PERFORMANCES INDIV$STUTTERERS IMPLICATIONS $RESEARCH |
| 6304 | COMPARISON PROCEDURES SCALING$SEVERITY$STUTTERING |
| 6304 | PALMAR$SWEAT INVEST DISFLUENCY EXPECTANCY$ADAPTATION |
| 6304 | PALMAR$SWEAT INVEST DISFLUENCY EXPECTANCY$ADAPTATION |
| 6304 | RATINGS$STUTTERING AUDIO$VISUAL$AUDIOVISUAL$CUES |
| 6304 | STABILITY CONSISTENCY$MEAS STUTTERING |
| 6304 | STABILITY ADAPTATION ORAL$PERFORMANCE STUTTERERS |
| 6304 | STUTTERING$SYNDROME |
| 6313 | AUD$VISUAL$IMPERCEP STUTTERERS |
| 6403 | ACCEPTABILITY STUTTERING CONTROL$PATTERNS |
| 6403 | COMPARISONS GOALS PARENTS$STUTTERERS NONSTUTTERERS CHIL |
| 6403 | DISFLUENCY$INDEX |
| 6403 | RECOVERY STUTTERING |
| 6403 | STANDARD$DEFINITION STUTTERING |
| 6403 | STUDY GOAL-SETTING$BEHAVIOR PARENTS$STUTTERERS PARENTS $NONSTUTTERE |

6403    STUTTERING BLIND$PARTIALLY$SIGHTED$CHIL
6404    IDENTIFICATION STUTTERERS RECORDED$SAMPLES FLUENT
        $SP
6404    STUTTERING AUD$CNS
6404    STUTTERING NORMAL$SP
6409    STUTTERING$RESEARCH
6413    RESULTS EXAM STUTTERERS CLUTTERERS
6503    INVEST LISTENER$REACTION SP$DISFLUENCY
6503    SELF-RECOVERY STUTTERING
6503    SENSORY$FEEDBACK STUTTERING
6503    STUTTERING INFO$LOAD R$STRENGTH
6504    COMPARISON REACTION$TIMES STUTTERERS WORD$ASSOC$TEST
6504    EFFECT SITUATIONAL$DIFFICULTY STUTTERING
6504    MIDDLE$EAR$ACTIVITY SP STUTTERERS
6504    PERCEIVED$SITUATIONAL$DIFFICULTY STUTTERING$FREQ
6510    MAGNITUDE-ESTIMATION$JUDGMENTS STUTTERING$SEVERITY
6510    STUTTERERS$ESTIMATE NORMAL$APPREHENSION SPEAKING
6513    SELF-ALIENATION$STUTTERING
6603    CHARACTERISTICS LINGUISTIC$OUTPUT STUTTERERS
6603    STUTTERING$ADAPTATION LEARNING RELEVANCE ADAPTATION
        $STUDIES
6604    BEHAVIORAL$RIGIDITY STUTTERERS
6604    EEG$ANALYSIS STUTTERING
6604    PROSODY STUTTERING$ADAPTATION
6604    PROTENSITY$EST STUTTERERS
6604    REL STUTTERING WORD$LENGTH WORD$FREQ
6604    SPONTANEOUS$RECOVERY STUTTERING
6605    OBSERVATIONS INCIDENCE$STUTTERING SPECIAL$CULTURE
6609    BIBLIOTHERAPY STUTTERERS CASE$HISTORIES
6704    ADAPTATION CONSISTENCY DISFLUENT$SP STUTTERERS
6704    EFFECTS LISTENING$INSTRUCTIONS ATTENTION MANNER$CONTENT
        $STUTTERING
6704    LINGUISTIC$FACTORS STUTTERING
6704    MEAS STUTTERING$SEVERITY
6704    REL ANTICIPATION CONSISTENCY STUTTERED$WORDS
6704    SLURVIAN$SKILL STUTTERERS
6704    STUTTERERS$PROJECTION LISTENER$REACTION
6704    STUTTERING WORD$LENGTH
6713    IMPERCEPTIVITY$STUTTERERS
6713    PROBLEMS DEV$TONUS$STUTTERING
6713    SEVERITY$STUTTERING CINE$RECORDINGS PHYSIOLOGICAL
        $OBSERVATIONS
6713    SIMILARITIES$DIFFERENCES CLUTTERING$STUTTERING
6804    DISFLUENCY$BEHAVIOR SCH$STUTTERERS ADAPTATION$EFFECT
6804    INTERREL FLUENCY$PRODUCING$VARIABLES STUTTERED$SP
6804    NOTE SYNTACTIC$REL NONFLUENCY

6804   PRIMARY$STUTTERING ONSET$STUTTERING
6804   STUTTERING
6817   REL MASKING$NOISE SEVERITY$STUTTERING
6903   EFFECTS STUTTERING
6903   FEEDBACK$MODEL STUTTERING ENGINEERS$VIEW
6903   FEEDBACK$MODEL STUTTERING ENGINEERS$VIEW
6904   AFFECTIVE$MEANING$WORDS RATED STUTTERING$READERS
6904   ANTICIPATION STUTTERING PUPILLOGRAPHIC$STUDY
6904   ASSESSING COMM$ATTITUDES STUTTERERS
6904   DISFLUENCY$BEHAVIOR SCH$STUTTERERS CONSISTENCY$EFFECT
6904   GOAL$SETTING$BEHAVIOR PARENTS BEGINNING$STUTTERERS
6904   INFLUENCE PROSODY STUTTERING$ADAPTATION
6904   PERFORMANCE STUTTERERS DICHOTIC$LISTENING$TASKS CEREBRAL
       $DOMINANCE
6904   SOUND PATTERN ARTIFICIAL$FLUENCY
6904   SPECULATION VOCAL$ADAPTATION STUTTERERS
6904   SPECULATION VOCAL$ADAPTATION STUTTERERS
6904   STUDY REL LATENCY CONSISTENCY STUTTERING
6904   TEST SATIATION FUNCTION ADAPTATION$STUTTERING
6913   EFFECTS STUTTERING PROBLEM$SOLVING
6913   LANG$ABILITIES STUTTERING$CHIL
7003   CONCERN SCH$STUTTERERS STUTTERING
7003   CONCERN SCH$STUTTERERS STUTTERING
7003   STUTTERERS
7004   ANCHORING SEQUENCE$EFFECTS CATEGORY$SCALING STUTTERING
       $SEVERITY
7004   COMPUTATION CONSISTENCY$EFFECT STUTTERING
7004   EFFECT STUTTERING CHANGES$AUDITION
7004   EFFECT VERBAL$STIMULUS$WORDS DISFLUENCY$RATES STUTTERERS
7004   EFFECT VERBAL$STIMULUS$WORDS DISFLUENCY$RATES STUTTERERS
7004   EXPERIMENTAL$ANALOGUE ANXIETY$STUTTERING$REL
7004   STUTTERING DISAPPEARANCE
7013   SPINAL$CORD$REFLEX STUTTERING
7013   STUTTERING$CLUTTERING DYSRHYTHMIC$SP
7013   STUTTERING$CLUTTERING DIFFERENTIAL$DIAGNOSIS
7103   ADULT$FEMALE$STUTTERER
7104   COMMENT STUTTERING DISAPPEARANCE
7104   CORTICAL$EXCITABILITY PERSEVERATION STUTTERING
7104   DIFFERENCES DISFLUENCY MALE$FEMALE$NONSTUTTERING$CHIL
7104   FREQ$STUTTERING REPEATED$UNISON$READINGS
7104   IDENTIFICATION BRIEF$PAUSES FLUENT$SP STUTTERERS
7104   INFLUENCE ONSET$PHONATION FREQ STUTTERING
7104   OBJECT-NAMING$LATENCY STUTTERING$CHIL
7104   PHONETIC$ABILITY STUTTERING
7104   REPORTS PARENTAL$ATTITUDES STUTTERING CHIL
7104   ROLE RANDOM$BLACKOUT$CUES DISCRIM MOMENTS STUTTERING

7105   FEAR STUTTERING
7105   FLUENCY
7114   EVAL PRESCH$DISFLUENCY
7203   APPROACH CLASSIFICATION MEAS STUTTERING
7203   CLINICAL$NOTES FORCED$STUTTERING
7203   STUTTERING$SEVERITY$INSTRUMENT CHIL ADULTS
7204   ANALYSIS FLUENCY STUTTERED$SP
7204   BEHAVIORAL$DIMENSIONS STUTTERED$SP
7204   COMPARATIVE$ANALYSIS ITPA PPVT STUTTERERS
7204   DISFLUENCIES YOUNG$CHIL SPEAKING$SITUATIONS
7204   DISFLUENT$SP PRESCH$CHIL ADOL GER
7204   INTERAURAL$PHASE$DISPARITY STUTTERERS
7204   RECOVERY STUTTERING ADOL$POPULATION
7204   RECOVERY STUTTERING ADOL$POPULATION
7204   STUTTERING$SEVERITY AGE
7204   VOCAL$CHARACTERISTICS STUTTERERS
7208   SELF-RATINGS AMT$STUTTERING SCH$CHIL
7208   STUTTERING
7211   PATTERNS$CEREBRAL$DOMINANCE SOUNDS ADULT$STUTTERERS
7303   STUTTERING$CHRONICITY$PREDICTION$CHECKLIST
7304   CLUSTERING PRESCH SP$DISFLUENCY$FREQUENCY
7304   EFFECT REDUCED$READING$RATE STUTTERING$FREQ
7304   EFFECTS STUTTERING SYSTOLIC$BLOOD$PRESSURE
7304   PERSONALITY IMPROVEMENT REGRESSION STUTTERING
7304   SCH$STUTTERERS$NONSTTERERS OR
7304   SPONTANEOUS$RECOVERY NONSTUTTERERS$DISFLUENCY ADAPTATION
7304   STUTTERERS ADAPT
7304   STUTTERING DISFLUENCY R$CLASSES
7304   STUTTERING$CONSISTENCY VARIED$CONTEXTS
7313   STUTTERING SOCIAL$ISOLATION ROLE ADAPATION$EFFECT
7317   VERBAL$BEHAVIOR$PATTERNS SP$CLINICIANS STUTTERERS
7403   IMAGINAL$CUES STUTTERS
7403   RULES EARLY$STUTTERING
7403   STUTTERING NORMAL$SPEECH
7403   STUTTERING$BLOCK
7404   ADJACENCY PREDICTION SCH$STUTTERERS
7404   ADULT$STUTTERERS
7404   EFFECTS WHITE$NOISE STUTTERING
7404   EFFECTS NOISE SPEAKING$BEHAVIOR STUTTERERS
7404   RELATIONSHIP DISFLUENT$SP NORMAL-SPEAKING PRESCH PARENTS
7404   SOCIAL$POSITION SPEAKING$COMPETENCE STUTTERING$BOYS
7404   STUTTERERS$EXPECTATIONS
7405   STUTTERING
7406   PRELIMINARY$STUDY TIMING$REL SP STUTTERERS
7408   DISFLUENCY$BEHAVIOR SCH$STUTTERERS
7417   CONSIDERATION STUTTERING$THERAPY

7503   YOUNG PREVALENCE RECOVERY STUTTERING
7504   CONTURE INFLUENCE NOISE STUTTERS'$DISFLUENCY
7504   SILVERMAN FLUENCY$FLUCTUATIONS MENSTRUAL$CYCLE
7504   SILVERMAN WORD$ATTRIBUTES PRESCHOOLERS DISFLUENCY
7504   YOUNG OBSERVER$AGREEMENT STUTTERING
7513   JENSEN ORAL$SENSORY-PERCEP STUTTERERS
7513   SCHIAVETTI JUDGMENTS STUTTERING$SEVERITY TYPE LOCUS
       DISFLUENCE
7527   BURKE STUTTERER'S INITIAL$REACTIONS DAF
7527   HUTCHINSON ORAL$SENSORY DEPRIVATION STUTTERING
7604   ADAMS STUTTERERS + NONSTUTTERERS PHONATION VOWEL
7604   CROSS PRESUMED$FLUENCY$RF$STIMULI
7604   HEALEY REDUCTION STUTTERING SINGING
7604   JAMES DURATION EFFECTS TIME-OUT SPEAKING
7604   MANNING AUD$ASSEMBLY STUTTERING$CHILDREN
7604   PERKINS STUTTERING PHONATION ARTIC RESPIRATION
7604   REED PUNISHMENT STUTTERING GSR
7604   RONSON WORD$FREQ STUTTERING SENTENCE$STRUCTURE
7604   STARKWEATHER  LATENCY VOCALIZATION$ONSET STUTTERERS
7604   TORNICK STUTTERING SENTENCE$LENGTH
7604   WOODS TRAITS STUTTERING FLUENT$MALES
7611   YAIRI EFFECTS BINAURAL AND MONAURAL$NOISE STUTTERING
7627   ANDREWS PERCEP AUD$COMPONENTS STUTTERED$SP
7627   FELDMAN SELF-DISCLOSURE PARENTS STUTTERING$CHILDREN
7627   HUTCHINSON JAW$MECHANICS STUTTERING
7627   KROLL TASK$PRESENTATION INFORMATION$LOAD ADAPTATION
       STUTTERERS NORMAL
7627   MANNING DISFLUENCIES PHONATORY$TRANSITIONS STUTTERED
       $SP
7627   MONTGOMERY PERCEP$ACOUS$ANALYSIS REPETITIONS STUTTERED
       $SP
7628   HOOD COMMUNICATIVE$STRESS FREQUENCY FORM-TYPES DISFLUENT
       $BEHAVIOR
7628   ICKES PALMAR$SWEAT$MEASURE EFFECT DRUGS STUTTERING
7628   MANNING JUDGEMENTS FLUENCY
7628   OELSCHAEGER RESPONSE-CONTINGENT$POSITIVE$STIMULATION
       STUTTERERS
7628   OTTO SP$DISFLUENCIES DOWN'S$SYNDROM
7628   RITTERMAN INTER-DIGITAL$VARIABLIITY PALMAR$SWEAT$INDICES
       STUTTERERS
7628   TREON EFFECTS GSR$BIOFEEDBACK DELAYED$DAF STUTTERING
7629   EPSTEIN EFFECT ARTIC$COMPLEXITY ADAPTATION STUTTERED
       $SPEECH
7632   MOORE BILATERAL$TACHISTOSCOPIC$WORD$PERCEP STUTTERERS
       NORMAL
7704   CONTURE LARYNGEAL$BEHAVIOR STUTTERING

7704    COOPER TIMING$CONTROL$ACCURACY NORMAL$APEAKERS STUTTERERS
7704    GARBER EFFECTS NOISE INCREASED$VOCAL$INTENSITY STUTTERING
7704    INGHAM LISTENER$JUDGEMENT STUTTERERS$NONSTUTTERED
        $SP READING CONDITION
7704    MARTIN EFFECT VICARIOUS$PUNISHMENT STUTTERING$FREQUENCY
7704    WINGATE CRITERIA STUTTERING
7704    WONG EFFECT ADJACENCY DISTRIBUTION STUTTERING READINGS
7728    BONFANTI FLUENCY INSTITUTIONALIZED$RETARDED$ADULTS
7728    CROSS ELECTROMYOGRAPHIC$BIOFEEDBACK FREQUENCY STUTTERING
7728    CURRAN INSTRUCTIONAL$BIAS LISTENER$RATINGS DISFLUENCY
        CHIL
7728    CURRAN LISTENER$RATINGS SEVERITY DISFLUENCY CHIL
7728    DEAN PREVALENCE STUTTERING USA
7728    GRONHOVD FLUENT$ORAL$READING$RATES STUTTERERS NONSTUTTERERS
7728    HUTCHINSON AUDITORY$STIMULI FREQUENCY STUTTERING$BEHAVIORS
7728    MILLER ADAPTATION$EFFECT NONFLUENT$SP CONTROLLED$STUTTERERS
7728    YONOVITZ ELECTROPHYSIOLOGICAL$MEASUREMENT TIME-OUT
        $PROCEDURE STUTTERER
7729    YOVETICH EFFECT DYSFLUENCIES ATTENTION STUTTERERS
        NON-STUTTERERS
7804    BRAYTON NOISE RHYTHMIC$STIMULATION SP STUTTERERS
7804    BRUCE MOTOR$PRACTICE STUTTERING$ADAPTATION
7804    DALY STUTTERING OPERANT$BEHAVIOR$EFFECTS VERBAL$STIMULI
        DISFLUENCY
7804    FREEMAN LARYNGEAL$MUSCLE$ACTIVITY STUTTERING
7804    HALL CENTRAL$AUDITORY$FUNCTION STUTTERERS
7804    HOROVITZ STAPEDIAL$REFLEX ANXIETY DISFLUENT$SPEAKERS
7804    INGHAM EFFECTS STUTTERING SELF-RECORDING$FREQUENCY
        $STUTTERING
7804    MCFARLANE NEURAL$RESPONSE$TIME STUTTERERS ORAL$MOTOR
        $TASKS
7804    TOSCHER CENTRAL$AUD$PROCESSES SYN$SENT$IDEN
7827    HANSON CONTINGENT$LIGHT-FLASH STUTTERING ATTENTION
7827    HAYNES DISFLUENCY FUNCTION LINGUISTIC$COMPLEXITY
7827    SCHMITT FUNDAMENTAL$FREQUENCIES ORAL$READING STUTTERING
        MALE$CHIL
7829    ST LOUIS MOTOR$SP$AWARENESS STUTTERING


                          0804


5804    CHIL REACTIONS NONFLUENCIES ADULT$SP
6009    STUTTERING SYMPOSIUM
6013    THERAPY$CLUTTERING
6104    DISFLUENCY NORMAL$SPEAKERS RF

6114    COMPARATIVE$STUDY HESITATIONS
6305    ASSESSING CULTURAL$SP$FLUENCY$EXPECTATIONS
6413    PGSR$STUTTERERS
6904    EPHPHATHA ADVICE STAMMERERS
6904    LOCI DISFLUENCIES SP NONSTUTTERERS
6904    LOCI DISFLUENCIES SP NONSTUTTERERS
7013    AUD$DISABILITY CLUTTERING$CHIL
7013    CLUTTERING
7013    CLUTTERING
7013    INVES INCIDENCE$SYMPTOMATOLOGY$CLUTTERING
7014    FUNCTIONS HESITATIONS SP FAMILIES SCHIZOPHRENICS
7406    PRELIMINARY$OBSERVATIONS TEMPORAL$COMPENSATION SP
        CHIL
7413    PHONATORY$REFLEX$MECHANISMS STAMMERING
7504    INGHAM COVERT+OVERT$ASSESSMENT STUTTERING$THERAPY
        $EVALUATION
7504    YOUNG OBSERVER$AGREEMENT STUTTERING
7508    WOODS TEACHERS$PREDICTIONS SOCIAL$POSITION COMP STUTTERING
7513    DUFFY FOUR$TYPES DISFLUENCY LISTENERS$REACTIONS
7526    BUTTERWORTH HESITATION SEMANTIC$PLANNING SP
7529    MARTIN DISFLUENCIES CHILD PRIVATE$SP CONVERSATION
7603    ADAMS PROBLEMS EXPERIMENTS STUTTERING
7603    TROTTER STUTTERER CONTEMPORARY$LITERATURE
7605    CULATTA FLUENCY
7628    STARKWEATHER BASE$RATE COMPARISONS TIME-DEPENDENT
        $BEHAVIOR
7703    BLOODSTEIN STUTTERING
7703    HALL DISFLUENCIES LANG-DISORDERED$CHIL
7705    MOWRER REVIEW ARTICLES STUTTERING
7705    VAN RIPER PUBLIC$SCHOOLS$SPECIALIST STUTTERING
7727    CROWE PARENTAL$ATTITUDES KNOWLEDGE STUTTERING
7728     FELDMAN WOMEN'S$LIBERATION, STUTTERING FLUENCY
7728    CONTURE READING SCHOOL-AGE$STUTTERERS
7728    CULATTA ACQUISITION LABEL "STUTTERING" SCHOOLCHIL
7728    DEAN PREVALENCE STUTTERING USA
7728    HAYNES LANG$DISFLUENCY$VARIABLES NORMAL$SPEAKING$CHIL
7728    MURRAY LANG$ABILITIES PRESCHOOL$STUTTERING$CHIL
7728    RECORDS HANDEDNESS STUTTERING
7728    STOCKER AUDITORY$RECALL DYSFLUENCY YOUNG$STUTTERERS
7728    THOMPSON SUGGESTIONS RESEARCH YOUNG$STUTTERERS
7827    HAYNES DISFLUENCY FUNCTION LINGUISTIC$COMPLEXITY


                          0901


5418    A

5503   SCH$SP$THERAPIST
5703   CHIL GUIDES$TEACHING
5803   APPRAISAL$FORM SP$HNG$THERAPISTS
5813   PHONIATRIC$PRACTICE NEW$YORK
5815   AUDIOLOGIST RESIDENTIAL$SCH
5815   PREPARATION AUDIOLOGIST RESPONSIBILITIES RESIDENTIAL
       $SCH DEAF
5903   PRIVATE$PRACTICE SCH$THERAPISTS INDIANA
5904   REL AUD$SP$THR
5905   PROBLEMS REL SP$HNG$SPECIALISTS MEDICAL$PROFESSION
6003   SP$PATHOLOGIST INTERESTS ACTIVITIES ATTITUDES
6005   SP$PATH$A
6103   SELF-JUDGMENTS SP$ADEQUACY JUDGMENTS TRAINED$OBSERVERS
6105   PRIVATE$PRACTICE SP$PATH FULL-TIME$SERVICE UNIVERSITY
       $FACULTY
6105   PRIVATE$PRACTICE SP$PATH$A
6105   SP$CLINICIANS$ROLE COMMUNITY
6107   SCH$SP$HNG$SERVICES SCH$CLINICIAN
6117   ROLE SP$THERAPIST TEACHER SP$IMPROVEMENT
6118   THERAPIST MEDICAL$SPECIALISTS
6120   THERAPIST LISTENER
6215   ROLE AUDIOLOGIST SCH$DEAF
6315   AUDIOLOGIST HA$DISPENSER
6403   PERSONAL$REPORT CLINICAL$EXPERIENCE$RESEARCH RECOMMENDATION
       $THERAP
6505   SP$CLINICIAN SCH
6517   SP$PATHOLOGIST FANTASY
6603   DEFENSIVE$SP$CLINICIANS SCH
6615   VIDEO$TAPE TEACHING CLINICAL$SKILLS
6703   PRACTICAL$A
6703   SP$CLINICIAN
6705   VOCATIONAL$INTERESTS WOMEN SP$PATH$A
7008   ACCOUNTABILITY CLINICIAN$SCH
7008   FUNCTION SCH$CLINICIAN
7008   PROGRAM TRNG SP$CLINICIANS SCH$PROGRAMS
7008   SERVICES FUNCTIONS SP$HNG$SPECIALISTS SCH
7017   OHIO SCH$SP$HNG$THERAPISTS REPORT EVAL TRNG
7017   SEMANTIC$APPRAISAL EVAL SP$PATH$A
7103   RESPONSIBILITIES SP$HNG$CLINICIAN SCH
7103   SP$CLINICIANS$CONCEPTS BOYS$MEN STUTTER
7106   REPORT$STRATEGIES
7208   ROLE SCH$SP$CLINICIAN INNER-CITY$CHIL
7208   SP$LANG$CLINICIAN LEARNING$CENTER$TEAM
7220   MICROTHERAPY STUDY BEHAVIORS SP$CLINICIAN
7303   BASES SP$PATH$A THERAPY$MODEL
7303   BASES SP$PATH$A EVAL

```
7313   PERCEP$SKILLS CLINICAL$MANAGEMENT NASALITY
7315   AUDIOLOGIST EUDC$ENVIRONMENT
7315   AUDIOLOGIST EDUC$ENVIRONMENT
7403   METHOD QUANTIFICATION DESCRIPTION CLINICAL$INTERACTIONS
7405   ORTHOPHONISTE
7405   SPEECH$PATHOLOGIST READING$PROCESS
7408   SP$CLINICIAN CHIL$ABUSE
7408   SP$CLINICIAN LANG$CLINICIAN
7408   SP$PATHOLOGIST RESOURSE$TEACHER LANG$LEARNING$DISABILITIES
7408   SPEECH$PATHOLOGISTS LANG$CLASSROOM$TEACHER
7408   TEACHER$ORANIZATION SCH$CLINICIANS
7408   TRAINING$PROGRAM PUBLIC$SCH$SP$CLINICIANS
7505   CULATTA CLINICAL$SUPERVISORS+TRAINEES
7505   CURLEE INCOMES SP+HRING$PROFESSION JANUARY
7505   CURLEE MANPOWER$RESOURCES$NEEDS SP$PATHOLOGY$AUD APRIL
7505   CURLEE TRAINING FORIGN$STUDENTS SP$PATHOLOGY$AUD US
       $COLLEGES
7505   GARRARD SP$PATHOLOGIST EARLY$CHILDHOOD$EDUC HANDICAPPED
7505   MELROSE PROFESSIONAL$LEADERSHIP$WOMEN SP$PATHOLOGY+AUD
       SEPTEMBER
7505   NICOLAIS STATE$LAWS$LICENSING$SP$PATHOLOGISTS+AUDIOLOGISTS
7505   PANNBACKER BIBLIOGRAPHY SUPERVISION
7505   SCHUBERT CLINICAL$SUPERVISORS UNIVERSITY$TRAINING
       JULY
7505   SHRIBERG WISCONSIN$PROCEDURE APPRAISAL CLINICAL$COMPETENCE
7505   WEPMAN HORIZONS SP+HRING$SPECIALISTS JANUARY
7508   DOPHEIDE SP$LANG$SERVICES CLIN-TEACHER$INSERVICE
7508   MOWRER SP$CLIN SC'$MONEY
7508   SCHUBERT HIGHER$EDUC SCH CLIN
7508   SCHUCKERS PROFESSIONAL$IMAGERY CLIN SCH
7512   SCHUBERT NONVERBAL$BEHAVIORS CLINICIANS$DURING$THERAPY
7520   IRWIN VERBAL BEHAVIORS SUPERVISORS SP$CLINICIANS
7527   LASS EFFECTS PRETESTING$INFO EVAL SP$CLINICIANS
7605   CULATTA COMPETENCY-BASED$SYSTEM TRAINING SP$PATHOLOGISTS
7605   CULATTA CONTENT+SEQUENCE$ANALYSIS SUPERVISORY$SESSION
7605   CURLEE CHARACTERISTICS ASHA$MEMBERS
7605   MILLER AUDIOLOGIST OCCUPATIONAL$HEARING$CONSERVATION
7605   PICKERING BILINGUAL+BICULTURAL$EDUCATION SP$PATHOLOGIST
7605   VAN HATTUM SP$CLINICIAN SCHOOLS
7627   ORATIO CRITERIA EVAL$STUDENT$CLINICIANS
7627   RITTERMAN THERAPIST$HABITUATION CLIENT$PROGRESS ARTIC
       $THERAPY
7705   ALEO TIME$ALLOCATION PROFESSIONAL$FEES SP-LANG$PATHOLOGISTS+AUDIO
7705   GERSTMAN SUPERVISORY$RELATIONSHIPS DYNAMIC$COMMUNICATION
7705   MARTIN PARENT$COUNSELING SP$PATHOLOGIST SOCIAL$WORKER
7705   MILLER AUDIOLOGISTS TESTIMONY GOVERNMENT$REPRESENTATIVES
```

7705    SHRIBERG PERSONALITY$CHAR ACAD$PERF CLIN$COMPETENCE
        COMM$DIS$MAJORS
7705    VAN RIPER PUBLIC$SCHOOLS$SPECIALIST STUTTERING
7708    BALDES SUPERVISION STUDENT$SP$CLINICIANS
7708    BASKERVILL SP-LANG$PATHOLOGIST STANDARD$ENGLISH
7708    MADRID STAFF$ASSIGNMENTS SCHOOLS
7729    HANSON SP$PATHOLOGIST ORAL$MYOLOGY
7805    GARSTECKI SCHOOL$AUDIOLOGISTS
7812    ORATIO INTERREL PERSONAL$TECHNICAL$SKILLS STUDENT
        $CLINICIANS
7912    ORATIO INTERPERSONAL+TECHNICAL SKILLS STUDENT$CLINICIANS


                                    0902

5409    BUILDING BALANCED COMM$PROGRAM
5503    MOBILE$UNIT$SP$THERAPY$PROGRAM
5615    FACILITIES LOS$ANGELES$SCH
5709    SP$CORRECTION SCH
5803    ELEMENTS SP$HNG$CENTER$OPERATION
5815    MEXICAN$INSTITUTE HNG$SP
5815    REL SP$HNG$CENTER PARENT DEAF$CHIL
5915    ALBANY PRESCH*TESTING
5918    SP$CLUBS SP$THERAPY
6003    SP$CORRECTION USSR
6005    CLINIC-LAB$DESIGN PURDUE$UNIV
6005    GALLAUDET HNG$SP$CENTER
6005    PLANNING MULTI-PURPOSE SP$HNG$FACILITY
6005    SP$HNG$REHAB JAPAN
6005    SP$PATH$A$CENTERS EUROPE
6005    STUDY SCH$SP$HNG$SERVICES
6016    RESEARCH$FACILITIES NORTHWESTERN$UNIV
6018    SP$THERAPY EUROPE
6105    COMMUNITY$SP$HNG$CENTER PROFESSION
6105    COUNTY$SP$SERVICES CLINICAL$PROGRAM SCH
6105    OPPORTUNITIES CLINICAL$TRNG MEDICAL$CENTER SP$HNG
        $CLINIC
6105    ORGANIZING HOSPITAL$PROGRAM COMM$DIS
6105    SP$PATH LOGOPEDICS USSR
6105    SP$THERAPY GREAT$BRITAIN
6107    SCH$SP$HNG$SERVICES SP$IMPROVEMENT
6107    SCH$SP$HNG$SERVICES CLINICAL$PRACTICE REMEDIAL$PROCEDURES
6107    SCH$SP$HNG$SERVICES PROFESSIONAL$STANDARDS$TRNG
6107    SCH$SP$HNG$SERVICES
6107    SCH$SP$HNG$SERVICES

6107 SCH$SP$HNG$SERVICES RECRUITMENT$CAREERS SP$PATH$A
6107 SCH$SP$HNG$SERVICES CLINICAL$PRACTICE DIAGNOSIS MEAS
6117 VETERANS$ADMINISTRATION A$SP$PATH$PROGRAM OHIO
6305 SP$THERAPY CAMP$SETTING GROWTH$DEV SP$HABILITATION
     $CENTER
6403 DEMONSTRATION$PROGRAM HNG$TESTS DAY$CARE$CENTERS
6405 SP$THERAPY GERMANY
6405 TREATMENT$SP$DIS DENMARK
6516 SAN$FERNANDO$VALLEY$STATE$COLLEGE
6605 STATE-WIDE$SP$HNG$PROGRAM MR$MENTALLY$ILL
6717 SCH$SP$THERAPY OHIO
6805 INFORMATIONAL$GAPS CLINICAL$SERVICES
6817 SUGGESTIONS RESEARCH SCH$SP$HNG$THERAPY OHIO
6903 INNOVATIVE$SCH$PROGRAMS OAKLAND$SCH$PLAN
7008 INNOVATIVE$SCH$PROGRAMS OAKLAND$SCH$PLAN
7008 RECOMMENDATIONS HOUSING SCH$SP$SERVICES
7008 ROTATIONAL$SYSTEM SUMMER$SP$PROGRAM
7008 SCH$SP$HNG$PROGRAMS
7105 SP$PATH$A ISRAEL
7205 SP$PATH BELGIUM
7208 SP$CORRECTION SCH
7215 ST.LOUIS$COUNTY$HNG$PROGRAM
7217 SCH$SP$HNG$THERAPY
7305 SP$HNG$SERVICES MALAYSIA
7317 REL SP$CLINICIANS$CONCEPT VERBAL$BEHAVIOR
7405 SP$SCIENCE SP$PATH SWEDEN
7405 STATUS SP$PATH$AUD KOREA
7408 OAKLAND$SCH$PREVENTION PLAN
7408 PROBLEMS SCH
7505 BAR DECREASING$NO-SHOW URBAN$SP+HRING$CLINIC JULY
7505 CURLEE CLINICAL$FACILITIES$SURVEY JULY
7505 IVEY SINGAPORE SP+HRING$PROGRAM OCTOBER
7505 SCHUBERT CLINICAL$SUPERVISORS UNIVERSITY$TRAINING
     JULY
7508 DAUM PRESCHOOL$COMM$SERVICES
7508 WORK ACCOUNTABILITY SCH$SP LANG$PROGRAM
7605 HARLAN COMPUTER$PROCESSING STUDENTS'$CLINICAL$HOURS
7605 KAMARA COMPUTER$BILLING SERVICE$ANALYSIS FINANCIAL
     $REPORTING
7605 VAN HATTUM SP$CLINICIAN SCHOOLS
7705 BOUCHARD MEDICAL$RECORD SP+HNG$PROFESSION
7705 CHAPEY LANG$SP$+HNG$SERVICES COMMUNITY$COLLEGES
7705 GARBEE CALIFORNIA AUDIOLOGY SCHOOLS
7705 O'NEILL SP$PATHOLOGY+AUDIO INDIA
7705 STRANDBERG HOSPITAL$SP$PATHOLOGY$SERVICES
7708 TRAYWICK RURAL SP$LANG$PROGRAM

**0902 (CONT.)**


7716    NORTH CAROLINA$LEGISLATURE RESPONDS NEEDS OF DEAF
7829    ZINK DELIVERY SP$SERVICES SCHOOL


## 0903


5406    SHORT-TERM$AUTOCORRELATION$ANALYSIS CORRELATOGRAMS
        SPOKEN$DIGITS
5706    CONSTANT$RATIO CONFUSION$MATRICES SP$COMM
5814    REL FUNCTIONAL$BURDENING$PHONEMES FREQ$OCCURRENCE
5904    LATIN$SQUARE$DESIGN SP$HNG$RESEARCH
6006    STATISTICAL$DETECTION$THEORY
6105    DATA$PROCESSING AUDIO-LINGUISTIC$PROBLEMS
6106    MULTIVARIATE$STATISTICAL$COMPUTER$PROGRAMS APPLICATION
6314    MULTIVARIATE$ANALYSIS LATIN$ELEGIAC$VERSE
6514    LEXICALITY STATISTICAL$REFLECTION
6706    PEST EFFICIENT$ESTIMATES PROBABILITY$FUNCTIONS
6706    TESTING SEQUENTIAL$DEPENDENCIES
6804    TESTING$SIGNIFICANCE AGREEMENT$OBSERVERS
6807    DATA VERBAL$SIGNALIZATION
7104    OPERANT$MANIPULATION VOCAL$PITCH NORMAL$SPEAKERS
7106    RELIABILITY RATINGS AUD SIGNAL-DETECTION EXPERIMENT
7304    STANDARDIZATION$TESTS
7306    LOGISTIC$DISTRIBUTION APPROXIMATION NORMAL$CURVE
7314    SIMULTANEOUS$INTERPRETATION TEMPORAL$QUANTITATIVE
        $DATA
7406    CONSTRAINED$ARRAY$OPTIMIZATION PENALTY$FUNCTION$TECHNIQUES
7406    PEST NOTE REDUCTION VARIANCE$THR$ESTIMATES
7527    KROLL COMM$DIS POWER$ANALYTIC$ASSESSMENT RECENT$RESEARCH
7604    YOUNG REGRESSION$ANALYSIS RESEARCH SP$PATHOLOGY
7606    CERMAK MULTIDIMENSIONAL$ANALYSES JUDGEMENTS TRAFFIC
        $NOISE
7611    BLACK RELIABILITY ONE$LISTENER
7706    GREY MULTIDIMENSIONAL$PERCEPTUAL$SCALING MUSICAL$TIMBRES
7833    GANDOUR DIMENSIONS TONES MULTIDIMENSIONAL$SCALING


## 0904


5403    EXPERIMENTAL$STUDY DISORGANIZATION SP MANUAL$R
5415    DIRECT$TONE TEST CHEWING$METHOD
5503    EARLY$ORTHODONTIA
5503    LATERALIZATION CEREBRAL$FUNCTION
5515    CLINICAL$PSYCHOLOGY

5515    EURHYTHMICS
5606    EFFECTS MESSAGE-STORAGE$SCHEMES COMM PROBLEM-SOLVING
        $GRPS
5606    PITCH-SYNCHRONOUS$PROCESSING SP
5615    EXPRESSIONS SP UNDERSTANDING USE
5616    NEBRASKA$TEST$LEARNING$APTITUDE
5703    BLUEMEL$COLLECTION STUTTERING
5703    CHIL GUIDES$TEACHING
5803    BIBLIOGRAPHY STETSON
5803    FILMS A ANNOTATED$LIST
5803    GEORGE$FORTUNE
5803    IBIS$FUISTIS
5804    MENTAL$IMAGERY
5806    SP COMM
5810    GENERAL$REASONING
5814    ANALYSIS STRUCTURED$CONTENT APPLICATION ELECTRONIC
        $COMPUTER$RESEAR
5814    SP$ANALYSIS MENTAL$PROCESSES
5815    LIMITATIONS USE INTELLIGENCE$SCALES MENTAL$AGES CHIL
5903    COMM$SKILLS INTELLIGENCE HEMIPLEGICS
5903    TONGUE$THRUST MONOZYGOTIC$TWINS
5913    SP$LANG NORMAL$ABNORMAL DUTCH$SCH$CHIL
5914    PEOPLE WHISTLE
6004    ARTIC$COMPETENCY READING$READINESS
6005    FULBRIGHTER NORWAY
6005    PROGRESS RESEARCH NEUROLOGICAL$SENSORY$DIS
6006    WORD$FREQ EFFECTS LEARNING UNKNOWN$MESSAGE$SETS
6014    ORGANIZATION RUSSIAN-ENG$STEM$DICTIONARY MAGNETIC
        $TAPE
6103    TONGUE-THRUST$SWALLOW ARTIC AGE
6105    THEORETICAL$CONSIDERATIONS SELF-CONCEPT BODY-IMAGE
6106    SEISMOMETER$SOUNDS
6114    LIKE-RATINGS PREDICTION HUMAN$BEHAVIOR
6203    INTERACTION USF METALINGUAL$FACTORS CHRONIC$SCHIZOPHRENIC
6203    TONGUE$THRUSTING CLINICAL$HYPOTHESIS
6206    INFLUENCE BEHAVIOR LINEAR$DYNAMICAL$SYSTEM IMPOSED
        RAPID MOTIONS
6209    PROPOSAL LISTENING$TRNG
6215    STUDY INTELLIGENCE ACHIEVEMENT CHIL$WAARDENBURG$SYNDROME
6303    F$MATHIAS$ALEXANDER SP$CLINICIAN HISTORICAL$NOTE
6303    JUDGMENTS PSYCHOSIS VOCAL$CUES
6303    OBSERVATIONS TONGUE-THRUST$SWALLOW PRESCH$CHIL
6303    PRACTICAL$METHOD SCREENING$VISUAL-PERCEP$MOTOR$PERFORMANCE
6304    EVAL CONTEXTUAL$SP$MATERIAL
6304    TEST$TRNG$STIMULI
6306    ARTIC$EFFECTIVENESS MEAS PROCESSED$SP

6306    PHYSICS$STUDENTS STUDY ACOUS
6314    PRELIMINARY$STUDIES MACHINE$GENERATED$INDEX$VOCABS
6315    MONTESSORI$EDUC
6404    COMPARISON GRAMMAR$CHIL FUNCTIONALLY$DEVIANT$SP
6404    INFLUENCE MOTOR$PERFORMANCE SIMULTANEOUS$DELAYED$SYNCHRONOUS
6404    INTELLIGIBILITY STM REPETITION DIGIT$STRINGS
6404    SEMANTIC$COMPONENTS QUALITY PROCESSED$SP
6406    MODIFICATION NOY$TABLES
6413    LOGOPEDIC$OBSERVATIONS MENTAL$HOSPITAL
6413    VIRILIZATION VOICE ANABOLIC$STEREOIDS
6503    TONGUE-THRUST INF
6503    TONGUE-THRUST DEGLUTITION ANATOMICAL PHYSIOLOGICAL
        NEUROLOGICAL
6503    TONGUE-THRUST$SWALLOW ALARYNGEAL$VOICE$TRNG CASE$REPORT
6504    AUDIO-VISUAL$TEST EVAL ABILITY$RECOGNIZE$PHONETIC
        $ERRORS
6505    HISTORICAL$VIGNETTES LEADERS APHASIA STUTTERING
6505    HISTORICAL$VIGNETTES LEADERSHIP SP$HNG SP$PATH
6506    MANNER$PRESENTATION
6507    UPPER$RESPIRATORY$ACTIONS INF
6511    INTRODUCTION RESEARCH$PLAN
6515    NATURE$INTELLIGENCE
6517    PROGRAMMED$LEARNING DECIBEL
6603    NATL$SP$HNG$SURVEY
6604    MASCULINITY-FEMININITY$DIMENSION
6606    FINITE-DIFFERENCE$METHOD INVEST VIBRATIONS SOLIDS
        EVAL
6614    MEM$GIST VARIABLES
6614    PREDICTABILITY DISRUPTION SPONTANEOUS$SP
6614    SERIAL$POSITION$EFFECT PREPARATION$ABSTRACTS
6703    MEAS NYSTAGMUS ENG
6703    MEAS NYSTAGMUS ENG
6703    SUGGESTIONS THERAPY TONGUE$THRUST
6706    INTERACTION AUD$VISUAL$SENSORY$MODALITIES
6706    REL INDUCED$TINNITUS PHYSICAL$CHARACTERISTICS INDUCING
        $STIMULI
6706    VARIATIONS MARILLS$DETECTION$FORMULA
6709    BAEDEKER SP$PATH
6711    METHOD STUDYING$ANIMAL$BEHAVIOR
6715    FILMS HNG$DEAFNESS
6806    MLD PHASE$ANGLE$ALPHA
6806    STRUCTURE CONFUSIONS SHORT-TERM$MEM ENGLISH$CONSONANTS
6807    PHONOLEXY KINESTHESIOLEXY
6807    RECORDING VERBAL$GRAPHIC$CONDITIONED$REACTIONS STUDY
        DERMOLEXY
6815    CONTROL VIRAL$INFECTIONS

6816    INTELLECTUAL$SOCIAL$COMM$FUNCTIONING
6904    KNOWLEDGE$GRP$RESULTS
6906    OBSERVATIONS LESHOWITZ RAAB
6909    ASSESSMENT QUANTITATIVE$RESEARCH SP
6909    EGO-INVOLVEMENT VARIABLE SP-COMM$RESEARCH
6911    EFFECTS CONCURRENT$MOTOR$TASKS
7003    TARDIVE$DYSKINESIA
7006    HEAD$EYE$MOVEMENTS
7006    REGULATION VOICE$COMM SENSORY$DYNAMICS
7007    DEGLUTITION REVIEW TOPICS
7014    PARALINGUISTIC$KINESIC$CUES WORD$ASSOCIATION
7015    IMPORTANCE COMM
7015    VOLUNTEER$TUTORING HANDICAPPED$CHIL
7017    DIAGNOSIS TREATMENT ABNORMAL$SWALLOWING
7103    TONGUE$THRUSTING CLINICAL$OBSERVATIONS
7104    LOMBARD$SIGN ROLE HNG SP
7106    MOSSBAUER$TECHNIQUE
7107    CRANIAL$ANALYSIS FUNCTIONAL$MATRIX
7107    DEGLUTITION
7107    INTERPRETIVE$SURVEY$LITERATURE
7108    WRITTEN$VS$ORAL$CONTACT CLASSROOM$TEACHERS
7111    NONLINEAR$DISTORTION PREFERRED$FREQUENCY$RANGE MUSIC
7112    PROJECTION ROLE-TAKING
7112    STUDY INTERPERSONAL$ATTRACTION
7113    FEDERAL$REPUBLIC$GERMANY
7113    MEDICAL$CARE SINGERS$ACTORS GREAT$BRITAIN
7113    MEDICAL$CARE SINGERS$ACTORS ITALY
7113    MEDICAL$CARE SINGERS$ACTORS NEW$YORK$CITY
7114    EFFECTS TRANSLATION READABILITY
7116    EFFECTS VERBAL$LOAD ACHIEVEMENT$TESTS
7204    DIFFERENTIAL$EFFECTIVENESS INFORMATION-INPUT$PROCEDURES
7206    MEAS MECHANICAL$IMPED SKIN EFFECTS STATIC$FORCE SITE
        $STIMULATION
7206    PHYSIOLOGICAL$NOISE MASKER LOW$FREQ CARDIAC$CYCLE
7215    GROUP$CONM
7303    OLIGODONTIA TAURODONTIA SPARSE$HAIR$GROWTH
7310    PHONETIC$TRANSCRIPTION$TEST DESCRIPTION EVAL
7311    EFFECTS LISTENING COMPRESSED$SP INTELLECTIVE$PROCESSES
        CHIL
7311    LOCUS
7315    EURHYTHMICS AUD
7316    CONTRIBUTION LOWER$AUDIBLE$FREQS RECOGNITION$EMOTIONS
7403    TONGUE$THURST$CONTROVERSY
7406    SIMPLE$FORM AUD$RUNNING-AVERAGE$HYPOTHESIS APPLICATION
7408    VIDEOTAPED$SELFCONFRONTATIONS
7408    WORD-FINDING$PROBLEMS NUMERICAL$CONCEPTS SCH$BOYS

7413  LONGEVITY VOCAL$CAREERS
7414  SIMULTANEOUS$TRANSLATION
7418  COMPARISON METHODS TEACHING LISTENING$COMPREHENSION
7504  WINGATE EXPECTENCY SHORT-TERM$PROCESS
7526  NATALE MARKOVIAN$MODEL OF ADULT$GAZE$BEHAVIOR
7526  PERFETTI DISCOURSE THEMATIZATION TOPICALIZATION
7526  POLLIO ANOMALY
7526  STEINGART PSYCHOLOGICAL$DIFFERENTIATION LANG$BEHAVIOR
7527  GILBERT SP MINERS BLACK$LUNG$DISEASE
7533  KAHN CULTURAL$DETERMINANTS PHONETIC$SEX-TYPING
7603  GANG DIAGNOSTIC$UTILITY ROLLOVER$PHENOMENON
7603  HANSON TONGUE$THRUST
7604  HAMLET DENTAL$PROTHESIS SPEAKER-SPECIFIC$CHARACTERISTICS
7605  SHOWALTER PURDUE$INTERACTIVE$TELEVISION$COLLOQUIUM
7605  SMOSKI TTY DEAF
7605  VAUGHN GERONTOLOGY
7605  VAUGHN TEL-COMMUNICOLOGY$HEALTH-CARE COMMUNICATIONS
      $DIS
7606  CHANAUD POROUS$BLADES FANS$NOISE
7629  PRIDEAUX RECOGNITION AMBIGUITY
7633  KOERNER FRENCH$LINGUISTICS DUFRICHE-DESENETTES
7703  MADISON COMMUNICATIVE COGNITIVE$DETERIORATION DIALYSIS
      $DEMENTIA
7705  CAIN HEW$REGULATIONS NONDISCRIMINATION HANDICAPPED
      SECTION$
7705  KNOPF ASHA$JOURNAL$SURVEY
7705  MARTIN PARENT$COUNSELING SP$PATHOLOGIST SOCIAL$WORKER
7705  MOWRER CORRESPONDENCE$COURSES SP$PATHOLOGY+AUDIO
7724  FARKAS ANTHROPOMETRY LATERAL$FACIAL$DYSPLASIA
7724  FARKAS ANTHROPOMETRY LATERAL$FACIAL$DYSPLASIA
7725  JOHNSON DICHOTICALLY-STIMULATED$EAR$DIFFERENCES MUSICIANS
7725  JOHNSON VERBAL$MUSICAL,TASKS UNIMANUAL$SKILL
7733  FONAGY PHONOSTYLISTICS
7803  HAYNES CLIENTS$PERCEP THERAPEUTIC$EFFECTIVENESS
7803  TRAVIS NEUROPHYSIOLOGICAL$DOMINANCE
7825  AGNETTI ICTAL$PROSOPAGNOSIA EPILEPTOGENIC$DAMAGE DOMINANT
      $HEMISPHERE
7825  SADICK LATERAL$FUNCTIONS READING$ABILITY

## 0905

5403  GRADUATE$THESES SP$HNG$DIS
5416  MEDICAL$SCH PERSONNEL SP$HNG$PROBLEMS
5503  GRADUATE$THESES SP$HNG$DIS

```
5603   GRADUATE$THESES SP$HNG$DIS
5603   PROFESSIONAL$TRNG SP$CORRECTION CLINICAL$A
5603   UTILIZATION STAFF$TIME SCH$SP$CORRECTION
5616   MEDICAL$SCH$PERSONNEL SP$HNG$PROBLEMS
5703   GRADUATE$THESES SP$HNG$DIS
5703   PROGRESS$GOALS ASSOCIATION
5803   PROFESSIONAL$UNITY
5804   GRAD$THESES SP$HNG$RESEARCH
5804   SP$HNG$RESEARCH
5815   CHANGING$CONCEPTS A
5903   PROFESSION
5903   SP$CORRECTION CERTIFICATION
5903   SP$THERAPY SCH STATE$LEGIS$CERTIFICATION
5904   GRAD$THESES SP$HNG$RESEARCH
5905   ASHA PROFESSIONAL$GROWTH
5905   ISSUES MEMBERSHIP
5907   RESEARCH$NEEDS SP$PATH$A BASIC$RESEARCH
5907   RESEARCH$NEEDS SP$PATH$A PROBLEMS ADMINISTRATION
6005   AMERICAN$SP$HNG$FOUNDATION
6005   ASHA
6005   ASHA HISTORICAL$PERSPECTIVE
6005   ASHA$CONVENTION
6005   ATTENDING$CONVENTIONS
6005   CLINICAL$PRACTICE
6005   EXAM ADVANCED$CERTIFICATION$HNG
6005   NEEDS PROFESSION
6005   PROFESSION SP$HNG$DIS
6005   PROGRAM$COMMITTEE ASHA$CONVENTION
6005   PROSPECTUS PROFESSIONAL$STATURE
6005   PROSPECTUS PROFESSIONAL$STATURE TRNG
6005   REFLECTIONS EDITORIAL$POLICY
6005   REPORT DIRECTORS ABESPA
6005   REPORT MEMBERSHIP
6005   REPORT TESTIMONY CONGRESSIONAL$HNG
6005   REPORT WHITE$HOUSE$CONFERENCE CHIL$ADOL
6005   WHITE$HOUSE$CONFERENCE CHIL$ADOL
6017   ETHICS CLINIC STUDENT$TRNG
6103   REPORT INDIA
6105   ASHA MEMBERS
6105   CHALLENGE$COMPETENCE
6105   CONTRIBUTIONS ASHA$MEMBERS ASHA$JOURNALS SP$HNG$LITERATURE
6105   DIAGNOSTIC$TRNG$OPPORTUNITIES
6105   PHILOSOPHY PROFESSIONAL$BEHAVIOR
6105   PROFESSIONAL$SELF-IMAGE SP$PATH THERAPY
6105   SP$HNG$CERTIFICATION NY$STATE
6105   STATE$APPROVAL$ACCREDITATION SCH
```

```
6105    STUDENTS SCHOLARS GRAD$RESEARCH
6105    TRENDS PROFESSION
6216    OFFICE$VOCATIONAL$REHAB RESEARCH$PROGRAM
6404    EDITORIAL$POLICY
6405    VOLUNTEERS SP$PATH$A$CLINIC MEDICAL$SETTING
6511    RESEARCH$PROCEDURES
6603    PROFESSIONAL$EXPERIENCE
6603    TOOL CLINICAL$SUPERVISION
6620    EMPLOYMENT$OPPORTUNITIES SP$PATH$A
6703    ANNUAL$REVIEW JSHR$RESEARCH
6803    ANNUAL$REVIEW JSHR$RESEARCH
6805    PREPROFESSIONAL$EDUC SP$PATH$A
6805    PREPROFESSIONAL$EDUC SP$PATH$A
6805    STATE$CERTIFICATION$REQUIREMENTS SP$HNG
6815    FEDERAL$LEGIS HANDICAPPED
7005    COMM$AIDE
7005    READING JOURNALS SP$PATH$A OHIO
7005    SUPPORTIVE$PERSONNEL SP$CORRECTION SCH
7005    THIRD$PARTY$PAYMENT$PLAN
7005    USE AUDIOVISUAL$FILMS SUPERVISED$OBSERVATION
7008    GUIDELINES ROLE TRNG SUPERVISION COMM$AIDE
7008    PROFESSION SP$PATH$A
7008    TASK$FORCES$ORGANIZED
7017    SEMANTIC$APPRAISAL EVAL SP$PATH$A
7105    EXECUTIVE$BOARD
7105    OPERATIONALLY$WRITTEN$THERAPY$GOALS SUPERVISED$CLINICAL
           $PRACTICUM
7117    DELIVERY$SERVICES
7208    COMM$AIDE PILOT$PROJECT
7208    SCH$SP$TECHNICIANS MINNESOTA
7208    SUPERVISION SP$HNG$LANG$PROGRAMS SCH
7215    LEGIS EXCEPT$CHIL
7305    ANSI
7405    COMPETENCE PROFESSION
7405    DEV OCCUPATIONAL$ASST
7405    IMPLICATIONS PSRO INDEPENDENT$HEALTH$PROFESSIONS
7405    INTERNATIONAL$INVOLVEMENT SP$PATH$AUDIO
7405    PSRO QUALITY MEDICAL$HEALTH$CARE
7405    REQUIREMENTS CLINICAL$SUPERVISORS
7405    SP$HNG$LANG$SERVICES PROFESSIONAL$TRAINING USSR POLAND
7405    SUPERVISION SCH$SP$HNG$LANG$PROBLEMS
7405    SUPERVISORS CFY$EXPERIENCE
7405    SURVEY TRAINING$PROGRAM SP$PATH$AUD
7408    PROBLEMS$CATEGORIZATION STATE$LAWS$REGULATIONS
7415    SP$HNG$SCREENING TRAINED$VOLUNTEERS
7505    CULATTA CLINICAL$SUPERVISORS+TRAINEES
```

7505 CURLEE INCOMES SP+HRING$PROFESSION JANUARY
7505 CURLEE MANPOWER$RESOURCES$NEEDS SP$PATHOLOGY$AUD APRIL
7505 CURLEE TRAINING FORIGN$STUDENTS SP$PATHOLOGY$AUD US
     $COLLEGES
7505 KLAR NATIONAL$HEALTH$INSURANCE
7505 MARTIN EDUC SP+HRING$PROFESSION JUNE
7505 MELROSE PROFESSIONAL$LEADERSHIP$WOMEN SP$PATHOLOGY+AUD
     SEPTEMBER
7505 NICOLAIS STATE$LAWS$LICENSING$SP$PATHOLOGISTS+AUDIOLOGISTS
7505 SEIGAL ACCOUNTABILITY
7505 SHRIBERG WISCONSIN$PROCEDURE APPRAISAL CLINICAL$COMPETENCE
7505 WEPMAN HORIZONS SP+HRING$SPECIALISTS JANUARY
7505 YANTIS AUDIO ASSOCIATION OCCUPATIONAL$HRING$CONSERVATION
7505 YANTIS ANTITRUST$LITIGATION ASSOCIATION
7505 YANTIS ASSOCIATION$GOVERNANCE
7505 YANTIS ECONOMICS ASSOCIATION$PROGRAMS
7505 YANTIS PROFESSIONAL$STANDARDS PUBLIC$ACCOUNTABILITY
7524 STARK MISSED$APPOINTMENTS CLEFT$LIP PALATE$CLINIC
7526 AARONSON ABSTRACTS PSYCHOLINGUISTICS$CIRCLE
7526 CARTON PSYCHOLINGUISTICS EDUCATION
7526 SANDBERG MIND$RULES COGNITIVE$BIN FOREIGN LANG TEACHING
7527 REES
7534 OBRIEN SP THERAPY IRELAND
7605 CULATTA CONTENT+SEQUENCE$ANALYSIS SUPERVISORY$SESSION
7605 CULATTA COMPETENCY-BASED$SYSTEM TRAINING SP$PATHOLOGISTS
7605 CURLEE CHARACTERISTICS ASHA$MEMBERS
7605 DEMPSEY HEALTH$PLANNING
7605 GRIFFIN QUALITY$ASSURANCE PATIENT-CARE$AUDIT
7605 HARLAN COMPUTER$PROCESSING STUDENTS'$CLINICAL$HOURS
7605 KAMARA COMPUTER$BILLING SERVICE$ANALYSIS FINANCIAL
     $REPORTING
7605 LAVOR HISTORY LEGISLATION CHILDREN LEARNING$DISABILITIES
7605 MUELLER CLINICAL$RECORD-KEEPING
7605 STRYKER PROCEDURES MEDICARE THIRD-PARTY$PAYMENTS
7605 VAUGHN GERONTOLOGY
7605 VAUGHN TEL-COMMUNICOLOGY$HEALTH-CARE COMMUNICATIONS
     $DIS
7703 ABKARIAN DISCIPLINE
7705 ALEO TIME$ALLOCATION PROFESSIONAL$FEES SP-LANG$PATHOLOGISTS+AUDIO
7705 BOUCHARD MEDICAL$RECORD SP+HNG$PROFESSION
7705 CAIN HEW$REGULATIONS NONDISCRIMINATION HANDICAPPED
     SECTIONS
7705 CHAPEY CONSUMER$SATISFACTION SP-LANG$PATHOLOGY
7705 CULATTA CONTENT+SEQUENCE$ANALUSIS SUPERVISORY$SESSION
7705 GERSTMAN SUPERVISORY$RELATIONSHIPS DYNAMIC$COMMUNICATION
7705 GOATES THIRD-PARTY$COVERAGE SP-LANG$PATHOLOGY+AUDIO

7705    HARDEN COMPUTER$PROGRAM CLINICAL$ENROLLMENT
7705    LUDLOW EVAL EDUCATION$DISTRICT$SERVICES DATA$SYSTEMS
7705    LUDLOW EVAL EDUCATION$DISTRICT$SERVICES PLAN DATA
        $SERVICES
7705    MILLER AUDIOLOGISTS TESTIMONY GOVERNMENT$REPRESENTATIVES
7705    PETERSON COMPUTER-ASSISTED$RECORD$KEEPING
7705    PICKERING CONCEPTS SUPERVISORY$PROCESS
7705    SHRIBERG PERSONALITY$CHAR ACAD$PERF CLIN$COMPETENCE
        COMM$DIS$MAJORS
7705    VAN HATTUM COMMUNICATING COMMUNICATIVELY$HANDICAPPED
7705    VAN HATTUM COMMUNICATING PROFESSIONAL$HORIZONS
7708    CHAPEY SUPERVISION CASE$STUDY
7716     CHALLENGE PROFESSION
7803    VOLZ INTERPERSONAL$COMM$SKILLS SP-LANG$PATHOLOGY$UNDERGRADS
7805    CARACCIOLO ROGERIAN$ORIENTATION SP-LANG$PATHOLOGY
        $SUPERVISORY$RELATION
7805    CARACCIOLO PERCEIVED$INTERPERSONAL$COND PROF$GROWTH
        MA$LEVEL
7805    CHAPEY AVAILABILITY SERVICES DAY-CARE$CENTERS
7805    DUBLINSKE PL$
7805    DUBLINSKE DEVELOPING IEP
7805    FELDMAN COMPETENCE-BASED$TEACHER$EDUCATION SP + HEARING
        $HANDICAPPED
7805    GARON CLINICAL$SP-LANG$PATHOLOGIST'S COMMUNICATION
        $DISORDERS
7805    KRICOS NONTRADITIONAL$SERVICES DEAF SP$HEARING$CENTERS
7805    LENTZ DISPENSING$HEARING$AIDS UNIVERSITY$PROGRAM
7805    LEVITT COMPUTER-BASED$TECHNIQUES ENHANCEMENT CLINICAL
        $TECHNIQUES
7805    LUBINSKI COMPETENCY-BASED$TEACHER$CERTIFICATION SP-LANG
        $PATHOLOGY
7805    ORATIO PERCEPTIONS THERAPEUTIC$EFFECTIVENESS STUDENT
        $SUPERVISORS
7805    VANHATTUM ACHIEVING$POTENTIAL
7820    LARSON CONVENTION$EVAL
7827    BLACK JOURNALS THESES


                         0906


5506    NOTE OBSERVATION TARTINI$PITCH
5513    PSYCHOLOGICAL$REL ONE'S$OWN$VOICE
5515    EXPERIMENTAL$PSYCHOLOGY
5706    PERFORMANCE VIGILANCE$TASK NOISE$QUIET
5814    INCIDENTAL$LEARNING NAMES$DEFINITIONS

```
6013   PSYCHOLOGY CASTRATO$VOICE
6114   EFFECT LEARNING SP$PERCEP DISCRIM$DURATIONS$SILENCE
6216   USE ARTHUR$ADAPTATION LEITER$INTERNATIONAL$PERFORMANCE
       $SCALE
6314   DOUBLING$HALVING$TECHNIQUE MEAS CAUSATION OPINIONS
6314   EFFECTS HIGH$LOW$SENTENCE$CONTINGENCY LEARNING ATTITUDES
6403   RRLJ NEW$TECHNIQUE NONCOOPERATIVE$PATIENT
6406   OHMS$ACOUS$LAW SHORT-TERM$AUD$MEM
6503   BEHAVIOR$THERAPY SP$PHOBIA STAGE$FRIGHT
6614   EFFECT WORD$RECOGNITION FREQ WORD$ASSOCIATION
6617   BEHAVIORISTS$APPROACH LEARNING
6703   APPLICATIONS BEHAVIOR$PRINCIPLES CLINICAL$SP$PROBLEMS
6703   SP$PATH EXPERIMENTAL$ANALYSIS BEHAVIOR
6704   EFFECT DISTINCTIVE$FEATURE$PRETRNG PHONEME$DISCRIM
       $LEARNING
6704   EFFECTS CS-US$INTERVALS CONDITIONING R$DECAY
6717   DEVIATION SAE$THOUGHT$PATTERNS
6804   REL PROSODIC$VARIATIONS EMOTIONS NORMAL$AMERICAN$ENG
       $UTTERANCES
6807   RETENTION$TEST CONDITIONED$REACTIONS RETROGRADE$ACTIVITY
       SIGNAL$SY
6814   AMORPHOUSNESS R$FORM FACTOR VERBAL$CONDITIONING
6903   VOCAL$CONDITIONING INF
6903   VOCAL$CONDITIONING INF
6916   PERFORMANCE$SCALE COGNITIVE$CAPACITY DEAF
7004   PSYCHOLOGICAL$CORRELATES SP$CHARACTERISTICS SOUNDING
       $DISADVANTAGED
7007   PSYCHOSOCIAL$DEV MODIFICATION
7007   RF$PROCEDURES FUNCTIONAL$SP BRAIN-INJURED$CHIL
7007   RF$PROPERTIES TV$PRESENTED$LISTENER
7007   USE OPERANT$PROCEDURES REDUCE$RATES$READING$SPEAKING
7011   EFFECT TRNG FREQ$DISCRIM SCH$CHIL
7011   MONAURAL$AL EFFECTS FEEDBACK INCENTIVE INTERSTIMULUS
       $INTERVAL
7012   SP$PATH BEHAVIOR$MODIFICATION
7014   STYLOSTATISTICS PSYCHIATRIC$GRPS
7015   RF LEARNING CONSIDERATIONS PROGRAMMED$INSTRUCTION
7017   MODIFICATION MR$CHIL CLASSROOM$BEHAVIOR POSITIVE$RF
       AVERSIVE$CONTR
7103   EARLY$MOTOR$UNIT$DISEASE PSYCHOGENIC$BREATHY$DYSPHONIA
7103   TOKEN$LOSS SP$IMITATION$TRNG
7103   USE OPERANT$PROCEDURES THEORETICAL$CONCEPTS TREATMENT
7104   EFFECTS DELAY RF PROBABILITY$LEARNING
7104   OPERANT$MANIPULATION VOCAL$PITCH NORMAL$SPEAKERS
7107   PSYCHOLOGICAL$DEV
7107   PSYCHOLOGICAL$DEV
```

7114    PSYCHOLOGICAL$VARIABLES ABILITY PRONOUNCE SECOND$LANG
7114    ROLE UNDERDETERMINACY REFERENCE SENTENCE$RECALL CHIL
7116    PERFORMANCE HI$CHIL NON-VERBAL$PERSONALITY$TEST
7120    REGIONAL$VARIATIONS TEACHER$ATTITUDES CHIL LANG
7204    PHONETIC$INTERFERENCE MOTOR$RECALL
7206    MISSING$FUND PERIODICITY$DETECTION HNG
7206    R-CONTINGENT$MEAS PROPORTION$CORRECT
7214    CONSTRAINTS EYE-VOICE$SPAN EMBEDDED$SENTENCES
7214    INDEX CONTINGENCY CRITIQUE
7215    BEHAVIOR$MODIFICATION DEAF CLASSROOM$TECHNIQUE
7217    R$TIME EXPANDED$SP PRESBYCUSIC$MALES
7304    EFFECTS COMM$FAILURE SPEAKER$LISTENER$BEHAVIOR
7306    PERCEP PERSONALITY SP EFFECTS MANIPULATIONS ACOUS
        $PARAMETERS
7311    R$DELAY$EFFECTS DURATION$JUDGMENTS
7316    BEHAVIOR$MODIFICATION DEAF$CLASSROOM
7404    DISTINCTIVE$PHONETIC$FEATURES SP$DISCRIM$LEARNING
7405    BEHAVIOR$MODIFICATION TRAINING$SPEECH$CLINICIANS PROCEDURES
        IMPLIC
7406    RULE-SYNTHESIS SP WORD$CONCATENATION
7512    BARRETT INFORMATION RELEVANCE NEURAL$SYSTEMS
7526    DRAPER R$CONTINGENT$CONSEQUATION ARTIC$R
7526    PERFETTI DISCOURSE THEMATIZATION TOPICALIZATION
7603    BOLLINGER RESPONSE-CONTINGENT$SMALL-STEP$TREATMENT
7603    MANNING VERBAL$VS$TANGIBLE$REWARD CHIL STUTTER
7708    PETERS EFFECT POSITIVE$REINFORCEMENT FLUENCY
7727    MALAC PROGRAM SYNTAX LANG$DELAYED$CHILDREN
7727    WEBSTER MANIPULATION SP STUTTERERS
7827    BLACHE CLINICAL$PROTOTYPE AUD$MEMORY$SPAN
7829    GUESS BEHAVIORAL$APPROACH SP$DEFICIENT$CHILD

## 0907

5403    CLASSROOM$TEACHER$ATTITUDES$ACTIVITIES SP$CORRECTION
5403    RORSCHACH$PROGNOSIS PSYCHOTHERAPY SP$THERAPY
5403    SOCIAL$POSITION SP$DEFECTIVE$CHIL
5407    DEFECTIVE$SPEAKING$CHIL
5409    SP$CORRECTION PRINCIPLES METHODS
5409    SP$HNG$THERAPY
5409    SP$THERAPY BOOK$READINGS
5418    SP$CORRECTION SURVEY$TESTING
5420    PRACTICE GRP$SP$THERAPY
5503    SOCIAL$REL SP$DEFECTIVE$CHIL
5503    SP$THERAPY LANG$ARTS SCH

```
5515    HANDICAPPED$CHIL MAINSTREAM
5519    DEFECTIVE$SP
5603    ANALYSIS GAMES$TECHNIC
5603    PEER$EVAL CHIL SP$CORRECTION$CLASS
5609    HANDBOOK SP$IMPROVEMENT CHIL
5609    HANDBOOK SP$IMPROVEMENT
5613    CHEWING$THERAPY
5615    DEPARTURE FORMAL$TEACHING COMM$SKILLS
5703    BEHAVIORAL$RIGIDITY SP-HANDICAPPED$CHIL
5703    FREQUENCY DURATION TREATMENT$SESSIONS
5703    PARENTAL$DIAGNOSIS CHILD
5703    PROGRESS SP$THERAPY REL PERSONALITY
5709    SP$DIS PRINCIPLES THERAPY
5713    EEG$DIAGNOSING SP$DISORDERS CHIL
5715    HOME$HELP SP
5716    ATTITUDES SP$DEFECTIVES HUMOR$BASED$ON$SP$DEFECTS
5718    SP$THERAPY SP$IMPROVEMENT
5803    CHIL SPEECHLESS SCH SOCIAL$LIFE
5804    FUNCTIONAL$SP$DIS PERSONALITY SURVEY RESEARCH
5804    FUNCTIONAL$SP$DIS PERSONALITY METHODOLOGICAL$THEORETICAL
        $CONSIDERA
5809    DEV SP$DIS CHIL
5809    SP$REHAB
5815    GUIDE$PARENTS
5816    DIFFERENTIAL$CLASSIFICATION DIS$COMM CHIL
5816    MULTIPLE$HANDICAPS REHAB
5903    ADULT$EDUC$PROGRAM MOTHERS CHIL$SP$HANDICAPS
5903    BINAURAL$SP$THERAPY
5903    CARRY-OVER SP$PALS
5903    COMM$CENTERED SP$THERAPY
5903    CREATIVE$DRAMATICS SP$CORRECTION
5903    EFFECTIVENESS TRAINED$PARENTS SP$THERAPISTS
5903    EFFICIENCY TEACHER$REFERRALS SCH$SP$TESTING
5903    GRP$INTERVIEW INITIAL$PARENTAL$CONTACT
5903    SERVO-MODEL SP$THERAPY
5903    SP PLAY$THERAPY
5903    TESTING$PRESCH$CHIL
5910    CHARACTERISTICS ADULTS SP$HNG$THERAPY
5915    DIAGNOSTIC$TEACHING
5917    PHYSIOLOGICAL$CONSIDERATIONS DIAGNOSIS TREATMENT SP
        $DIS
5918    PERSONALITY$CHARACTERISTICS SP$THERAPY
5918    SP$CORRECTION CALIFORNIA
5918    SP$IMPROVEMENT SP$THERAPIST
5920    HYPNOSIS DIAGNOSIS THERAPY
5920    SURVEY SP$HNG$DEFECTIVENESS
```

| | |
|---|---|
| 6003 | COMM THERAPY$SESSIONS |
| 6003 | MOTIVATION SP$THERAPY |
| 6003 | RADIOGRAPHY SP$PATH |
| 6003 | UNIT$TEACHING SP$HNG SCH |
| 6004 | ARTIC$COMPETENCY READING$READINESS |
| 6004 | EFFECTS LISTENER$SOPHISTICATION RATING SP$BEHAVIOR |
| 6005 | REHAB ADULT SP$HNG$PROBLEMS |
| 6013 | DIFFERENTIAL DIAGNOSIS CHIL COMM$DIS |
| 6103 | HYPNOSIS SP$PATH$A |
| 6103 | METHODS SP$CORRECTION |
| 6103 | PSYCHOTHERAPEUTIC$TOOLS PARENTS |
| 6104 | SOCIAL$VARIABLES SP$DIS |
| 6105 | SP$DIS |
| 6105 | SP$IMPAIRED |
| 6117 | SP$HNG$THERAPY PRESCH$CHIL |
| 6203 | CATEGORIZATION SP$LANG$COMM$DIS |
| 6203 | FACTORS EFFECTIVENESS MOTHERS TRAINED SP$CORRECTION |
| 6203 | FACTORS EFFECTIVENESS MOTHERS TRAINED SP$CORRECTION |
| 6203 | SP$RATINGS DISMISSAL$THERAPY |
| 6203 | SP$RATINGS DISMISSAL$THERAPY |
| 6205 | SURVEY EUROPEAN$LITERATURE SP$VOICE$PATH |
| 6206 | TEACHING$MACHINE |
| 6215 | AUD$TRNG SP |
| 6215 | DIAGNOSIS EDUC$PLANNING |
| 6303 | MEAS SP$DISTURBANCE ANXIOUS$CHIL |
| 6303 | SCREENING$INTELLIGENCE |
| 6305 | SP$IMPROVEMENT SP$THERAPY SCH |
| 6305 | TEACHING$MACHINE SP$PATH$A |
| 6306 | ARTIC$EFFECTIVENESS MEAS PROCESSED$SP |
| 6315 | COMM REVIEW CURRENT$RESEARCH |
| 6315 | SP$THER |
| 6403 | SP$CORRECTION |
| 6403 | SP$CORRECTION |
| 6405 | DEV COMM$EVAL$CHART |
| 6415 | CLASSROOM$DISCIPLINE |
| 6415 | DEV PRESENTATION CLASSROOM$OBSERVATION |
| 6415 | RESEARCH APPLICATION$CLASSROOM |
| 6504 | TRNG TRANSFER$TASKS |
| 6510 | EFFECT MISPRONUNCIATION SPEAKING$EFFECTIVENESS |
| 6513 | APPLICATION LANG$PREDICTION SP$HNG |
| 6516 | CLASSROOM$RESEARCH |
| 6603 | CARRYOVER |
| 6603 | CASE$SELECTION SCH |
| 6603 | CASE$SELECTION SCH |
| 6603 | EEG STUDY DEV$DIS$COMM |
| 6603 | ORAL$MANOMETER DIAGNOSTIC$TOOL CLINICAL$SP$PATH |

6603    PARENT$COUNSELING SP$PATH$A
6603    SUCCESS FAILURE SP$THERAPY
6604    EFFECTIVENESS GRP$INDIV$THERAPY
6604    SOCIAL$STATUS SPEECH$HANDICAPPED$CHIL
6605    ORIGINS STATUS SP$THERAPY SCH
6609    REACTIONS PATH$SP
6614    GRAMMATICAL$CONSTRAINT PATH$SP
6617    GOAL$DIFFERENTIATION SP$REHAB
6703    INTERPERSONAL$APPROACHES STUDY COMM$DIS
6703    INTERPERSONAL$APPROACHES STUDY COMM$DIS
6703    SPONTANEOUS$SP PRIMARY$SOURCE THERAPY$MATERIAL
6704    LESSON$SERIES$TESTING
6705    REHAB SP$HNG$LANG$DIS EXTENDED$CARE$FACILITY
6715    DIAGNOSTIC$EVAL PLACEMENT$RECOMMENDATIONS
6717    PARENT$CONFERENCE
6719    COUNSELING SP$CORRECTION
6803    CASE$SELECTION SCH ADDENDUM
6803    PROCEDURES GRP$PARENT$COUNSELING SP$PATH$A
6810    DIFFERENT$POPULATIONS
6815    COMM$PROBLEMS PRESCH$CHIL
6816    OBSERVATIONS MONOSYLLABLE$PROD DEAF$SPEAKERS DYSARTHRIC
        $SPEAKERS
6817    COUNSELOR SP$PATH$A
6820    INTERVIEWING SP$PATH$A
6903    CAUSALITY SP$PATH
6903    DEV STANDARD$CASE$RECORD$FORMS
6903    SP$PATH SYMPTOM$THERAPY INTERDISCIPLINARY$TREATMENT
6903    USE STORAGE$OSCILLOSCOPE SP$THERAPY
6904    IMPARTING$DIAGNOSTIC$INFO MOTHERS COMPARISON METHODOLOGIES
6904    OBSERVER$AGREEMENT CUMULATIVE$EFFECTS REPEATED$RATINGS
        SAME$SAMPLE
6904    OBSERVER$AGREEMENT CUMULATIVE$EFFECTS RATING$MANY
        $SAMPLES
6907    CITIZENS$VIEW
6907    COMMUNITY$SURVEYS
6914    EFFECTS DST SP$APHASICS DYSARTHRICS MR
7003    CONTINGENCIES CONSEQUENCES SP$THERAPY
7003    TREATMENT EXTENSION DIAGNOSTIC$FUNCTION
7004    MAINTENANCE DIAGNOSTIC$INFO IMPARTED METHODS
7005    ANALYSIS MOTIVATIONAL$TECHNIQUES SP$THERAPY
7005    TAPE$RECORDER CLINICAL$PRACTICE
7007    IMPLICATIONS FUNCTIONAL$APPROACH SP$HNG$RESEARCH$THERAPY
7007    IMPLICATIONS FUNCTIONAL$APPROACH SP$HNG$RESEARCH$THERAPY
7008    APPLICATION TEACHING$MACHINE SP$PATH$A
7008    PARENT$COUNSELING SP$PATH$A
7013    INHERITANCE$SP$DEFECTS

7015   APPLICATION PROGRAMMED$INSTRUCTION CLASSROOM$INSTRUCTION
7015   APPROACH COMM$DIS
7015   EARLY$CASE$FINDING CHIL COMM$PROBLEMS
7017   PROJECTIVE$TESTING SP$PATH
7103   FOSTER$HOME$APPROACH SP$THERAPY
7103   FUNCTIONAL$SP$DIS PERSONALITY RESEARCH
7103   INFORMATIONAL$SPECIFICITY CORRELATE VERBAL$OUTPUT
       DIAGNOSTIC$INTER
7103   PARENT$EDUC SCH SP$THERAPY
7105   REHAB$COUNSELORS$PERCEP SP$DIS
7107   OBSERVATIONS DENTAL$RESEARCH
7108   ORGANIC$IMPAIRMENTS SCH
7108   PRESCH$PROGRAM CHIL COMM$PROBLEMS
7112   SYMPTOM$SUBSTITUTION
7117   APPLICATION GENERAL$SEMANTICS SP$THERAPY
7117   DATA COMM$DIS
7117   MEAS EFFECT CARRYOVER$TECHNIQUE
7203   INTERROGATION MODEL IMPLICATIONS
7204   FACTORS PROGRAMMED$APPROACH$THERAPY
7205   CONTENT$SEQUENCE$ANALYSES SP$HNG$THERAPY
7205   PARENTAL$EVAL
7207   CASE$PRESENTATION DISCUSSION
7207   COLLABORATIVE$RESEARCH DENTISTRY SP$PATH$A
7208   PARENTAL$R PARENT$COUNSELING
7212   USE DISTINCTIVE$FEATURES$MODEL SP$PATH
7215   AUD SP METHODOLOGY
7215   EDUC COMM
7303   EVAL PRE-SCH$CHIL RADIO$TELEMETRY
7303   IMITATIVE$SP OPERANT$TECHNIQUES GROUP$SETTING
7303   PILOT$TRNG$PROGRAM PARENT-CLINICIANS
7303   PROGRAMMING$ANTECEDENT$EVENT THERAPY
7303   VIBROTACTILE$STIMULATION CLINICAL$TOOL SP$PATHOLOGISTS
7304   COMM$SKILLS CHIL HIGH-RISK$NEONATAL$HISTORIES
7304   SP$PROB HIGH$SCH
7305   SOCIOLINGUISTICS SP$LANG$PATH
7313   PERSONALITY$CORRELATES COMM$DIS PROJECTIVE$ASSESSMENT
       VERBAL$EXPRE
7405   PREVALENCE RECOVERY SP$DISORDERS FRESHMEN UNIVERSITY
       $ALABAMA
7408   CASE$STUDIES STRUCTURING$REMEDIATION
7408   COUNSULING$WITH$TEACHERS
7408   DIAGNOSTIC$INFORMATION PLACEMENT$TREATMENT
7408   REACTION TEACHER
7408   STRUCTURING$REMEDIATION
7408   STRUCTURING$REMEDIATION SELF-CONTAINED$CLASSROOM
7503   HELTMAN RE-EDUCATION$TECHNIQUES SP$CORRECTION

7503   PANNBACKER DIAGNOSTIC$REPORT$WRITING
7505   GARRARD SP$PATHOLOGIST EARLY$CHILDHOOD$EDUC HANDICAPPED
7508   BLUE MARGINAL$COMM
7508   CLAUSON TEACHER$ATTITUDES+KNOWLEDGE SP$PROGRAMS
7508   MARTIN TEACHERS REFER
7508   SEATON COMM$DIS SCH$PSY
7508   WERTZ TEACHER SP$CLIN SEVERITY$RATINGS
7603   BOLLINGER RESPONSE-CONTINGENT$SMALL-STEP$TREATMENT
7603   PARKER DISTINCTIVE$FEATURES SP$PATH
7603   PRUTTING IMITATION
7703   COSTELLO PROGRAMMED$INSTRUCTION
7703   DIRKS PERFORMANCE-INTENSITY$FUNCTIONS DIAGNOSIS
7704   SILVERMAN CRITERIA ASSESSING$THERAPY$OUTCOME SP$PATH+AUDIO
7704   YOUNG INDEX OBSERVER$AGREEMENT
7708   PHELPS ATTITUDES TEACHERS LD$SPECIALISTS PRINCIPALS
       SP$LANG$PROGRAMS
7708   RATUSNIK BIRACIAL$TESTING CLINICIANS'$INFLUENCE CHILDREN'S
       $PERF
7708   SIMON PARTNERSHIP LD$TEACHER SP-LANG$PATHOLOGIST
7708   ZEMMOL CASE-LOAD$SELECTION
7727   MERCURIALIS DISEASES OF CHILDREN
7727   ORATIO PREDICTORS ACHIEVEMENT SP THERAPY
7803   PRUTTING CLINICIAN-CHILD$DISCOURSE
7804   BROOKSHIRE SAMPLING SP$PATHOLOGY$TREATMENT SAMPLING
       $PROCEDURES

## 0908

5703   SP$CHIL REMOVAL$TONSILS$ADENOIDS
5813   PHONIATRIC$PRACTICE NEW$YORK
6005   AMA$COMMITTEE REL MEDICINE ALLIED$HEALTH
6013   PSYCHOLOGY CASTRATO$VOICE
6303   SJOGREN$LARSSON$SYNDROME HISTIDINEMIA HEREDITARY$BIOCHEM
       $DISEASES
6507   DENTAL$RESEARCH
6807   VERBAL$METHOD DETERMINING STATE$MANS$HIGHER$NERVOUS
       $ACTIVITY
7004   SOUND$PRESSURE EAR$CANALS SURGERY
7007   DEV FACIAL$COMPLEX
7104   UPPER$CERVICAL$SPINE$ANOMALIES OSSEOUS$NASOPHARYNGEAL
       $DEPTH
7107   SKELETAL$DENTAL$IRREGULARITIES REL NEUROMUSCULAR$DYS=UNCTIONS
7206   SP TEMPORAL$LOBECTOMY
7207   DENTAL$MATURATION

7503    PASHAYAN BASIC$CONCEPTS MEDICAL$GENETICS
7512    GOTTLIEB MEDICATIONS SCHOOL$PROBLEMS
7513    ARNOTT DYSARTHRIA STEELE-OLZEWSKI-RICHARDSON SYNDROME
7513    GOULD VOICE$FUNCTION MICROLARYNGOLOGY
7513    LOOS BRONCHUS$ANOMALIES SEDLACKOVA$SYNDROME
7513    ONDRACKOVA COMPENSATORY$PRONUNCIATION VELAR$CONSONANTS
7606    SCHACHT BIOCHEMISTRY NEOMYCIN$OTOTOXICITY
7613    MICHELSSON CRY$ANALYSIS CONGENITAL$HYPOTHYROIDISM
7613    OKAMURA INVOLUNTARY VOCALIZATION GILLES DE LA TOURETTE'S
        DISEASE
7713    DARBY SP PATTERNS DEPRESSIVE$PATIENTS
7713    DORDAIN VOICE SP WILSON'S$DISEASE
7713    HIROSE EUNUCHOIDISM VOICE PITCH
7724    BERKOWITZ OROFACIAL$GROWTH DENTISTRY
7724    KOCH SURGICAL$ASPECTS MANAGEMENT
7727    COMSTOCK STAMMERING$SYSTEM$ELOCUTION
7727    MERCURIALIS DISEASES OF CHILDREN
7727    MORGAGNI CAUSES OF DISEASES LONDON
7727    SIEGEL SP DURING ORAL ANESTHESIA

## 0909

5406    INTENSITY$DISCRIM$THR PSYCHOPHYSICAL$PROCEDURES
5406    SUBJECTIVE$MUSICAL$PITCH
5406    TECHNIQUE SCALE LOUDNESS$MEAS
5406    TIME$FACTORS PITCH$DETERMINATION
5503    SCALE MEAS PARENTAL$ATTITUDES
5506    HALVING$DOUBLING LOUDNESS WHITE$NOISE
5506    MEAS LOUDNESS
5506    RATINGS$SCALE$METHOD LOUDNESS$MEAS
5610    REL VOCAL$CHARACTERISTICS MEN RATINGS VOCAL$CHARACTERISTICS
        OTHER$
5706    ABSOLUTE$JUDGMENTS MUSICAL$TONALITY
5706    EFFECT TIME PITCH$DISCRIM$THR PSYCHOPHYSICAL$PROCEDURES
        COMPARISON
5706    LOUDNESS$FUNCTION
5706    THR$HNG EQUAL-LOUDNESS$REL PT LOUDNESS$FUNCTION
5804    FREQ-INTEN$REL OPTIMUM$PITCH$LEVEL
5806    ADVANTAGES DISCRIMINABILITY$CRITERION LOUDNESS$SCALE
5806    DIFFRACTION$EFFECTS ULTRASONIC$FIELD PISTON$SOURCE
5806    PSYCHOPHYSICAL$MEAS
5906    INDICES SIGNAL$DETECTABILITY PSYCHOPHYSICAL$PROCEDURES
5906    MULTIPLE$OBSERVERS MESSAGE$RECEPTION RATINGS$SCALES
5906    OPERATING$CHARACTERISTICS BINARY$DECISIONS RATINGS

5906    PHYSICAL$CORRELATES PSYCHOLOGICAL$DIMENSIONS SOUNDS
5906    PSYCHOPHYSICAL ESTIMATE VELOCITY TRAVELING$WAVE
5906    PSYCHOPHYSICAL ESTIMATE VELOCITY TRAVELING$WAVE
5906    VALIDITY LOUDNESS$SCALE
6006    PREDICTION FORCED-CHOICE PHENOMENAL-REPORT THR
6006    PSYCHO-ACOUS
6006    PSYCHOACOUS DETECTION$THEORY
6006    SCALING PITCH$INTERVALS
6011    NYSTAGMUS$AUDIOCINETIQUE
6011    NYSTAGMUS$AUDIOCINETIQUE
6014    EFFECTS DELAYED$VISUAL$CONTROL WRITING DRAWING TRACING
6014    RECURRENTLY$IMPULSED$RESONATORS SP PSYCHOPHYSICAL
        $STUDIES
6014    WORD$SCALES
6106    FACTORS ESTIMATION LOUDNESS
6106    OPERATING$CHARACTERISTICS SIGNAL$DETECTABILITY METHOD
        $FREE$R
6106    PSYCHOACOUS DETECTION$THEORY
6114    PREDICTION WORD-RECOGNITION$THR STIMULUS$PARAMETERS
6204    LOWER$LIMITS PITCH MUSICAL$PITCH
6206    CALCULATION LOUDNESS$LEVELS MUSICAL$SOUNDS
6206    EXTENSION THEORY$SIGNAL$DETECTION MATCHING$PROCEDURES
        PSYCHOACOUS
6206    FRACTIONAL$MULTIPLE$JUDGMENTS LOUDNESS
6206    LOUDNESS RECIPROCALITY PARTITION SCALES
6206    MAG$EST LOUDNESS CLICKS
6206    MAGNITUDE$EST PITCH
6306    BASIS PSYCHOPHYSICAL$JUDGMENTS
6306    EXPERIMENTS PITCH$PERCEP
6306    RATIO$SCALES CATEGORY$SCALES VARIABILITY PROD LOUDNESS
6306    SINGLE ESTIMATES PITCH$MAGNITUDE
6306    SINGLE ESTIMATES PITCH$MAGNITUDE
6314    DURATION$EXCERPT
6314    REACTION$TIMES UNKNOWN$WORDS NOISE
6314    REL IDENTIFICATION DISCRIM SP$NON-SP$CONTINUA
6406    EQUIVALENCE VECTOR AUTOCORRELATION PITCH$DETECTORS
6406    INDIVIDUAL LOUDNESS$FUNCTIONS
6406    JUDGMENTS RELATIVE$PITCH
6406    LOUDNESS DETECTABILITY SCALING BANDPASS-FILTERED SHORT
        $TONES
6406    NEUTRALIZATION STIMULUS$BIAS AUD$RATING$SCALES
6406    NOTE VARABILITY$HYPOTHESIS CATEGORY$SCALING
6413    READING$DIFFICULTY LANG$TYPE
6506    RATING$SCALES TWO-STATE$THR$MODELS
6506    RATING$SCALES DETECTION$EXPERIMENTS
6506    THEORY PSYCHOPHYSICAL$LEARNING

```
6514   PREFERENCES PHONETIC$STIMULI
6606   INFORMATION MULTIDIMENSIONAL$SOUNDS
6606   OPERATING$CHARACTERISTICS YES-NO FORCED-CHOICE PROCEDURES
6606   REFERENCE$CONDITIONS SP$PREFERENCE$TESTS
6606   TWO-STATE$THR$MODEL RATING-SCALE EXPERIMENTS
6606   WEBERS$LAW POWER$LAW INTERNAL$NOISE
6614   NAMING$SEQUENTIALLY$PRESENTED$LETTERS$WORDS
6704   COMFORT$LEVEL LOUDNESS$MATCHING CONTINUOUS$INTERRUPTED
       $SIGNALS
6704   PHYSICAL$PSYCHOLOGICAL$CORRELATES SPEAKER$RECOGNITION
6706   CEPSTRUM PITCH$DETERMINATION
6706   MATCHING$FUNCTIONS EQUAL-SENSATION$COUTOURS LOUDNESS
6711   MEANING MUSICAL$DYADS
6804   PERCEP DAF SUBJECTIVE$EST DELAY$MAGNITUDE
6806   IDENTIFYING MEANINGLESS$TONAL$COMPLEXES
6806   RECOGNITION$PERFORMANCE FUNCTION DETECTION$CRITERION
6806   REFERENCE$SIGNAL SIGNAL$QUALITY STUDIES
6811   SCALING$INTENSITY NOISE PIGEONS
6906   MULTIDIMENSIONAL$ANALYSIS CIRCUIT$QUALITY$JUDGMENTS
6906   MULTIPLE$RATINGS SOUND$STIMULI
6911   CROSS-MODALITY$MATCHING DECISION$MAKING
6911   EFFECTS CONCURRENT$MOTOR$TASKS
7004   SENSITIVITY TONGUE ELECTRICAL$STIMULATION
7006   ELIMINATION BIASES LOUDNESS$JUDGMENTS TONES
7006   EXPERIMENTS PITCH$PERCEP DIPLACUSIS HARMONIC AM$SIGNALS
       PITCH
7006   FIXED-SCALE$MECHANISM ABSOLUTE$PITCH
7006   FREQ$INCREMENTS
7106   ACOUS$LEVEL VOCAL$EFFORT CUES LOUDNESS SP
7106   EFFICIENCY PSYCHOPHYSICAL$MEAS
7111   NONLINEAR$DISTORTION PREFERRED$FREQUENCY$RANGE MUSIC
7206   EFFECTS STIMULUS$BANDWIDTH LISTENER$JUDGMENTS VOCAL
       $LOUDNESS$EFFOR
7206   EQUAL$LOUDNESS$CONTOURS SENSORY$MAGNITUDE$JUDGMENTS
7206   PSYCHOPHYSICAL$EVIDENCE LATERAL$INHIBITION HNG
7206   RANK$ORDER$PROCEDURE AUD$STIMULI
7211   PSYCHOACOUSTICS LOMBARD$VOICE$R
7214   STABILITY SPECIFIC$MEANINGS TERMS NONE-ALL$SCALE$OF
       $AMOUNT
7306   PSYCHOPHYSICS
7306   STEVENS$OPERATIONISM
7311   INSTABILITY AUD$PERCEP$EXPERIENCES SPONTANEOUS$SHIFTS
       PITCH LOUDNE
7311   OCULAR$R AUD$STIMULATION OCULAR$MOVEMENTS
7406   NON-METRIC$SCALING$LOUDNESS
7406   PSYCHOPHYSICAL$VERIFICATION PREDICTED$INTERAURAL$DIFFERENCES
```

7414    SUBJECTIVE$ESTIMATES CONSONANT$PHONEME$FREQS
7506    HALL NONMONOTONIC$BEHAVIOR DISTORTION$PRODUCT
7506    OSMAN SIGNAL-NOISE$DURATION INTERAURAL$CONFIGURATION
        PSYCHOMETRIC$FUNC
7511    RUSSEL LOUDNESS$BALANCING COMPLEX$SOUND$LOCALIZATION
7526    FRENCH MEAS AFFECT GRAPHIC$DIFFERENTIAL
7526    JAMES MEMORY ACTIVE PASSIVE$SENTENCES
7526    MCLEOD UNCERTAINTY$REDUCTION READING$COMP
7529    BEASLEY INTRA-ORAL$DURATION INTERVAL$MEAS ORAL$STEREOGNOSIS
7606    BERGLUND SCALING$LOUDNESS NOISINESS ANNOYANCE COMMUNITY
        $NOISES
7606    BRAUN TIME-DOMAIN$FORMULATION DOPPLER$EFFECT
7606    HEFFNER PERCEP MISSING$FUNDAMENTAL CATS
7606    HOUTGAST SUBHARMONIC$PITCHES PT LOW$S/N$RATIO
7606    ISHIZAKA INPUT$ACOUSTIC-IMPEDANCE$MEAS SUBGLOTTAL
        $SYSTEM
7606    JOHNSON ENERGY$SPECTRUM$ANALYSIS MODEL ECHOLOCATION
        $PROCESSING
7606    MCGEE PSYCHOPHYSICAL$TUNING$CURVES CHINCHILLAS
7606    SANTON NUMERICAL$PREDICTION ECHOGRAMS INTELLIGIBILITY
        SP$IN$ROOMS
7606    STEVENS EQUAL-SENSATION$FUNCTIONS MAGNITUDE$ESTIMATION
7606    YONEYAMA FURTHER CALCULATION RAYLEIGH$WAVE$DIFFRACTION
        ELASTIC$WEDGES
7629    GILBERT HEMISPHERECTOMIZED$SUBJECTS DICHOTIC$BINAURAL
        $FREQ$FUSION
7706    BOONEN PSYCHOPHYS$ELECTROPHYSIO COMBINATION$TONES
        PERCEP PHASE$CHANGES
7706    HOWARD PSYCHOPHYSICAL$STRUCTURE UNDERWATER$SOUNDS
7827    GIVENS DISCRIM SP$INTENSITY VIBROTACTILE$STIMULATION
7829    BENNETT RELATIONSHIPS SP$DISCRIM COMFORTABLE$LISTENING
        $LEVELS


                            0910


5506    MESSAGE$RECEPTION FUNCTION TIME$OCCURRENCE$EXTRANEOUS
        $MESSAGES
5606    RESEARCH SINGING$VOICE
5606    RESULTS ANALYSIS SINGING$VOICE
5606    STUDY MAYDAY$SOS RADIOTELEPHONY$DISTRESS$SIGNALS
5606    TECHNIQUE CODING$SP$SIGNALS TRANSMISSION DIGITAL$CHANNEL
5806    MESSAGE$PROCEDURES UNFAVORABLE$COMM$CONDITIONS
5906    MESSAGE$UNCERTAINTY MESSAGE$RECEPTION
5906    MESSAGE$REPETITION MESSAGE$RECEPTION

5914   PEOPLE WHISTLE
6014   MESSAGE$UNCERTAINTY MESSAGE$RECEPTION
6406   MESSAGE$PROBABILITY MESSAGE$RECEPTION
6614   SOUND-MEANING$CORRELATIONS ENG$WORDS
6906   PERCEP VOCODER$SP PATTERN$MATCHING
6906   RESPIRATORY$VOLUMES NORMAL$SP INTRAORAL$PRESSURE DIFFERENCES
6907   MESSAGE$CONSTRAINTS INDUSTRIAL$SP$COMM
7014   PARALINGUISTIC$KINESIC$CUES WORD$ASSOCIATION
7106   ON-LINE$RECOGNITION$SYSTEM SPOKEN$DIGITS
7111   TIME$PERIODS$GREATER$THAN$
7313   SOURCE$SPECTRUM SINGING
7413   RESPIRATORY$TRNG SINGER
7512   TOWNER MISSPELLINGS READING$RATE RECALL
7513   MATSUSHITA VIBRATORY$MODE VOCAL$FOLDS EXCISED$LARYNX
7513   MURRY AIR$FLOW$ONSET VARIABILITY
7526   HOFFMAN BIDIRECTIONAL JUDGMENTS SYNONYMY
7526   WOLF COGNITIVE$MODEL MUSICAL$SIGHT-READING
7606   CERMAK MULTIDIMENSIONAL$ANALYSES JUDGEMENTS TRAFFIC
       $NOISE
7606   KERR DESIGN$APPROACH QUADRATURE SAMPLED DIGITAL$BANDPASS
       $FILTERS
7620   PELC SYLLABLE$ASYMMETRY SENTENCE$PRODUCTION (SUMMER
7706   BILSEN PITCH NOISE$SIGNELS EVIDENCE CENTRAL$SPECTRUM
7706   COLWILL SURFACE-WAVE$SIMULATOR STUDY JET-NOISE$SOURCES
7706   HOWARD PSYCHOPHYSICAL$STRUCTURE UNDERWATER$SOUNDS
7706   KATHURIYA MEASUREMENT ACOUSTICAL$IMPEDANCE BLACK$BOX
       LOW$FREQUENCIES
7706   PIERCY REVIEW NOISE$PROPAGATION ATMOSPHERE
7706   ROTHENBERG VIBROTACTILE$FREQUENCY ENCODING SP$PARAMETER
7706   ROTHENBERG FILTERING$TECHNIQUE ESTIMATING GLOTTAL-AREA
       $WAVEFORM
7727   KIRK STUTTERING IN GA
7733   KEMPGEN SYNTAGMATIC$TYPOLOGY PHONEMES


                          0911


5403   THEORY SP$MECHANISM SERVOSYSTEM
5406   ACOUS COMM
5506   CALCULATIONS MODEL$VOCAL$TRACT VOWEL LARYNX
5509   COMM$THEORY EXTENSION INTRAPERSONAL$BEHAVIOR
5509   COMM$THEORY EXTENSION INTRAPERSONAL$BEHAVIOR
5703   PREDICTION MISSING$WORDS SENTENCES
5709   ORAL$COMM
5806   DYNAMIC$ANALOG$SP$SYNTHESIZER

5814    PREDICTABILITY$WORDS$IN$CONTEXT LENGTH$PAUSES
6006    MODEL SP$RECOGNITION
6014    MODEL SP$UNIT$DURATION
6104    ACOUS$THEORY VOWEL$PROD IMPLICATIONS
6106    STIMULUS$VERSUS$R$UNCERTAINTY RECOGNITION
6111    SENSORY$FEEDBACK MOTOR$PERFORMANCE
6118    CYBERNETICS SP$HNG$RESEARCH
6206    COMPARISON ROC MESSAGES EAR EYE
6304    SP$MONITORING VERBAL$LEARNING
6306    PARTIALLY-CORRELATED$INPUTS
6307    EFFECTS FEEDBACK$MODIFICATION VERBAL$BEHAVIOR
6314    EFFECTS FEEDBACK ORAL$ENCODING
6406    ARTIC*TEST CONTROL CIRCUITS
6509    INTRODUCTION CYBERNETICS INFORMATION$THEORY
6606    ACOUS$DESCRIPTION SYLLABIC$NUCLEI INTERPRETATION DYNAMIC
        $MODEL$ART
6613    MOVEMENTS SOUND$GENERATIONS MODEL
6704    NOMOGRAM ARTIC$PROD
6706    EFFECTS TRANSMISSION$DELAY ACCESS$DELAY EFFICIENCY
        VERBAL$COMM
6706    MODEL$SECONDARY$RESIDUE$EFFECT PERCEP COMPLEX$TONES
6706    NUMERICAL$MODEL$COARTIC
6804    CONSIDERATION KINESTHETIC$FEEDBACK$RESEARCH
6804    PARAMETERS VOICE$PROD MECHANISMS REGULATION$PITCH
6810    SP$PROCESS CASE$STUDY
6814    EFFECTS FEEDBACK$AVAILABILITY GENERATION$SENTENCE
        $STRUCTURES
6903    PHONOLOGICAL$MODEL CHIL$ARTIC
6906    COMPARISON ROC$CURVES INTERVAL$RATING$SCALE$PROCEDURES
6906    PERCEP VOCODER$SP PATTERN$MATCHING
6906    UNCERTAINTY
7004    LATERALITY$DIFFERENCES AUD$FEEDBACK$CONTROL SP
7011    PREDICTABILITY$WORDS SENTENCES
7106    PATTERN$REVERSAL AUD$PERCEP
7204    OBSERVATIONS ARTIC LABIAL$SENSORY$DEPRIVATIONS
7214    RANDOM$GENERATION SP$RHYTHMS
7304    EFFECTS COMM$FAILURE SPEAKER$LISTENER$BEHAVIOR
7306    ARTIC$MODEL STUDY SP$PROD
7306    CORRELATION$MODEL BINAURAL$DETECTION INTERAURAL$AMPLITUDE
        $RATIO
7306    OPTIMUM$PROCESSOR$THEORY CENTRAL$FORMATION PITCH COMPLEX
        $TONES
7309    COMM$MODEL
7406    CATEGORICAL$NONCATEGORICAL$MODES SP$PERCEP VOICING
        $CONTINUUM
7406    MODEL WAVE$PROPAGATION LOSSY VOCAL$TRACT

```
7406   MYNAH$BIRD IMITATE HUMAN$SP
7410   VISUALIZATION VERBALIZATION MEDIATORS THOUGHT
7509   GROSSBERG COMM$THEORY
7509   HAWES BUILDING SCIENCE COMM
7512   HELMICK STIMULUS$FORM CONCEPT$IDENTIFICATION
7512   TOWNER MISSPELLINGS READING$RATE RECALL
7519   DALY QUALITY LISTENING UNDERSTANDING VOCAL$ACTIVITY
7526   CATLIN SEMANTIC$REPRESENTATIONS VERIFICATION
7526   FIGUEROA MEANING: SEMANTIC NETWORKS
7526   POWERS CONTROL-SYSTEM THEORY PERFORMANCE
7526   WINKLEMAN SEMANTIC$REPRESENTATIONS$OF$KINSHIP$SYSTEMS
7526   WOLF COGNITIVE$MODEL MUSICAL$SIGHT-READING
7527   CAIRNS PHONETIC$FEATURE$THEORY LINGUIST SP$SCIENTIST
       $PATHOLOGIST
7527   STUDDERT-KENNEDY ACOUSTIC$SIGNAL PHONETIC$MESSAGE
7606   SACHS PHENOMENOLOGICAL$MODEL TWO-TONE$SUPPRESSION
7609   SMITH COMM THEORY
7610   CLEMENT FEEDBACK HUMAN$COMM
7610   CRONEN AFFECTIVE$RELATIONSHIP SPEAKER LISTENER
7706   EGOLF MATHEMATICAL$MODELING PROBE-TUBE$MICROPHONE
7706   HALL SPATIAL$DIFFERENTIATION AUD$SECOND$FILTER ASSESS
       MODEL BAS$MEM
7706   HALL TWO-TONE$SUPPRESSION NONLINEAR$MODEL BASILAR
       $MEMBRANE
7706   IVEY ACOUSTICAL$SCALE$MODEL ATTENUATION WIDE$BARRIERS
7706   KUHN MODEL INTERAURAL$TIME$DIFFERENCES AZIMUTHAL$PLANE
7706   VILLCHUR ELECTRONIC$MODELS SENSORY$DISTORTIONS SP
       $PERCEPTION DEAF
7706   YUND MODEL RELATIVE$SALIENCE PITCH PURE$TONES PRESENTED
       DICHOTICALLY
7709   BOCHNER COMM$THEORY
7709   LITTLEJOHN SYMBOLIC$INTERACTIONISM HUMAN$COMM
7710   FISHER COMPLEX$COMM$SYSTEMS
7710   MULAC EFFECTS AMERICAN REGIONAL DIALECTS AUDIENCE
       MEMBERS
7727   ORATIO PREDICTORS ACHIEVEMENT SP THERAPY
7733   MARCHAL VOT BOUROUCHASKI
7806   FUNNELL MODELING CAT$EARDRUM FINITE-ELEMENT$METHOD
7806   SONDHI COMPUTING$MOTION TWO-DIMENSIONAL$COCH$MODEL
7821   BUCKINGHAM NEURAL$MODEL LANG SP
```

0912

```
5406   INSTRUMENTATION MEAS HEAD$MASTOID$IMPED
```

| 5506 | DEV SEMIPLASTIC$EARPHONE$SOCKET |
| 5506 | DEV SEMIPLASTIC$EARPHONE$SOCKET |
| 5606 | EARPHONE PROBE$TUBE$MICROPHONY AUDIOMETRIC$ZERO |
| 5606 | MULTICHANNEL$COMM |
| 5606 | NATURALNESS DISTORTION SPEECHPROCESSING$DEVICES |
| 5706 | EFFECTS LOUDSPEAKERS ECHO-FREE$CONDITIONS |
| 5706 | TWO-LOUDSPEAKER$SYSTEMS |
| 5804 | VOICE-MESSAGE$STORAGE |
| 5806 | POWER CLIPPING$SP AUDIO$BAND |
| 5806 | SOUND$SYNTHESIZER OPTICAL$CONTROL |
| 5806 | SP$ANNUNCIATOR$WARNING$INDICATOR$SYSTEM |
| 5904 | SP$PICKUP CONTACT$MICROPHONE HEAD$NECK$POSITIONS |
| 6006 | AIR$DAMPED ARTIFICIAL$MASTOID |
| 6006 | STEREOPHONIC$QUASI-STEREOPHONIC$REPRODUCTION |
| 6006 | SUGGESTION STANDARDIZATION LOUDNESS-BALANCE$DATA TELEPHONICS $TDH- |
| 6013 | MODERN$INSTRUMENTATION |
| 6103 | DEVICE FREE-FIELD$MONITORING DSF |
| 6103 | USE SHORT$LOOPS RECORDING$TAPE |
| 6104 | VARIABLE$PHASE$SHIFTER |
| 6106 | PHASOR$ANALYSIS STEREOPHONIC$PHENOMENA |
| 6106 | PHONETIC$TYPEWRITER |
| 6106 | SUPRA-AURAL$CUSHIONS AUDIOMETRY |
| 6206 | EARPHONE$R ONSET$TIME |
| 6206 | SP$SYNTHESIZER |
| 6306 | ECHO SP$CIRCUITS LONG$DELAY |
| 6306 | ELECTROSTATIC$MICROPHONES ELECTRET$FOIL |
| 6306 | MULTI-CHANNEL THR AUDIO-NOISE-REDUCTION$CIRCUIT |
| 6306 | OUTPUT$PROBABILITY$DISTRIBUTION CORRELATION$DETECTOR |
| 6306 | OUTPUT$PROBABILITY$DISTRIBUTION MULTIPLIER-AVERAGER |
| 6403 | EVAL ARTIFICIAL$MASTOID INSTRUMENT CALIBRATION AUDIOMETER $BC |
| 6403 | INSTRUMENT PTS$DAF |
| 6403 | TRIOPTOPHON THREE-DIMENSIONAL$PHONETIC$MIRROR AMPLIFIER |
| 6405 | AUDIOMETRIC$DESIGN STABILITY |
| 6405 | AUDIOMETRIC$DESIGN STABILITY |
| 6406 | EFFECT NOISE LISTENING$LEVELS  CONFERENCE$TELEPHONY |
| 6406 | FREQ$MULTIPLEX$SYSTEM |
| 6406 | INSTRUMENTATION |
| 6406 | SPECTRALLY$FLATTENED$PITCH-EXCITED$CHANNEL$VOCODER |
| 6406 | TRANSIENTFREE$SWITCHES |
| 6507 | RESEARCH$TECHNIQUES$INSTRUMENTATION EMG |
| 6606 | EARCANAL$PRESSURE EARPHONES |
| 6606 | EARCANAL$PRESSURE CIRCUMAURAL$SUPRAAURAL$EARPHONES |
| 6606 | EQUIVALENT$THR SPL TDH |
| 6606 | EQUIVALENT-CIRCUIT$CHARACTERISTICS PIEZOELECTRIC$RESONATORS |

6606    LOUDSPEAKER$COMM
6606    POWER-GRP$TRANSFORMATIONS GLARE MASKING RECRUITMENT
6606    STUDY ISOPREFERENCE$METHOD CIRCUIT$EVAL
6606    STUDY ISOPREFERENCE$METHOD CIRCUIT$EVAL
6606    STUDY ISOPREFERENCE$METHOD CIRCUIT$EVAL
6704    INSTRUMENT PT$DAF
6704    REAL$EAR ARTIFICIAL$MASTOID METHODS CALIBRATION$BC
        $VIBRATORS
6704    REAL$EAR ARTIFICIAL$MASTOID METHODS CALIBRATION$BC
        $VIBRATORS
6706    ATTENUATION PROVIDED FINGERS PALMS TRAGI V
6706    ATTENUATION PROVIDED FINGERS PALMS TRAGI V
6706    LIMITATIONS USE CIRCUMAURAL$EARPHONES
6706    OPTIMUM$LINEAR$FILTER SP$TRANSMISSION
6706    OPTIMUM$LINEAR$FILTER SP$TRANSMISSION
6706    ZWISLOCKI$BRIDGE
6804    REL VIBRATOR$SURFACE$AREA STATIC$APPLICATION$FORCE
6804    VIBRATOR-TO-HEAD$COUPLING
6806    DISTORTION COMPENSATING CONDENSER-EARPHONE PHYSIOLOGOCAL
        $STUDIES
6806    DISTORTION COMPENSATING CONDENSER-EARPHONE DRIVER
        PHYSIOLOGICAL$ST
6806    EFFECT SAMPLING$PROCEDURE PERFORMANCE ELECTRICAL$MODEL
        AUD$DETECT1
6806    VALIDITY LARYNGEAL$PHOTOSENSOR$MONITORING
6806    VOCODER$FILTER$DESIGN
6807    SIGNAL$SYSTEMS PHASIC$REL ULTRA-PARADOXICAL$PHASE
        EFFECTOR$REACTIO
6811    SOUND$TRANSDUCER INTRAUTERINE$USE PREGNANT$HUMANS
6813    APPLICATION MINIATURIZED$PRESSURE$TRANSDUCER
6813    APPLICATION MINIATURIZED$PRESSURE$TRANSDUCER
6904    USE HOOKED-WIRE$ELECTRODES EMG
6906    EMG ELECTRODE DIAPHRAGM
6906    FREE$FIELD$CALIBRATION EARPHONES
6906    MULTIDIMENSIONAL$ANALYSIS CIRCUIT$QUALITY$JUDGMENTS
6906    SP$ANALYSIS-SYNTHESIS$SYSTEM HOMOMORPHIC$FILTERING
6919    DEVICE AUTOMATIC$MODIFICATION VOCAL$FREQ$INTENSITY
7006    AUDIOMETER$EARPHONE$MOUNTING IMPROVE INTERSUBJECT
        $RELIABILITY
7006    AUDIOMETER$EARPHONE$MOUNTING IMPROVE INTERSUBJECT
        $RELIABILITY
7006    CUSHION$FIT$RELIABILITY
7006    EFFECT AMBIENT-NOISE$LEVEL THR$SHIFT MEAS EAR-PROTECTOR
        $ATTENUATIO
7011    AUDIOMETRIC$ACOUS$COUPLER$COMPARISONS CIRCUMAURAL
        $EARPHONES

7011    AUDIOMETRIC$ACOUS$COUPLER$COMPARISONS CIRCUMAURAL
        $EARPHONES
7103    RESPIROMETER DIAGNOSTIC$CLINICAL$TOOL SP$CLINIC
7104    USE CIRCUMAURAL$EARPHONES AUDIOMETRY
7105    ANSI$SPECIFICATIONS AUDIOMETERS
7105    ANSI$SPECIFICATIONS AUDIOMETERS
7106    NEED STANDARDIZATION MEAS SP$LEVEL
7106    REAL-EAR$ATTENUATION AUDIOMETRIC$RECEIVER$ENCLOSURES
7106    REAL-EAR$ATTENUATION AUDIOMETRIC$RECEIVER$ENCLOSURES
7206    AREA$PROBE
7206    COMPARABILITY COMMERCIAL$ARTIFICIAL$MASTOIDS
7206    COMPARABILITY COMMERCIAL$ARTIFICIAL$MASTOIDS
7206    COUPLER REAL-EAR$MEAS SUPRAAURAL-$AND$INSERT-TYPE
        $EARPHONES
7206    EXTERNAL$SOUND EARPHONES
7208    STABILITY PORTABLE$AUDIOMETERS
7211    INFLATABLE$EARPLUG ATTENUATION$CHARACTERISTICS
7304    CALIBRATION$DATA
7311    PT$AUDIOMETRY NOISE-BARRIER$HEADSETS
7404    COMPARSION INDIVIDUAL$UNITS ARTIFICAL$MASTOID
7404    COMPARSION INDIVIDUAL$UNITS ARTIFICAL$MASTOID
7405    AMERICAN$STANDARD$SPECIFICATION ARTIFICIAL$HEAD$BONE
7406    AUDIOMETER$RISE$TIME
7406    AUDIOMETER$RISE$TIME
7406    CALIBRATION$METHODS
7406    MODIFICATION DIF$SUMMATING$POTENTIAL STIMULUS$BIASING
7406    PSYCHOACOUSTIC$CALIBRATION TELEX$
7406    PSYCHOACOUSTIC$CALIBRATION TELEX$
7408    STABILITY PT$AUDIOMETERS IDENTIFICATION$AUDIOMETRY
7418    COMPARISON METHODS TEACHING LISTENING$COMPREHENSION
7504    STEVENS ACCELEROMETER GLOTTAL$WAVEFORMS NASALIZATION
7506    MERMELSTEIN AUTOMATIC$SEGMENTATION SP SYLLABIC$UNITS
7513    TANABE HIGH-SPEED$MOTION$PICTURES VOCAL$FOLDS
7519    BEHNKE TIME-COMPRESSED$SP COMPREHENSION
7603    NICKERSON COMPUTER-AIDED$SP$TRNG DEAF
7604    DIRKS BONE$CONDUCTION$THR NORMAL$LISTENERS
7605    FELLENDORF BELL'S$AUDIOMETER
7605    SMOSKI TTY DEAF
7606    DRAGSTEN INTERFEROMETER VIBRATION$MEAS AUD$ORGANS
7606    KILLION NOISE EARS MICROPHONES
7606    KLEINMAN PHOTOPHONE OPTICAL$TETEPHONE$RECEIVER
7606    KLEINMAN PHOTOPHONE PHYSICAL$DESIGN
7606    MICHAEL CALIBRATION$DATA CIRCUMAURAL$HEADSET HNG$TESTING
7606    NELSON PHOTOPHONE$PERFORMANCE
7606    PATTERSON AUD$FILTER$SHAPES NOISE$STIMULI
7606    STUMPF INSTRUCTIONAL-LAB$EXPERIMENT TEMP$DEPENDENCE
        TRANSDUCER$IMPED

298                          0912 (CONT.)


7606   VOGEN COMPARISON RELIABILITY AURALDOME$HEADSET STANDARD
       $HEADSET PT THR
7624   HOLLIEN INSTRUMENTATION CRANIOFACIAL$RESEARCH
7704   BILLINGS CALIBRATION$FORCE FOR BONE$VIBRATORS
7704   BURKHARD SOUND$PRESSURE INSERT$EARPHONE$COUPLERS REAL
       $EARS
7704   MARGOLIS MEAS TEMPORAL$CHAR FILTER$R IMPEDANCE$INSTRUMENTS
7704   MUSKET CIRCUMAURAL$ENCLOSURES CHILD
7706   EGOLF ANALYZING DYNAMIC$BEHAVIOR ELECTROACOUS$TRANSDUCERS
7706   EGOLF MATHEMATICAL$MODELING PROBE-TUBE$MICROPHONE
7706   HRUSKA ENVIRONMENTAL$EFFECTS MICROPHONES VARIOUS$CONSTRUCTIONS
7706   MICHAEL REAL-EAR$COMPARISONS EARPHONE METEL$OUTER
       $SHELL PLASTIC SHELL
7706   MILLER ACOUSTIC$MEASUREMENTS INSTRUMENTATION
7706   NAKATANI COMPUTER-AIDED$SIGNAL$HANDLING SP$RESEARCH
7706   PATTERSON STIMULUS$VARIABILITY AUDITORY$FILTER$SHAPE
7727   KATZ PATENTED$ANTI-STUTTERING$DEVICES
7803   OLSEN SIGNAL$MONITOR AUDIOMETRY
7804   WATKIN ULTRASONIC-EMG$TRANSDUCER BIODYNAMIC$RESEARCH


                          1001


5403   PARENT$TRNG$PROGRAM CP
5413   CP$CHIL
5413   TREATMENT CP REFLEX$INHIBITION MANUAL$FACILITATION
       SP
5503   PHONETIC$EQUIPMENT SPASTIC$ATHETOID$CHIL
5603   ADJUSTMENT$PROBLEMS CP
5603   CONSONANTS SP CP$CHIL
5603   SHORT$TEST CP$CHIL
5703   BIBLIOGRAPHY PUBLICATIONS SP$HNG CP
5703   CP MONOVULAR$TWINS
5713   PREPARATION$SP CP$CHIL
5716   CP$DEAF
5803   CP$SP$CORRECTION CLINICAL$TEAM
5803   EFFECTS INTERMEDIATE$MIDBRAIN$CRUSTOMY SP ATHETOID
       $CP
5804   PREDICTING$INTELLIGIBILITY CP$SP
5813   LANG$DEV SPASTIC$CHIL
5903   DYSARTHRIA CP
5903   NEUROPHYSIOLOGICAL$ORIENTATION CP$HABILITATION
5903   SITUATIONAL$SP$THERAPY MR$CP$CHIL
5903   SP$LANG$DEV ATHETOID$SPASTIC$CHIL
5907   SP$VOICE$PROBLEMS CP

5909    CP$CHIL GUIDE$PARENTS
5918    REHAB SP CHIL$CP
6003    SP$REHAB CP
6004    BOBATH$PRINCIPLES CP$HABILITATION
6103    BREATHING$THERAPY CP
6103    INTRAORAL$BREATH$PRESSURE CP
6103    SURGICAL$MANAGEMENT PALATAL$PARESIS SP$PROBLEMS CP
        PRELIMINARY$REP
6117    EDUC CP
6303    DEV ELECTRICAL$STIMULATION MODIFYING$RESPIRATORY$PATTERNS
        CHIL CP
6304    MOTOR$ABILITIES ATHETOID$SPASTIC$PATIENTS
6403    RESTRICTED$MOTILITY SP$ARTICULATORS CP
6504    STUDY LANG$DISABILITIES CP
6603    PROBLEMS LANG$COMPREHENSION USE CHIL KERNICTERIC$ATHETOSIS
6903    MANAGEMENT VELO$DYSFUNCTION CP
7203    TREATMENT CP$HI
7303    COMM$BOARDS CP$CHIL
7303    NONVERBAL$COMM CHIL CEREBRAL$PALSY
7303    NONVERBAL$COMM CHIL CP
7311    AUD$DURATION$DISCRIM CP
7317    DIAGNOSIS COMM$DEFICITS CP
7713    ANDREWS INTELLIGIBILITY CEREBRAL PALSIED SP
7713    KEITH ACOUS REFLEX CHILDREN CEREBRAL PALSY
7713    PRUSZEWICZ HNG$VOICE SP EXTRAPYRAMIDAL CEREBRAL PALSY
7803    KENT ARTIC$ABNORMALITIES ATHETOID$CP
7804    LARSON EFFECTS CEREBELLAR$LESIONS MONKEY$JAW$FORCE
        $CONTROL
7813    PLATT MEAS SP$IMPAIRMENT CP
7821    FARMER EFFECTS AUDITORY$MASKING CEREBRAL$PALSIED$SPEAKERS
7822    SMITH FAMILIAL$MYOCLONIC$EPILEPSY ATAXIA NEUROPATHY


                        1002

5403    FAMILIAL$INCIDENCE CLP
5403    INTELLIGIBILITY CLP$SP
5403    POST-OPERATIVE$VELO$MOVEMENTS CLP
5503    ASSESSING NASAL$QUALITY CLP$CHIL
5503    CLP$HABILITATIVE$PLANNING
5503    STUDY FACTORS OCCURRENCE CLP
5513    CLP INCOMPETENT$PALATOPHARYNGEAL$CLOSURE
5603    ARTIC CHIL$CLP
5603    CIRTERIA SP$APPLIANCE
5603    TEAMWORK CLP$PROGRAM

```
5718   CLINICAL$APPROACH CLP$SP$THERAPY
5718   IMPORTANCE DENTISTS$APPROACH CLP$CHIL
5718   ROLE PSYCHOLOGIST CLP$TEAM
5718   ROLE SURGEON CLP$HABILITATION
5718   SCH$THERAPIST CLP$TEAM
5718   TEAM$APPROACH CLP$REHAB
5803   CLINICAL$PSYCHOLOGIST HABILITATION CLP
5803   PHARYNGEAL$FLAP ROLE SP$THERAPIST
5803   SP$THERAPY PRESCH$CLP
5804   ARTIC NASALITY CLP
5804   ARTIC$PROBLEMS CLP$ADULTS
5804   LANG$SKILLS CHIL CLP
5903   GLOTTAL$STOPS SP CHIL$CLP
5904   INTELLIGIBILITY PHYSIOLOGICAL$FACTORS CLP
5904   NASALITY ISOLATED$VOWELS CONNECTED$SP CLP
5904   PITCH INTENSITY CLP$VOICE$QUALITY
5904   VELO$CLOSURE ORAL$BREATH$PRESSURE CHIL$CLP
5907   RESEARCH$NEEDS SP$PATH$A CLP$SP
5913   NASAL$LATERAL$DEFECTS ARTIC CLP
6003   ARTIC$SKILLS ADOL ADULTS CLP
6003   BULB$APPLIANCE PALATOPHARYNGEAL$CLOSURE
6003   SP$ANALYSIS CLP
6004   CONSONANTAL$NASAL$PRESSURE CLP
6004   MMPI$DIFFERENCES PARENTS CHIL$CLP
6004   PERSONALITY$TEST$DIFFERENCES PARENTS CHIL$CLP
6004   PHARYNGEAL$WALL$PALATAL$MOVEMENTS POST-OPERATIVE$CLP
6005   CLP$CONFERENCE
6013   SP$IMPROVEMENT PALATOPLASTY ELONGATED$PHARYNGEAL$FLAP
6017   DENTAL$PROBLEMS CLP$THERAPY
6017   ROLE ORTHODONTIST CLP$THERAPY
6103   ARTIC$SKILL PHYSICAL$MANAGEMENT CLASSIFICATION CHIL
       CLP
6103   PALATAL$FUNCTION CLP$SP
6103   TAPE$RECORDINGS CLP$SP
6104   INTELLECTUAL$IMPAIRMENT CHIL$CLP
6104   SUBJECT$CLASSIFICATION ARTIC CLP
6203   IMITATED$ENG$CLP$SP NORMAL$SPANISH$SPEAKING$CHIL
6203   MULTIPLE$APPROACH EVAL VELO$COMPETENCY
6204   CINE$INVEST ARTIC$MOVEMENTS CLP
6204   COMM$SKILLS CHIL CLP
6204   SP PHARYNGOPLASTY POSTOPERATIVE$CLP
6303   INCIDENCE CLEFT$LIP CLP MONTANA$INDIANS
6303   PROSTHETIC$FACILITATION PALATOPHARYNGEAL$CLOSURE
6317   REHAB CHIL$CLP
6403   EFFECTS PHARYNGEAL$FLAP SP CLP$ADULTS
6503   CLINICAL$ASSESSMENT PALATOPHARYNGEAL$CLOSURE
```

6503 COMPENSATORY$TONGUE-PALATE-POSTERIOR$PHARYNGEAL$WALL
     REL CLP
6507 A$PROBLEMS CLP
6507 CLP
6507 PSYCHOSOCIAL$ASPECTS CLP
6507 TECHNIQUE CLP$SURGERY
6603 ARTIC$SKILLS BREATH$PRESSURE CLP$CHIL
6603 CLP
6603 TEFLON$INJECTION VELO$INSUFFICIENCY
6605 MENTAL$HEALTH CLP REVIEW$LITERATURE PARENTS
6613 STUDY ORAL$CONDITIONS OSCILLOGRAPHIC$ANALYSIS VOWEL
     $SOUNDS REPAIRE
6704 INTERREL ORAL$BREATH$PRESSURE$RATIOS ARTIC$SKILLS
     CLP
6803 PSYCHOLINGUISTIC$CONSIDERATIONS MANAGEMENT CHIL$CLP
6803 PSYCHOLINGUISTIC$CONSIDERATIONS MANAGEMENT CHIL$CLP
6804 CONSONANT$INTELLIGIBILITY PROCEDURE EVAL SP ORAL$CLEFT
     $SUBJECTS
6804 DURATION ORAL$PORT$CONSTRICTION CLP$SP
6906 CRY$CHARACTERISTICS CLP$INF
6913 COMPARISON PALATAL$MOVEMENTS CLP$PATIENTS
7003 STIMULABILITY$TEST CLP$CHIL
7004 COMPARISON RESULTS PRESSURE$ARTIC$TESTING VARIOUS
     $CONTEXTS CLP
7004 NASAL$AIR$FLOW SP PROSTHETICALLY$MANAGED$CLP$SPEAKERS
7013 LINGUAL$POSITIONS CLP$PATIENTS VELO$CLOSURE
7103 MANAGEMENT PATIENT VELO$INCOMPETENCY CLINICAL$REPORT
7103 OBSERVATIONS HNG$LEVELS PRESCH$CLP
7103 SP$AID VELO$INCOMPETENCY
7103 USE BILATERAL$SP$APPLIANCE PHARYNGEAL$FLAP CASE$REPORT
7113 NASALITY$RATINGS WORDS$PHRASES$RUNNING$SP CLP$CHIL
7207 DEGENERATION DENTAL$OROFACIAL$STRUCTURES
7313 STUDY VELO$MECHANISM CLP PROD VOWEL$PLOSIVE SENTENCE
7404 SP$PATHOLOGISTS$ROLE OBDURATOR$WEARING$SCH$CHIL
7417 LINGUISTIC$ABILITIES CHIL SURGICALLY$REPAIRED$CLP
7524 BISHARA SP$PRODUCTION ORO-FACIAL$STRUCTURES
7524 BLOCKSMA DEFORMITY CLEFT$PALATE$REPAIR NORMAL$LIP
7524 CHRISTIANSEN HABILITATION CRANIOFACIAL$ANOMALIES
7524 DALSTON PRIMARY$NASOPALATAL$PHARYNGOPLASTY
7524 DICKSON RESEARCH CLEFT$LIP$PALATE ANATOMY$PHYSIOLOGY
7524 HUNTER CLEFTING CROWNROOT$LENGTH$ERUPTION
7524 KAPETANSKY TRANSVERSE$PHARYNGEAL$FLAPS
7524 KAPLAN OCCULT$SUBMUCOUS$CLEFT$PALATE
7524 KROGMAN CRANIOFACIAL$GROWTH$PATTERN CHILDREN CLP
7524 LANDIS ARTICULATION INTELLIGIBILITY VIETNAMESE$CHIL
     UNOPERATED$CLEFTS

7524    LAWRENCE TELEFLUOROSCOPIC LINGUAL$CONTACTS PALATAL
        $DEFECTS
7524    MOCERI VIABLE$MUSCLE$TISSUE REPAIR CLEFT$LIP
7524    NEIMAN DELAYED$PHARYNGEAL$FLAP$SUCCESS
7524    ONIZUKA PALATAL$ARCH UNILATERAL$CLEFT$LIP PALATE$SURGERY
7524    PANNBACKER ORAL$LANG ADULT$CLEFT$PALATE
7524    PARADISE ME$PROBLEMS CLEFT$PALATE
7524    PETER SOCIOLOGICAL$ASPECTS CLEFT$PALATE$ADULTS VOCATIONAL
        $ECONOMIC
7524    RANALLI GROWTH CLEFT$CHIL
7524    SKOLNICK VELOPHARYNGEAL$CLOSURE REPAIRED$CLEFT$PALATE
        NORMAL$SP
7524    SOUDIJN CLEFT$PALATES ME$EFFUSIONS BABIES
7524    STARR MISSED$APPOINTMENTS CLEFT$LIP PALATE$CLINIC
7524    VANDEMARK PREDICTION VELOPHARYNGEAL$COMPETENCY
7524    WADA GROWTH$CHANGES MAXILLARY$ARCH UNILATERAL$CLEFT
        $LIP$PALATE$CHIL
7524    WEINBERG ACOUSTIC$FEATURES PHARYNGEAL FRICATIVES CLEFT
        $PALATE
7624    BISHARA CEPHALOMETRIC$COMPARISONS WARDILLKILNER VON
        LANGENBECK
7624    BISHARA FACIAL$DENTAL$RELATIONSHIPS UNOPERATED$CLEFTS
7624    EHMANN UNOPERATED$CLEFT$LIPS$PALATES
7624    FALK SOCIAL$R ORAL$CLEFT
7624    GOLDEN "BASKET$SUSPENSION" TONGUE$FLAP
7624    HAYASHI CRANIOFACIAL$GROWTH COMPLETE$CLEFT$PALATE
7624    HIRSHOWITZ PHARYNGEAL$FLAP VELOPHARYNGEAL$INCOMPETENCE
7624    ISHIGURO MORPHOLOGICAL$CRANIOFACIAL$PATTERNS P-A$X-RAY
7624    KRAUSE RESULTS VON LANGENBECK V-Y$PUSHBACK
7624    KRISCHER MATHEMATICS TREATMENT$EVALUATION
7624    LATHAM EXPANSION$APPLIANCE CLEFT$PALATE$INFANTS
7624    LEWIN SPHENO-PHARYNGEAL$MENINGOCELE CLEFT$PALATE
7624    PANNBACKER PUBLICATIONS PARENTS CLEFT$PALATE$CHIL
7624    PETERSON-FALZONE CLEFT$PALATE MANDIBULOFACIAL$DYSOSTOSIS
7624    PODOL VISIBILITY PREPALATAL$CLEFT EVALUATION SP
7624    RICHMAN BEHAVIOR CLEFT$PALATE$CHIL
7624    ROGERS TREATMENT CLEFT$LIP$PALATE WAR
7624    RUTOWITSCH ORTHODONTIC-RETENTIVE$APPROACH PROSTHODONTIC
        $REHABILITATION
7624    SAFRA VALIUM ORAL$CLEFT$TERATOGEN
7624    SAWHNEY NASAL$DEFORMITY UNILATERAL$CLEFT$PALATE
7624    SMITH CLEFT NASAL$ALA
7624    WADA TREATMENT$PRINCIPLES CHANGING$ARCH$FORM COMPLETE
        $UNILATERAL$CLEFT
7624    WATSON PPVT INTELLIGENCE CHIL PALATAL$PROBLEMS
7629    BORLAK PHONETIC$CONTEXT HYPERNASALITY CLEFT$PALATE
        $SPEAKERS

```
7724    BARDACH CLEFT$LIP$REPAIR FACIAL$GROWTH LIP$PRESSURE
7724    BEHRENTS PRENATAL$MANDIBULOFACIAL$DYSOSTOSIS
7724    BRADLEY SP$LANG
7724    BRALLEY MAXILLARY$ADVANCEMENT SP SUBMUCOSAL$CLEFT
        $PALATE
7724    BURDI EPIDEMIOLOGY ETIOLOGY PATHOGENESIS CLP
7724    DEBIE DERMATOGLYPHIC$ANALYSIS CLP
7724    FLETCHER CLP$RESEARCH
7724    HIRSHOWITZ CORRECTION SP PHARYNGEAL$FLAP V-Y$ADVANCEMNT
7724    KOCH SURGICAL$ASPECTS MANAGEMENT
7724    LINDERMANN CLEFT$UVULA
7724    MAHER PALATAL + OTHER$ARTERIES CLEFT + NON-CLEFT
7724    SELLE CLP TWO$SYNDROMES
7724    STARR MENTAL$MOTOR SOCIAL$BEHAVIOR INFANTS CLP
7724    WITZEL VELOPHARYNGEAL$INSUFFICIENCY MAXILLARY$ADVANCEMENT
7724    ZOOK DETACHED$PROLABIUM
7803    DICKSON AERODYNAMIC$STUDIES P
7803    DICKSON AERODYNAMIC$STUDIES CLP$SP
```

## 1003

```
5503    SP$DIS BULBAR$POLIO
5603    RH$CHIL DEAF APHASIC PSYCHOLOGICAL$CONSIDERATIONS
5603    RH$CHIL DEAF APHASIC AUD$DIS
5613    CHOREATIC$QUADRIPLEGIA
5713    SUPRABULBAR$PARESIS SURGICAL$SP$THERAPEUTIC$ASPECTS
5803    SP MALPOSITIONED$CERVICAL$SPINE POLIOMYELITIS
5903    BRAIN$STEM$DAMAGE SP PSYCHOLOGICAL$FACTORS
5903    COMM$SKILLS INTELLIGENCE HEMIPLEGICS
6003    EFFECT ISONIAZID SP MULTIPLE$SCLEROSIS
6003    SP$PROBLEMS MULTIPLE$SCLEROSIS
6003    VELAR$FACIAL$PARALYSIS
6103    SP MUSCULAR$DYSTROPHIC
6113    CONGENITAL$SUB-GLOTTIC$BARS
6115    REHAB BRAIN-DAMAGED$CHIL
6205    PROGRAM GERIATRIC$PATIENT
6303    SP PARKINSONS$DISEASE INTENSITY PITCH DURATION
6403    CASE$REPORT ENDENTULOUS$APHASIC$LARYNGECTOMEE
6403    PITCH$CHARACTERISTICS MONGOLOID$BOYS
6503    SP PARKINSONS$DISEASE PHYSIOLOGICAL$SUPPORT
6503    SP PARKINSONS$DISEASE ARTIC DIADOCHKINESIS SP$ADEQUACY
6503    SSF$CHARACTERISTICS MONGOLOID$GIRLS
6603    COMM$AIDS AMYOTROPHIC$LATERAL$SCLEROSIS
6703    COMM$DIS CHIL KERNICTERIC$ATHETOSIS AUD$DIS
```

6703   HYPERNASALITY SYMPTOM MYASTHENIA$GRAVIS
6704   SP$PROD PERCEP SEVERE$IMPAIRMENT SOMESTHETIC$PERCEP
       MOTOR$CONTROL
6704   VERBAL$EXTRAVERBAL$COMPONENTS LANG LATERALIZED$BRAIN
       $DAMAGE
6803   MYOTONIC$DYSTROPHY SP$DISABILITY
6804   SFF RATE$CHARACTERISTICS ADULT$FEMALE$SCHIZOPHRENICS
6807   AGNOSIA APRAXIA NEUROPSYCHIC$DISEASES CHIL
6807   BODY$IMAGE$DIS PATHOPHYSIOLOGICAL$MECHANISMS SP$DIS
       FOCAL$LESIONS
6807   STUDY PATHOPHYSIOLOGICAL$MECHANISMS SP$DIS FOCAL$LESIONS
6813   VALUE SP$AMPLIFICATION PARKINSON$DISEASE
6903   VISUAL-SPATIAL$NEGLECT BRAIN$INJURY
6904   LANG$SP$CORRELATES ANATOMICALLY$VERIFIED$LESIONS THALAMIC
       $SURGERY
6904   PARKINSONISM
6913   SP$PATH PATIENT$HEAD$INJURY
6913   WAVEFORM$MEAS MS
7004   PARKINSONS$DISEASE SP$DIS
7004   SFF MONGOLISM$CHIL
7012   ROLE$THEORY MENTAL$ILLNESS
7113   PARKINSONS$DISEASE MOTOR$SP$BEHAVIOR
7203   REHAB DYSPHAGIA$PARALYTICA
7204   EFFECTS ALCOHOL SP$ALCOHOLICS
7204   NEUROMUSCULAR$CONTROL$EXAM PARKINSONISM VOWEL$PROLONGATIONS
7317   SP$CHARACTERISTICS MS
7503   KENT ATAXIC$DYSARTHRIC$CINERADIOGRAPHIC$SPECTROGRAPHIC
       $OBSERVATIONS
7503   KENT CINERADIOGRAPHIC$ASSESSMENT ARTICULATORY$MOBILITY
       DYSARTHRIAS
7503   NETSELL ACCELERATION WEAKNESS PARKINSONIAN$DYSARTHRIA
7503   ROSENBEK SP$LANG CHRONIC$HEMODIALYSIS$PATIENT
7503   WEINBERG SP$FUNDAMENTAL$FREQUENCY PATIENTS$ACROMEGALY
7512   WARYAS PHONOLOGICAL DISCRIM HI$RETARDED CHILDREN
7513   ARNOTT DYSARTHRIA STEELE-OLZEWSKI-RICHARDSON SYNDROME
7516   ACHIEVEMENT$TEST$SCORES MULTIPLY$HANDICAPPED$CHILD
7527   WOLFE SP CHANGES PARKINSON'S TREATMENT L-DOPA
7622   FLOWERS MOVEMENT VOLUNTARY PARKINSONISM INTENTION
       $TREMOR
7622   YANAGISAWA SPASTIC$HEMIPLEGIA INHIBITION
7629   SLOTIUK DYSARTHRIA PARKINSONISM
7716   COPING$PATTERNS PARENTS DEAF-BLIND$CHILD
7724   MEYERSON NAGER$ACROFACIAL$DYSOSTOSIS
7727   KONSTANTAREAS SIMULTANEOUS$COMM AUTISTIC$DYSFUNCTIONAL
       $CHILDREN
7734   MARTIN DRAMA BRAIN-DAMAGED CHILDREN

7803 LOGEMANN FREQ COOCCURRENCE VOCAL$TRACT$DYSFUNCTION
PARKINSON$PATIENTS
7822 COMPSTON RISK MULTIPLE$SCLEROSIS PATIENTS OPTIC$NEURITIS
7822 FLOWERS FREQUENCY$RESPONSE PARKINSONISM PURSUIT$TRACKING
7822 FLOWERS PREDICTION MOTOR$BEHAVIOR PARKINSONISM
7822 ITO ACETYLCHOLINE$RECEPTORS ENDPLATE$ELECTROPHYS MYASTHENIA
$GRAVIS
7822 O'CONNELL TRIGEMINAL$FALSE$LOCALIZING$SIGNS CAUSATION
7827 ALTSHULER EMOTIONALLY$DISTURBED$DEAF$CHILD RESEARCH
THERAPY